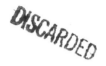

ANNUAL REVIEW OF
NURSING RESEARCH

Volume 19, 2001

C

T
Ce
Ne
New

Barb
Colle
Michi
East La

ANNUAL REVIEW OF NURSING RESEARCH

Volume 19, 2001

Women's Health Research

Joyce J. Fitzpatrick, PhD, RN, FAAN
Series Editor

Diana Taylor, PhD, RN, NP, FAAN
Nancy Fugate Woods, PhD, RN, FAAN
Volume Editors

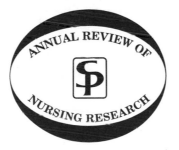

 SPRINGER PUBLISHING COMPANY

Order ANNUAL REVIEW OF NURSING RESEARCH, Volume 20, 2002, prior to publication and receive a 10% discount. An order coupon can be found at the back of this volume.

Springer Publishing Company, Inc.
536 Broadway
New York, NY 10012

01 02 03 04 05 / 5 4 3 2 1

ISBN-0-8261-1408-3
ISSN-0739-6686

ANNUAL REVIEW OF NURSING RESEARCH is indexed in *Cumulative Index to Nursing and Allied Health Literature* and *Index Medicus*.

Printed in the United States of America by Maple Vail.

Contents

Preface

We are rapidly approaching the end of two decades of publication of the *Annual Review of Nursing Research* (ARNR) series. This nineteenth volume follows a pattern established in the eighteenth, that is, the entire volume is devoted to one area of nursing research. In this nineteenth volume the focus is women's health. Drs. Diana Taylor and Nancy Woods, well-known scientists in women's health research, have served as volume editors. They selected the content as well as the authors; their editing created this comprehensive volume.

Drs. Taylor and Woods set the tone for the volume in their introductory chapter, "What We Know and How We Know It: Contributions from Nursing to Women's Health Research." Also in Part I is a chapter by Linda Andrist and Kathleen MacPherson. These authors explore the research on menopause as an example of nursing's contributions to feminist scholarship.

Part II includes three chapters focused on women's social roles. Angela Barron McBride and Cheryl Prohaska Shore review the research on women as mothers in chapter 3. Marcia Gruis Killien, in her chapter on women and employment, focuses on the past decade of research in this area. And in chapter 5 Margaret Bull describes research on women's roles as family caregivers.

Part III includes two chapters of research reviews focused on diversity and women's health. Linda Bernhard reviews research on lesbian health and health care and Karen Aroian describes immigrant women and their health.

In Part IV, the focus is on reviews of women's health and illness. Cheryl Cahill describes the research on women and stress in chapter 8. Kathryn Lee reviews sleep and fatigue in chapter 9. Chapter 10, authored by Janice Humphreys, Barbara Parker, and Jacquelyn Campbell, includes a review of research on intimate partner violence against women. And the final chapter includes a review of gender-based biological research by Nancy Reame.

As with previous volumes, the editors owe a significant debt to the scientists who contributed to the review of chapter drafts, and who helped us to hone the topics and chapters into the essence that appears in print. Also, we wish to recognize the many nurse-researchers whom the authors cite in their chapter reviews. We hope that we have done justice to your work. ARNR Advisory Board members have been loyal supporters of our continuing efforts to describe the "state of the science" no matter what the specialized topic chosen for the volume. We wish to recognize their contributions to the selection of topics and also the ongoing support that they have provided to the ARNR series editor.

JOYCE J. FITZPATRICK, PhD, RN, FAAN
Series Editor

Acknowledgments

We thank Dr. Joyce Fitzpatrick for her editorial encouragement and thoughtful review of every aspect of this project. We sincerely acknowledge Springer Publishing and editor Ruth Chasek. We especially thank Pamela Lankas, Production Editor, to whom we are indebted for extremely capable editorial assistance. In addition, we are grateful to Claudia Schumann at the UCSF School of Nursing for her assistance with manuscript preparation and coordination.

Contributors

Linda C. Andrist, PhD, RNC, WHNP
Associate Professor and Coordinator
Adult/Women's Health Nurse
  Practitioner Program
MGH Institute of Health
  Professions
Boston, MA

Karen J. Aroian, PhD, RN, CS, FAAN
Professor, College of Nursing
Adjunct Professor, Department of
  Anthropology
Katherine E. Faville Professorship
  in Research
Wayne State University
Detroit, MI

Linda A. Bernhard, PhD, RN
Associate Professor of Nursing and
  Women's Studies
The Ohio State University
Columbus, OH

Margaret J. Bull, PhD, RN, FAAN
Professor
Marquette University
Milwaukee, WI

Cheryl A. Cahill, RN, PhD
Amelia Peabody Endowed Professor
  of Nursing Research
MGH Institute of Health
  Professions
Co-Director of the Clinical Core
Partners/Fenway/Shattuck Center for
  AIDS Research
Boston, MA

Jacquelyn C. Campbell, PhD, RN, FAAN
Anna D. Wolf Endowed Professor
  and Associate Dean for the PhD
  Program and Research
School of Nursing
Johns Hopkins University
Baltimore, MD

Janice Humphreys, PhD, RN, CS, NP
Assistant Professor
School of Nursing
University of California, San Francisco
San Francisco, CA

Marcia Gruis Killien, PhD, RN, FAAN
Professor and Co-Director
Center for Women's Health Research
Department of Family and Child Nursing
University of Washington
Seattle, WA

Kathryn A. Lee, RN, PhD, FAAN
Professor and James and Marjorie Livingston Chair in Nursing
School of Nursing
University of California, San Francisco
San Francisco, CA

Kathleen I. MacPherson, PhD, RN
Professor Emeritus
School of Nursing and Health Professions
University of Southern Maine
Gorham, ME

Angela Barron McBride, PhD, RN, FAAN
University Dean and Distinguished Professor
Indiana University School of Nursing
Indiana University-Purdue University at Indianapolis, IN

Annette M. O'Connor, PhD, RN
Professor, University of Ottawa School of Nursing
Senior Investigator, Ottawa Health Research Institute
Ottawa, Ontario, Canada

Barbara Parker, RN, PhD, FAAN
Director, Center for Nursing Research and Doctoral Program
School of Nursing
University of Virginia
Charlottesville, VA

Nancy King Reame, MSN, PhD, FAAN
The Rhetaugh Graves Dumas Professor of Nursing
and Research Scientist, Reproductive Sciences Program
The University of Michigan
Ann Arbor, MI

Marilyn L. Rothert, PhD, RN, FAAN
Dean and Professor
College of Nursing
Michigan State University
East Lansing, MI

Cheryl Prohaska Shore, PhD, MA, RN
Indiana University School of Nursing
Indiana University-Purdue University at Indianapolis, IN

PART I

Introduction

Chapter 1

What We Know and How We Know It: Contributions from Nursing to Women's Health Research and Scholarship

DIANA TAYLOR AND NANCY WOODS

ABSTRACT

In this first chapter, we trace the historical roots of nursing research and scholarship focused on protecting and promoting women's health. Beginning with Florence Nightingale, modern nursing's first researcher, who focused on the health impact of women's daily lives through her detailed observations of human behavior. More recently, nursing's contributions to women's health over the past 30 years have redefined women's health, proposed new frameworks for understanding women's health; provided reviews of the women's health literature across disciplines; developed communities of nurse scholars and researchers focused on new areas of women's health research; generated and expanded the knowledge base for women's health practice and education; promoted a global view of women's health; and proposed new models for women's health care delivery. Clearly, a community of nursing scholars, developed over the past 25 years, has contributed to advancing women's health knowledge and improving the health and well-being of women. Without the benefit of a crystal ball, we suggest that nursing will continue to provide leadership in the conduct and the application of research to improve women's health and women's lives.

Key words: feminist scholarship, nursing research, research methods, women's health

In this chapter we will highlight some of the historical contributions of nursing to women's health and women's health care with an emphasis on our contributions to women's health scholarship, and consider nursing's future contributions to women's health as a field of study. In the chapters to follow, 11 nurse-researchers have reviewed the knowledge base generated by the past decade of nursing research focused on an expanded view of women's health and illness. Clearly, nursing research in women's health has continued the shift in scholarship from "critique-to-assertion" described by Angela McBride in the early 1990s (McBride & McBride, 1993). The resulting chapters collectively demonstrate that nursing research for women's health is concerned about the overall wellbeing of women-as-women, their "dis-eases," and not only their diseases (Stevenson, 1977). And while this decade of nursing research uses critique in the development of new and relevant research questions, this body of research asserts an expanded foundation of science, theory and values toward the improvement of women's lives.

ORIGINS OF WOMEN'S HEALTH IN NURSING

Nurses have engaged in the work of women's health care since the time of Florence Nightingale. Indeed, Nightingale wrote *Notes on Nursing* as a text to guide women in their ministrations to their families, and in the process offered women an opportunity to harness their intellectual abilities to care for the sick. Nightingale was also the first nurse researcher to focus on the impact of women's daily lives on their health through her detailed observations of human behavior. Consider this quote, describing her observations of women's lives, from *Notes on Nursing* (ref date): "Why do they sit up so late or get up so early? Not because the day is not long enough but because they have no time in the day to themselves." As such, Nightingale's writings are an important part of the history of self-care, a movement that re-emerged in the 20th century and became linked to the contemporary women's health movement. Another of Nightingale's contributions, less well known than *Notes on Nursing*, is her essay "Cassandra." In her essay, Nightingale pointed out that women of her day had intellect but lacked the opportunity to use it! What we may not appreciate about Nightingale's vision was her attempt to broaden opportunities for women beyond those available to her contemporaries.

In the U.S. nursing's efforts to improve women's health can be traced to the care our profession provided to women and their children. Lillian Wald's work among the poor women of New York, Margaret Sanger's efforts to help women control their fertility, and Mary Breckenridge's efforts to provide maternity care in the rural Kentucky Hills are a few examples.

Nursing has also had a unique presence in the contemporary women's health movement, part of the feminist movement and the popular health movements of the 1960s and 1970s. We have been active critics of the health care system for women in the United States. We have been political and community activists in collaboration with feminist groups, self-help groups, and grass-roots organizations to revolutionize women's health. Few nurses, however, were visible in the early descriptions of the women's health movement. Instead, we were organizing, implementing, and advocating feminist positions, often from within the health care system. Not until the early 1980s did we see independent nursing voices emerge in the published literature. These nursing researchers of the 1980s were the social and political activists of the 1970s.

Nurses with a concern for women's health have historically included feminist approaches in their clinical practice as well as their scholarship. For example, the Boston Women's Health Book Collective authored *Our Bodies, Ourselves* in the late 1960s, early 1970s, depending on which version you count as first. There were a few nurses who have been part of that collective, e.g., Kathleen MacPherson, a leading feminist scholar of women's health, and Nancy Reame, a feminist physiologist and nurse. Along with the many members of the BWHBC, they helped to produce the feminist handbook to acquaint women with their bodies, empowering women by demystifying health care. The new *Our Bodies, Ourselves* is now in its fourth edition (Boston Women's Health Book Collective, 1973, 1998) and has become a classic treatise on women's health.

A feminist nurse-scholar and president of the National Organization for Women, Wilma Scott Heide, wrote about social responsibility and political activism as critical principles for all health professionals (Heide, 1985). In 1981, a group of feminist nurses published the first edition of a news journal titled *Cassandra: A radical feminist nurses newsletter and journal* with the goal to present feminist critiques and book reviews on nursing issues and provide a network for feminist nurses. A major goal of Cassandra was to support nursing research that employed feminist approaches and explored new dimensions of women's health.

Despite nurses' participation in many aspects of the women's health movement, some feminists, concerned with promoting opportunity for women, at times ignored their sisters in the traditional women's ghettoes and instead advocated for women in nontraditional occupations. When feminist scholars did focus on nurses, it was often with the same disdain they expressed toward physicians. The kinder critique of the 1990s has helped infuse our practice of women's health with a richer understanding of the intersection of gender, race, ethnicity, and class.

In the past decade, multidisciplinary efforts have increased our power to institute change in women's health status, building on the wisdom of early pioneers and combining the strength of all women's voices. Efforts to expand the knowledge of women's health and illness beyond the biomedical model began with clinicians and researchers closely associated with allopathic medicine—health psychologists, nursing and social scientists (Daly, 1978; Woods & Hulka, 1979; Marieskind, 1980; Verbrugge, 1980; McBride & McBride, 1981; Fee, 1983; Duffy, 1985; Lewin & Oleson, 1985; Shaver, 1985; Woods, 1985; Chinn & Wheeler, 1986; Zambrana, 1987; McBride, 1993; Dan, 1994; Woods & Fogel, 1995; Taylor & Woods, 1996). New paradigms have been proposed and are being implemented to enhance women's health from a biopsychosocial and cultural perspective. For example, in 1978, radical feminist scholar, Mary Daly had first used the term "Gyn/Ecology" to describe an alternative model of medical services for women, otherwise considered a "sado-ritual system." Building upon Daly's critique, Angela McBride, philosopher and nurse, proposed new theories for women's health in 1981 followed by a 1993 proposal for a "GYN-ecological practice-research agenda" for women's health. Theories have been operationalized as new models for women's health care delivery (Taylor & Woods, 1996). Nursing has challenged the profession to consider policy recommendations for nursing practice, education, and research for women's health. Clearly, women's health and women's health care have been stimulated by nursing scholars, nursing clinicians, and nursing activists.

NURSING CONTRIBUTIONS TO WOMEN'S HEALTH SCHOLARSHIP

Nursing's legacy of keen observation, combined with a focus on the multiple environmental factors that influence human health and illness, has been the foundation for contemporary nursing research in general and women's health research in particular. More recently, nursing's contributions to women's health over the past 30 years have: redefined women's health; proposed new frameworks for understanding women's health; provided reviews of the women's health literature across disciplines; developed communities of nurse scholars and researchers focused on new areas of women's health research; generated and expanded the knowledge base for women's health practice and education; promoted a global view of women's health; and proposed new models for women's health care delivery.

Developing Communities of Scholars and Researchers Focused on New Areas of Women's Health Research

Researchers and scholars at U.S. schools of nursing have provided leadership in the development of women's health research. In the early 1980s, faculty and students (lead by Beverly McElmurry and Carol Leppa) at the University of Illinois in Chicago launched a graduate concentration in women's health that provided critical reviews and synthesis of extant literature by women's health scholars. This group gave voice to nursing's contributions to women's health by naming the assumptions regarding the health care of women, for example: 1) the human body, mind, and spirit form a whole; 2) events and interactions in the family, community, and world affect and shape the health of women; 3) control over one's body is a basic right; 4) lived experiences are the starting point for future action; and 5) the health of all is improved by focusing on women's health (McElmurry & Huddleston, 1991). They furthered our understanding of nursing's contributions to women's health by labeling and categorizing our published work in the bi-monthly literature review, *Women's Health Nursing Scan* from 1985–91 followed by four volumes of women's health reviews (Leppa, Miller, 1988; Leppa, 1989; Leppa, 1990; McElmurry & Parker, 1993, 1995; 1997). These important reviews provided us with new visions and theoretical frameworks for subsequent empirical investigations, practice innovations, and new policy perspectives.

Nancy Woods, Joan Shaver, Margaret Heitkemper, Ellen Mitchell, and Martha Lentz started the first NIH-funded Center for Women's Health Research at the University of Washington in 1989. Each has developed independent programs of research in interrelated areas of women's health that have provided a foundation for doctoral and post-doctoral research training.

In the early 1990s, Alice Dan established the Center for Research on Women and Gender at the University of Illinois, Chicago campus, where she has provided postgraduate research training in women's health as well as providing a forum for interdisciplinary research collaboration and dissemination in new areas of women's health research.

Reviews of Women's Health Research & Scholarship: 1980–1996

Nursing scholars have provided some of the most extensive reviews of the literature related to women's health research over the past 15–20 years. We are fortunate to have this foundation of scholarship that combined feminist values, ethics, and sound methods of inquiry to improve women's health care and the education of women's health care providers and to encourage the marked growth of nursing research in women's health. Earlier reviews of women's health research included research across disciplines conducted by physicians, psychologists, sociologists, and health service researchers in addition to nurses.

The predecessors to this review of nursing's contributions to women's health research were Woods' (1988) review of women's health research in the seventh volume of the *Annual Review of Nursing Research*, published by Springer (Fitzpatrick, Taunton, & Benoliel, 1988); the three volumes on *Women's Health Perspectives: An Annual Review* published by Oryx Press (Leppa, Miller, 1988; Leppa, 1989; Leppa, 1990), and three volumes of the *Annual Review of Women's Health* edited by McElmurry and Parker (1993, 1995, 1997) published first by the National League for Nursing and subsequently by Jones and Bartlett Publishers.

In the seventh volume of the *Annual Review of Nursing Research* (Fitzpatrick, Taunton, & Benoliel, 1988), the review of women's health research by Nancy Woods was relegated to the last section titled, "Other Research" along with reviews on human information processing and nursing research in the Phillipines. In spite of defined inclusion criteria and few journals focused on women's health research, 175 research reports published between 1980 and 1985 were included in this review. In addition to providing a categorical analysis of the research, integrative reviews of two areas of women's health research in which significant contributions were made by nursing scholars were included (perimenstrual symptoms, women's roles and health). The focus of nursing research in the early 1980s was on: (1) women's lifespan or developmental issues (83 reports) with the majority dealing with young adult women; (2) wellness–illness dimensions such as health promotion needs (67% of the reports); (3) contributions to nursing science and practice with the majority extending nursing knowledge of how women adapt to health and illness states (59% of the reports); (4) the use of two major research paradigms—the positivist-empiricist and the historicist with only 39% of the reports including an emphasis on the context for women's health experiences; and (5) research measurement and methods for women's health research. Based on this extensive review, multiple recommendations were made that would provide the basis for nursing's agenda for women's health research in the 1990s. Building on nursing's scholarship in the previous 15 years, Dr. Woods provided a broad yet specific vision for future women's health research. This consisted of: (1) greater emphasis on adolescent, middle-aged, and elderly women using cross-theoretical perspectives of biological, psychological, and social development; (2) maintaining emphasis on health promotion and prevention and promoting greater emphasis on knowledge about women who are ill, disabled, or recovering from illness; (3) emphasizing greater understanding of the physical and social environments that support or damage women's health and the means by which they influence health; (4) expanding research paradigms beyond those rooted in logical positivism to include multiple modes of inquiry; (5) increased emphasis on clinical therapeutics for women as well as work on the contexts that promote women's health; (6) expanding the use of research methods to study dynamic processes such as the menstrual cycle and adjustment to chronic illness; and (7) focusing on experiential, dynamic analyses of women's lives, including transitions to and from parenthood and employment.

In the three annual reviews on women's health perspectives, Leppa and associates at the University of Illinois-Chicago School of Nursing pioneered a standard for subsequent literature reviews by establishing criteria and classification for the selection of topics and content that concerned women only or influenced them differently. Categories that summarized the literature reviewed were labeled women's characteristics, development across the life cycle, health promotion and maintenance, women as providers of health care, delivery of health care to women, health and work, reproductive health, physical diseases and health problems, mental health/illness, and therapeutic interventions (including drugs and devices). Additional categories included articles about research issues, theoretical perspectives, and ethical/economic/political/policy concerns of importance to women's health. Multidisciplinary perspectives were included in these reviews; authors represented scholars and clinicians from nursing as well as from biomedical, social, and behavioral disciplines. Theory and policy perspectives were reviewed in addition to research and clinical reports.

McElmurry and Parker have taken up where Leppa left off with the publication of the *Annual Review of Women's Health* in 1993 and two subsequent reviews in 1995 and 1997. These reviews of women's health continued to apply the classification framework established by the previous reviews. Contributors provided integrative reviews of the latest findings in some previously reviewed topics (childbearing, sexuality, mental health, and alcohol & drugs) and some emerging areas of concern (e.g., contraception, weight control, occupational issues, cardiovascular health, STDs, and midlife women's health). While the topics included in this annual review illustrate the content categories established by the University of Illinois-Chicago, there were some notable differences from the earlier *Women's Health Perspectives Annual Review*. For example, all contributors were nurses and all but one was from an academic setting. Clearly, by 1993 there were many nursing scholars who identified with a women's health focus, and nursing research on (and for) women's health had markedly increased. While some contributors reviewed a broad range of literature on a particular topic (books, audiotapes and pamphlets reviewed by Denise Webster in her review of women's mental health), most authors narrowed their review to the published, peer-reviewed, research-based literature. Most contributors, however, continued to apply a feminist framework in their literature critique and analysis. A few reviews recommended clinical changes (treatment of women with cardiovascular disease), policy changes (women and employment), or attention to methodological issues in women's health research.

In the second (1995) and third (1997) volumes of McElmurry's *Annual Review of Women's Health,* topics were expanded to focus on emerging women's health problems and the boundaries expanded to incorporate an international focus as well as the recognition of the impact of social environments (family, community, society, race, class, politics) on women's health. New contributions to the 1995 review included topics on health in older African American women, health promotion and maintenance, delivery of health care to women, HIV infection and AIDS, depression in Hispanic women, drug use and violence, and international reproductive rights. New topics in Volume III presented integrative reviews on sexual harassment, clinical trials in older women, menopause, violence against health workers, lesbian women's access to health care, community-based services for vulnerable populations, autoimmunity and gender effects, hypertension management, suicide in Latina female youth, domestic violence against women and children, and female circumcision. In total, these three volumes provided an overview and analysis of women's health research and scholarship conducted across multiple disciplines that spans almost two decades between the late 1970s and 1997.

The science of women's health, as shaped by nurse researchers, grew from the redefinition of women's health to proposing new conceptual frameworks for studying women and development of methodology and methods for studying women's health to the generation of new knowledge about several aspects of women's health.

Redefining Women's Health

The feminist critique has moved us to reconsider women's health and, in fact, to redefine it. Angela McBride's 1982 treatise on women's health and its philosophical underpinnings asserted that clinicians and researchers alike needed to concern themselves with health as well-being, not just women's diseases. She advocated that women's health was more than reproductive health, although reproductive health was a significant part of our health. McBride argued that the goals of attaining, regaining, and retaining health should frame our practice with women. She urged us to ground our understanding of health in women's lived experiences. In brief, McBride urged us to redefine women's health from gynecology (the study of women's diseases) to gyn-ecology (the study of women's health in the context of women's lives).

Moreover, nursing literature reflects a definition of health that is grounded in everyday life, with functional status, role performance, adaptation to environmental demands, and high-level wellness all dimensions worthy of study— not just clinical definitions of health such as risk factors and diseases (Woods et al., 1988). In addition, our broader definition of women's health has brought us into conversations about the critical intersection of gender with race, social class, and sexual orientation. We have also expanded the definition of who is a woman (Taylor & Woods, 1996; Taylor & Dower, 1997).

Although the NIH research agenda on women's health did not appear until 1991 (U.S.P.H.S., 1992), it is important to reflect on the fact that the nursing profession published significant works on women's health earlier. Indeed, the *Journal of Obstetrics & Gynecologic and Neonatal Nursing* was first published 29 years ago and the *Journal of Health Care for Women International* was first published 22 years ago.

Another important dimension of redefining women's health is appreciation of the developmental dimensions of health. Redefining health as having a developmental trajectory has encouraged many of us to engage women in longitudinal studies, for example, those focusing on the menopausal transition. Not surprisingly, Angela McBride's first book was entitled *The Growth and Development of Mothers*, a treatise focusing not only on the infant but also on the woman in the picture.

In this volume, Linda Andrist and Kathleen MacPherson review nursing's contributions to redefining women's health using women's transition through menopause as an example. In their review of nursing research over the past 15 years, these feminist nursing scholars demonstrate that nursing research has helped to refocus women's development and developmental transitions as normal rather than deficiency conditions that need medical treatment. Nursing's contribution to redefining women's health has also included women's diversity which is illustrated by their review of cross-cultural perspectives of women's midlife transitions. Feminist methods of inquiry have also been expanded by nurse researchers in their quest to redefine the "health" in women's health. They describe nurse investigators' use of methods such as researcher-in-relation, reflexivity, and social transformation to understand menopause within the context of women's midlife experiences. In their conclusion, Andrist and MacPherson chart a course for future investigations by proposing that women's lived experience should be the critical starting point for all scholarly efforts involving women's health as well as health care delivery.

Changing Conceptual Frameworks

New frameworks for studying women's health put women at the center of the inquiry, not on the periphery. Early studies of maternal child nursing had focused on the infant, with the mother a part of the context. Recent literature reflects the woman as the mother, the primary concern of the investigator.

Foundations of women's health research include theoretical models of human health, illness, therapeutics, and the interaction of the individual woman with physical, social, political, and cultural environments. Inherent in this theoretical framework are the values of health, holism, and person–environment interactions. An individual is recognized as a complex whole with multidimensional needs achieving a healthy state through a process of interaction and balance with a personal, physical, and social environment (Barnard, 1980; Hall, 1984). Many nurse theorists have proposed conceptual models to guide nursing practice, but validation of these models in the clinical setting has lagged behind development (Stevenson & Woods, 1986). Most studies on interventions and care for women's health have been non-experimental or have assessed single procedures and treatments. Few studies have assessed the impact of interventions on complex person–environment relationships.

Shaver's human ecological model (1985), providing an important theoretical framework for women's health research, is based upon the interaction of the individual with the environment and the influence of that interaction upon health-related behavior. Although this model improves understanding of environmental influences upon personal behavior, it does not explain the importance of the physical and sociopolitical elements of the environment that have significant impact upon the health of many women, especially the poor and disadvantaged. Williams (1989), in her feminist critique of health promotion in the United States, rejects the emphasis on individual behavior as the most important determinant of health.

A model of health adaptation incorporating multiple individual and environmental variables has been developed by Pender (1982; 1987) and includes polar constructs of health promotion and health protection. The domain of health protection includes individual behavior directed toward the regulation and maintenance of homeostasis and structural integrity. Health promotion is the actualization of inherent and acquired individual potential. Both health-protecting and health-promoting behaviors include physical, social, and self-care components.

Assumptions guiding Pender's model include concepts of personal choice and self-directed behavior. The assumption of personal suggests that change, self-actualization, or the capacity for change exists if the individual so chooses. A second assumption supposes that individual behavior is purposeful and motivated toward a goal. Purpose can only exist if choices are available and the individual is capable of making a choice. In a revision of this model, Pender has added a component of environmental modification that includes assessment and sociopolitical change. Environmental modification is considered along with personal change strategies for illness prevention and health promotion.

Another noticeable difference in the frameworks used to study women in nursing was the integration of the biological with psychosocial and cultural dimensions of health. New research about pregnancy (for example, early studies by Regina Lederman) focused on women's endocrine changes as well as the stressors in their lives. In addition, studies about premenstrual symptom and menopausal symptoms increasingly attempted to account not just for the role of ovarian hormones in symptoms but also to consider the context in which women lived their lives—the stressors and supports in their environments as well as stress arousal. Women with specific health problems such as irritable bowel syndrome (IBS) were studied in ways that allowed investigators to take into account ovarian steroids, stress arousal, and life stressors, and to identify that a history of sexual abuse was common in this group. Taylor (1996, 1999, 2000), building on the ecological health framework developed by Shaver and Pender, using a symptom management framework (UCSF Symptom Management Writing Group, 1995) as well as data from women's focus groups, developed and tested a symptom management package of nondrug strategies for perimenstrual symptom distress that has application to women's chronic illness management and general health promotion.

Including a view of the lifespan and development in the frameworks for studies has necessitated use of longitudinal designs in which women are studied over an extended period of time. This was the case in the studies of pregnancy and the postpartum done by Ramona Mercer, Marcia Killien, and Deborah Koniak-Griffin. Here the focus was on how women's health changed as a consequence of their changing biology during pregnancy and the postpartum as well as the changes that were ongoing in their lives, particularly the changes in the family relationships.

Continuing to focus on context for women's health has prompted nurses to include awareness of the social and physical environment in framing studies. Ethnicity and culture as well as education, occupation, and income become relevant parts of a framework for studying women when viewed from this vantage point (Meleis, Norbeck, & Laffrey, 1989). Racism, sexism, and classism have become part of the framework for understanding women's lives. Nursing's holistic perspectives have contributed to the advancement of innovative frameworks for new women's health services (Taylor & Woods, 1996) and also policy recommendations for women's health practice, education and research (Writing Group of the American Academy of Nursing Expert Panel on Women's Health, 1997).

Changing Methodology and Methods

In a review of women's health nursing research during the mid-1980s, Woods (1988) found that a empiricist paradigm predominated in research designs. The majority of studies during this 7-year review (1980–1986) were correlational in design, with five experimental or quasi-experimental study designs. Holistic designs were incorporated into subsequent studies—hermeneutics to study menopausal hot flashes (Levine-Silverman, 1989) and women's experiences of menopause (Dickson, 1990); an ethnographic descriptive study of women and self-care in weight management (Allan, 1989); and a phenomenological approach to psychological health and inner strength in older women (Rose, 1990). Studies related to women, health, and nursing practice during the 1980s have addressed attitudinal correlates of health promotion or risk screening behaviors such as motivation performance of breast self-examination, weight management behaviors, correlates of exercise performance, images of health, health beliefs, roles, coping, and social support. Cross-cultural studies were limited, but included those of depression, life stressors, and health practices or beliefs in poor Black or immigrant women (Johnson, Cloyd, & Wer, 1982; O'Brien, 1982; Powers, 1982; Muecke, 1983; Oakley, 1986). In a thorough review of the nursing literature between 1980 and 1985, only 3% of the published research in women's health examined older women specifically (Woods, 1988).

In 1992, Woods reviewed the then new NIH research agenda on women's health and worried that our efforts would not contribute much to understanding fully the dimensions of women's health if they merely reproduced contemporary mainstream science. Simply adding a cohort of women to a study designed to illuminate health issues from the perspective of "male as the norm" would not solve the problems of understanding and explaining health as women experienced it. Woods urged a re-examination of the nature of science that would foster a more complete understanding of the diverse populations of women in the U.S. and serve emancipatory ends (Woods, 1992).

A recent review of nursing research by Taylor (Olesen, Taylor, Ruzek, & Clarke, 1998) indicated that, by the 1980s, nurse researchers had made significant contributions to investigating cultural differences in women's health, especially aimed at diversity issues (age, culture, race/ethnicity, immigrant women, homeless women, culture-specific illness conditions, and developmental transitions). Many of these studies provided conceptual models and clinical recommendations that encompass changes in how clinicians contribute to the social construction of gender, race, class, health, and illness (Caroline & Bernhard, 1994). A number of studies depict health and illness experiences among diverse women in a variety of circumstances, including diverse ethnic groups (Mexican American, Native American, African American, Southeast Asian and Haitian women) as well as health behaviors of vulnerable groups such as homeless women and low-income working women of color. Several nursing studies departed from merely investigating women's situations and looked at women and their providers. Barriers to diverse women's access to health services have been studied from economic, psychological, and social perspectives by nurses. Nursing research on multiple diversities of women's health and illness has also applied multiple research methodologies and paradigms.

Since 1990, nursing research about women's health has expanded, both methodologically and substantively. Continuing to incorporate a holistic and biopsychosocial framework, nursing research has focused on multiple factors related to women's health and illness, in addition to women's lived experience. While empirical research has predominated in the study of women's health, nursing research has used a wide variety of qualitative and quantitative research methods. Descriptive and exploratory studies have used phenomenological, hermeneutical, or grounded-theory methodologies. Quantitative research designs have progressed well beyond the simplistic applying experimental, theory-testing approaches and participatory-action research designs to complex women's health conditions. Theoretical perspectives (feminist, political, social, or cultural theories) have provided critical foundations for these research endeavors.

The purposes of feminist science are to provide information *for* women rather than merely about women. As described in the review chapter by Andrist and Macpherson, there are now many nursing research programs that have generated explanations about women's health that are liberating, that have the capacity to be used by women for women's good. For example, we know that, regardless of the society, the most prevalent symptom during the postpartum is fatigue, among young adults and midlife women. We need to consider what context predisposes women to fatigue and what solutions or changes come about as a result of the research. Do the solutions really benefit most women? Or do they benefit the health care system?

Because concepts and methods shape our knowledge, they bear on the issues of diversity and commonality in women's health. In order to understand the complex realities of women's health in a wider social context, traditional epidemiological methods have been adapted to focus on health risks inherent to women's daily lives. Instead of identifying diseases and then searching for a cause, some nurse researchers have used both qualitative and quantitative methods to explain women's health risks within the context of their work, family and/or culture (Taylor, Woods, Lentz, Mitchell, & Lee, 1991; Woods & Mitchell, 1997).

Regardless of the difficulties inherent in both qualitative and quantitative research methods for investigation of differences originating from women's diverse contexts, new and developing methods have advanced our understanding. In quantitative research, when little is known about intra-individual variability of any particular phenomena, such as pain, fatigue, or perimenstrual symptom experience in different ethnic groups, a time-series methodology can answer questions of individual experience yet approximate the internal validity of experimental designs (Taylor, 1990). In addition, structural equation or hierarchical linear modeling strategies that better reflect the complexity of the dimensions compared with simple linear analytic models can analyze multiple indicators of diversity (ethnicity, race, occupation, income, class, education, etc.) as well as build and test complex theoretical models using multidimensional and longitudinal data that represent both the individual woman and her environment (social, political, cultural variables) (Taylor, Woods, et al., 1991). Further, some researchers have applied hybrid or triangulated designs (Mitchell, 1990) where both quantitative and qualitative methods are used in the investigation of women's diverse experiences. In qualitative research, advances in narrative and phenomenological analysis can facilitate deeper exploration of the meaning of women's diverse experiences (Bell, 1994; Stevens, Hall, & Meleis, 1992).

Realization that we, as researchers, are situated knowers means that we can have only a partial perspective of a problem based on our position. Only through multiple perspectives can multiple truths inform a topic. The need for a more complete understanding implies that investigators need to seek multiple perspectives in constructing their studies. Indeed, we collaborate with women in designing the projects, even at the point of selecting the important questions to study (Harraway, 1989). Regarding women as legitimate sources of knowledge means that women are valid informants on their own lives and health. Women's subjective perceptions are taken as valid, and the women are regarded as experts on their own lives. Who can tell us about symptoms other than the person experiencing them?

Notable in the review of nursing research literature of women's health are the articles of clinical recommendations. One of the unrecognized yet valuable types of nursing research is the report found in the clinical literature. Though not reported as case studies, which are in the style of medical journals, clinical reports nevertheless contain rich details about health care for diverse women (women of color, lesbian and bi-sexual women, women with disabilities, and women across the life span, such as young, middle-aged, and older women).

Because knowledge generation has the goal of benefiting participants, the participants have a stake in interpreting the findings. Many of us have consistently invited women who participated in our studies to have an opportunity to help interpret the results. Reflexivity involves looking at oneself as the researcher, examining one's own positions and values relative to the participants in a study (Reinharz, 1987). This is difficult. We as investigators need to examine our own biases at each point in the study, considering how they may have influenced our interpretations. We need to be willing to consider if the data analysis used women's experiences as the test of the adequacy of the problems, concepts, hypotheses, research design, data collection, and interpretation. We need to be honest about whether the research was done *for* women or for men and the institutions they control. We need to worry about whether we can place ourselves in the same class, race, culture, and gender sensitive critical plane as the women we study.

Other areas where nursing has contributed to changing methods and knowledge generation for women's health include the integration of public, political, scientific, and historical perspectives. We have dared to study how the society can make women sick. For example, interventions directed at individuals to change their health rather than community or population-oriented public health approaches negate the role of society in producing poor health and locate the responsibility for health only within the individual (Flynn, 1994).

Generating and Expanding New Knowledge for Women's Health

In this volume on nursing research in selected areas of women's health, we were challenged to be able to include all of the research conducted by nurses. Clearly, nurse researchers in the aggregate have contributed to women's health research. We have provided the leadership in many areas. We could have filled two volumes with reviews of nursing's contributions to generating and expanding women's health knowledge. In the following sections, we will describe the reviews included in this volume and highlight those areas that were not included which need further attention or have been reviewed elsewhere.

Nursing scholarship in women's health has expanded the knowledge of women's health and illness and also generated new knowledge across biopsychosocial and cultural domains. Most importantly, nurse researchers have included women in studies that generate information about health issues that matter to women; inform practice for a diverse groups of women, address differences in ethnic, racial, socioeconomic, sexual orientation groups; and have significant consequences for advancing the health of all women in the world. In choosing particular topics, we hoped to show the breadth and depth of research and scholarship by nurses that spans women's bodies and biology (menstrual cycle research), women's multiple roles (parenting, employment and caregiving), women's diversity (lesbian health and immigrant women's health), and cross-cutting and emerging areas of women's health and illness issues (violence, fatigue, stress, and health care decision-making).

Now, in 2001, 13 years after nursing research on women's health was reviewed in one chapter of the *Annual Review of Nursing Research* (Woods,

1988), we have one whole volume dedicated to women's health research conducted by nurses, and we struggled to delimit the topics for review due to the extensive contributions by nursing scholars. Building on previous reviews as well as emphasizing nursing's leadership in extending the knowledge base in women's health, 11 topical areas were selected. Topics were considered for inclusion that demonstrated some of the areas where nursing has provided leadership or demonstrated a significant contribution of research and scholarship. The following areas of new or expanding women's health knowledge generated by nurse researchers are included in this volume:

- Women's multiple roles, including parenting (Angela McBride & Cheryl Prohaska Shore), employment (Marcia Killien), and caregiving (Margaret Bull)
- Disparities in health, including differences among ethnic and social groups of women affecting their chances for health, such as lesbian health (Linda Bernhard) and immigrant women's health (Karen Aroian)
- Menstrual cycle research—a focus on Nursing's contributions (Nancy Reame and Cheryl Andrist)
- Stress and women's health and illness (Cheryl Cahill)
- Fatigue and sleep alterations affecting women's health and illness (Kathryn Lee)
- Violence against women and health care directed at assessing and caring for women who have survived male partner violence (Janice Humphreys)
- Women's health care decision-making (Marilyn Rothert and Annette O'Connor)

Some of the areas of significant contribution by nurse researchers that are not reviewed in this volume include reproductive health issues (fertility protection and prevention, menstruation, childbearing, and sexuality), women's mental health, women's health problems related to aging (incontinence and falls prevention), and comprehensive reviews of women's health disparities and diversity, symptoms and symptom management research (pain, dyspnea, altered mobility). The following areas of women's health knowledge have been reviewed by nurse researchers in recent publications.

- Sexuality (reviewed by Linda Bernhard, 1993; Catherine Fogel, 1999) and fertility protection and contraception (reviewed by Theresa McDonald & Susan Johnson, 1993)
- Menstrual cycle research (reviewed by Alice Dan, 1988; Nancy Woods, Ellen Mitchell & Diana Taylor, 1999)

- Childbearing and women's health (reviewed by Kathryn Barnard & Margo Neal, 1977; Marlene Mackey & Susan Brouse, 1988; Patricia Geary and associates, 1993)
- Infertility and women's responses to infertility diagnosis and therapy (reviewed by Ellen Olshansky, 1999)
- Disparities and diversities in women's health (reviewed by Virginia Oleson and Diana Taylor, 1997)
- Women's mental health and illness (reviewed by Denise Webster, 1988; 1993) and substance use and abuse in women (reviewed by Tonda Hughes, 1989; 1993)
- Problems of aging and older women's health, including mental health status, functional limitations, osteoporosis, managing incontinence, and supportive and non-supportive environments (reviewed by Bev McElmurry & Emily Zabrocki, 1988, 1990; Pat Archbold, 1999; Beverly Roberts, 1999; Linda Phillips & Martha Ayres, 1999; Cornelia Beck, Diane Cronin-Stubbs, Kathleen Buckwalter & Carla Rapp, 1999; Molly Dougherty & Linda Jensen, 1999)
- Problems of gender-specific diseases and physical health, such as auto-immunity and Lupus Erythematosus (reviewed by Ayhan Aytekin Lash, 1997), the management of hypertension in women (reviewed by Lynne Braun, Beth Staffileno, and Kathleen Potempa, 1997), women's cardio-vascular health (reviewed by Karyn Holm and Sue Penckofer, 1993), sexually transmitted diseases (reviewed by Catherine Fogel, 1993), women and cancer (reviewed by Tish Knobf, 1989), and osteoporosis (reviewed by Amy Clarke Olson, 1989)
- Symptom management research, such as pain, dyspnea, altered mobility, and nausea and vomiting (reviewed by Christine Miaskowski, 1997; Barbara Smith & Mary Macvicar, 1999; Ginger Carrieri-Kohlman & Susan Janson, 1999; and Peg Heitkemper, 1999)
- Occupational issues, such as women as health care providers (reviewed by Carol Leppa, 1988), violence against health care workers (reviewed by Carol Collins, 1997), and sexual harassment (reviewed by Judith Ross, 1997)

SUMMARY

The science of women's health, as shaped by nurse researchers, grew from the redefinition of women's health to proposing new conceptual frameworks for studying women, development of methodology and methods for studying women's health, and to the generation of new knowledge about several aspects of women's health. Clearly, a community of nursing scholars developed over the past 25 years has contributed to advancing women's health knowledge and improving the health and well-being of women. In subsequent reviews, the adequacy of women's health research in nursing will be demonstrated by future research that: includes women in studies that generate information about health issues that matter to women; informs practice for a diverse groups of women, addressing differences in ethnic, racial, socioeconomic, sexual orientation groups; and has significant consequences for advancing the health of all women in the world.

REFERENCES

Allan, J. D. (1989). Women who successfully manage their weight. *Western Journal of Nursing Research, 11,* 657–675.

Archbold, P. (1999). Older adults: Health and illness issues. In A. Hinshaw, S. Feetham, & J. Shaver (Eds.), *Handbook of clinical nursing research* (pp. 561–562). Thousand Oaks, CA: Sage.

Barnard, K. B. (1980). Knowledge for practice: Directions for the future. *Nursing Research, 29,* 208–212.

Barnard, K. B., & Neal, M. (1977). Maternal-child nursing research: Review of the past and strategies for the future. *Nursing Research, 26,* 193–200.

Beck, C., Cronin-Stubbs, D., Buckwalter, K., & Rapp, C. (1999). Managing cognitive impairment and depression in the elderly. In A. Hinshaw, S. Feetham, & J. Shaver (Eds.), *Handbook of clinical nursing research* (pp. 578–598). Thousand Oaks, CA: Sage.

Bell, R. (1994). Prominency of women in Navajo healing beliefs and values. *Nursing and Health Care, 15,* 232–240.

Bernhard, L. A. (1992). Consequences of hysterectomy in the lives of women. *Health Care for Women International, 13,* 281–291.

Bernhard, L. A. (1993). Women's sexuality. In B. I. McElmurry & R. S. Parker (Eds.), *Annual review of women's health* (pp. 67–93). New York: National League for Nursing Press.

Boston Women's Health Book Collective. (1973). *Our bodies, ourselves: A book by and for women* (1st ed.). Boston: New England Free Press.

Boston Women's Health Book Collective. (1998). *New our bodies, ourselves: A book by and for women for the new century* (4th ed.). New York: Simon & Schuster.

Bowles, G., & Klein, R. D. (Eds.). (1983). *Theories of women's studies.* Boston: Routledge & Kegan Paul.

Braun, L., Staffileno, B., & Potempa, K. (1997). The management of hypertension in women. In B. J. McElmurry & R. Parker (Eds.), *Annual review of women's health* (Vol. 3). New York: Jones & Bartlett.

Bullough, B., David, M., Whipple, B., Dixon, I., Allgeier, E. R., & Drury, K. C. (1984). Subjective reports of female orgasmic expulsion of fluid. *Nurse Practitioner, 9*(3), 55–56, 58 59.

Caroline, H., & Bernhard, L. (1994). Health care dilemmas for women with serious mental illness. *Advances in Nursing Science, 16,* 78–88.

Carrieri-Kohlman, V., & Janson, S. (1999). Managing dyspnea. In A. Hinshaw, S. Feetham, & J. Shaver (Eds.), *Handbook of clinical nursing research* (pp. 379–394). Thousand Oaks, CA: Sage.

Cassandra: A Radical Feminist Nursing Newsletter. 1(1), 1–12.

Chinn, P., & Wheeler, C. (1986). Feminism and nursing. *Nursing Outlook, 33*(2), 74–77.

Cohen, S., Hollingsworth, A., Rubin, M., Graff, B., Thomas, J., Linenberger, H., & Morgan, M. (1994). Issues of convalescence after hysterectomy. In N. F. Woods (Ed.), *Proceedings, 9th Conference, Society for Menstrual Cycle Research* (pp. 213–215). Seattle, WA: Hamilton and Cross.

Collins, C. (1997). Violence against healthcare workers. In B. J. McElmurry & R. Parker (Eds.), *Annual Review of Women's Health, Vol. 3.* New York: Jones & Bartlett.

Daly, M. (1978). *Gyn/ecology: The metaethics of radical feminism.* Boston, MA: Beacon.

Dan, A., & Leppa, C. (1988). Menstrual cycle research. In C. Leppa (Ed.), *Women's health perspectives: An annual review* (Vol. 1, pp. 143–160). Phoenix, AZ: Oryx.

Dickson, G. (1990). A feminist poststructuralist analysis of the knowledge of menopause. *Advances in Nursing Science, 12*(3), 15–31.

Dickson, G. (1991). Menopause: Language, meaning, and subjectivity: A feminist poststructuralist analysis. In A. Voda & R. Conover (Eds.), *Proceedings of the Society for Menstrual Cycle Research, Eighth Conference* (pp. 112–125). Scottsdale, AZ: Society for Menstrual Cycle Research.

Dougherty, M., & Jensen, L. (1999). Managing urinary and fecal incontinence. In A. Hinshaw, S. Feetham, & J. Shaver (Eds.), *Handbook of clinical nursing research* (pp. 407–424). Thousand Oaks, CA: Sage.

Duffy, M. E. (1985). A critique of research: A feminist perspective. *Health Care for Women International, 6,* 341–352.

Duffy, M., & Hedin, B. (1988). New directions for nursing research. In N. Woods & M. Catanzaro (Eds.), *Nursing research: Theory and practice* (pp. 530–539). St Louis: Moody.

Fee, E. (1983). Women and health care: A comparison of theories. In E. Fee (Ed.), *Women and health: The politics of sex in medicine* (pp. 17–34). Farmingdale, NY: Baywood.

Fitzpatrick, J., Taunton, R., & Benoliel, J. (Eds.). (1988). *Annual review of nursing research* (Vol. 6). New York: Springer Publishing Co.

Flaskerud, J. H., & Nyamathi, A. M. (1989). Black and Latina women's AIDS related knowledge, attitudes and practices. *Research in Nursing and Health, 12,* 339–346.

Flaskerud, J. H., & Rush, C. E. (1989). AIDS and traditional health beliefs and practices of Black women. *Nursing Research, 38,* 210–215.

Flaskerud, J. H., & Thompson, J. (1991). Beliefs about AIDS, health and illness in low-income White women. *Nursing Research, 49,* 266–271.

Flynn, B. (1984). An action research framework for primary health care: A conceptual approach to the study of primary health care in communities. *Nursing Outlook, 32,* 316–318.

Fogel, C. (1993). Sexually transmitted diseases. In B. J. McElmurry & R. Parker (Eds.), *Annual review of women's health* (Vol. 1, pp. 311–330). New York: National League for Nursing.

Fogel, C. (1999). Women and sexuality: Contributions from nursing research and practice recommendations. In A. Hinshaw, S. Feetham, & J. Shaver (Eds.), *Handbook of clinical nursing research* (pp. 517–534). Thousand Oaks, CA: Sage.

Fogel, C., & Woods, N. (Eds.). (1995). *Women's health care.* Thousand Oaks, CA: Sage.

Fontaine, K. L (1991). The conspiracy of culture: women's issues in body size. *Nursing Clinics of North America, 26,* 669–676.

Geary, P., Hastings-Tolsma, M., Voytko, D., Wahba, A., & Patrick, T. (1993). Childbearing. In B. J. McElmurry & R. Parker (Eds.), *Annual review of women's health* (Vol. 1, pp. 123–162). New York: National League for Nursing.

Griffin, F. N. (1994). The health care system: factoring in the ethnicity, cultural and health care needs of women and children of color. *American Black Nursing Journal, 5,* 130–133.

Grisso, J., & Watkins, K. (1992). A framework for a women's health research agenda. *Journal of Women's Health, 1,* 177–187.

Haraway, D. (1988). Situated knowledges: The science question in feminism and the privilege of partial perspective. *Feminist Studies 14,* 575–599.

Harding, S. (1991). *Whose science? Whose knowledge? Thinking from women's lives.* Ithaca, NY: Cornell University Press.

Hall, B. (1981). The change paradigm in nursing: growth versus persistence. *Advances in Nursing Science, 3*(4), 1–6.

Heide, W. S. (1985). *Feminism for the health of it.* Buffalo, NY: Margaretdaughters.

Heitkemper, M. (1999). Managing nausea and vomiting. In A. Hinshaw, S. Feetham, & J. Shaver (Eds.), *Handbook of clinical nursing research* (pp. 425–434). Thousand Oaks, CA: Sage.

Henderson, D. J., Boyd, C. J., & Whitmore, J. (1995). Women and illicit drugs: Sexuality and crack cocaine. *Health Care for Women International, 16,* 113–124.

Holm, K., & Penckhofer, S. (1993). Women's cardiovascular health. In B. J. McElmurry & R. Parker (Eds.), *Annual review of women's health* (Vol. 1, pp. 287–309). New York: National League for Nursing Press.

Hughes, T. (1989). Women, alcohol and drugs. In C. Leppa (Ed.), *Women's health perspectives: An annual review* (Vol. 2, pp. 17–35). Phoenix, AZ: Oryx.

Hughes, T. (1993). Research on alcohol and drug use among women: A review and update. In B. J. McElmurry & R. Parker (Eds.), *Annual review of women's health* (Vol. 1, pp. 243–286). New York: National League for Nursing.

Jemmott, L. S., & Jemmott, I. B. (1991). Increasing condom-use intentions among sexually active Black adolescent women. *Nursing Research, 40,* 273–279.

Jemmott, L. S., & Jemmott, I. B. (1992). Applying the Theory of Reasoned Action to AIDS risk behavior: Condom use among Black women. *Nursing Research, 41,* 229–234.

Johnson, F., Cloyd, C., & Wer, J. (1982). Life satisfaction of poor urban Black aged. *Advances in Nursing Science, 4,* 27–34.

Kauffman, K. S. (1994). The insider/outsider dilemma: Field experience of a White researcher "getting in" a poor Black community. *Nursing Research, 43,* 179–183.

Kearney, M., Murphy, S., & Rosenbaum, M. (1994). Learning by losing: Sex and fertility on crack cocaine. *Qualitative Health Research, 4,* 142–146.

Killien, M., & Brown, M. A. (1987). Work and family roles of women: Sources of stress and coping strategies. *Health Care for Women International, 8*(2/3), 169–184.

Klein, R. (1983). How to do what we want to do: Thoughts about feminist methodology. In G. Bowles & R. D. Klein (Eds.), *Theories of women's studies* (pp. 88–104). Boston: Routledge & Kegan Paul.

Knobf, T. (1989). Women and cancer. In C. Leppa (Ed.), *Women's health perspectives: An annual review* (Vol. 2, pp. 175–206). Phoenix, AZ. Oryx.

Koniak-Griffin, D., Anderson, N., Verzemnieks, I., & Brecht, M. (2000). A public health nursing early intervention program for adolescent mothers: outcomes from pregnancy through 6 weeks postpartum. *Nursing Research, 49,* 130–138.

Lather, P. (1991). *Getting smart: Feminist research and pedagogy with/in the postmodern.* New York: Routledge.

Lash, A. (1997). Autoimmunity and gender effects: Lupus Erythematosus. In B. J. McElmurry & R. Parker (Eds.), *Annual review of women's health* (Vol. 3). New York: Jones & Bartlett.

Lederman, R. (1986). Maternal anxiety in pregnancy. Relationship to fetal and newborn health status. *Annual Review of Nursing Research, 4,* 3–20.

Leppa, C. (1988). Women as health care providers. In C. Leppa (Ed.), *Women's health perspectives: An annual review* (Vol. 1, pp. 181–206). Phoenix, AZ: Oryx.

Leppa, C. (1988). *Women's health perspectives: An annual review* (Vol. 1). Phoenix, AZ: Oryx.

Leppa, C. (1989). *Women's health perspectives: An annual review* (Vol. 2). Phoenix, AZ: Oryx.

Leppa, C (1990). *Women's health perspectives: An annual review* (Vol. 3). Phoenix, AZ: Oryx.

Lethbridge, D. I. (1991). Choosing and using contraception: Toward a theory of women's contraceptive self-care. *Nursing Research, 40,* 276–280.

Levine-Silverman, S. (1989). The menopausal hot flash: A procrustean bed of research. *Journal of Advanced Nursing, 14,* 939–949.

Lewin, E., & Oleson, V. (1985). *Women, health & healing: New perspectives for women's health.* London: Tavistock-Methuen.

Lipson, J., & Miller, S. (1994). Changing roles of Afghan refugee women in the United States. *Health Care for Women International, 15,* 171–180.

Mackey, M., & Brouse, S. (1988). Childbearing. In C. Leppa (Ed.), *Women's health perspectives: An annual review* (Vol. 1, pp. 109–142). Phoenix, AZ: Oryx.

MacPherson, K. (1981). Menopause as disease: The social construction of a metaphor. *Advances in Nursing Science, 3,* 95–114.

MacPherson, K. (1990). Nurse researchers respond to the medicalization of menopause. In M. Flint, F. Kronenberg, & W. Utian (Eds.), *Multidisciplinary perspectives on menopause* (pp. 180–184). New York: New York Academy of Sciences Press.

Marieskind, H. (1980). *Women's health.* St. Louis: C. V. Mosby.

McBride, A. B. (1987). Developing a women's mental health research agenda. *Image, 19*(1), 4–8.

McBride, A. B. (1993). From gynecology to GYN-ecology: Developing a practice-research agenda for women's health. *Health Care for Women International, 14,* 315–325.

McBride, A. B., & McBride, W. L. (1993). Women's health scholarship: From critique to assertion. *Journal of Women's Health, 2,* 43–47.

McBride A. B., & McBride, W. L. (1981). Theoretical underpinnings for women's health. *Women & Health, 6*(1–2), 37–55.

McCraw, R. K. (1991). Psychosexual changes associated with the perimenopausal period. *Journal of Nurse Midwifery, 36*(1), 17–24.

McDonald, T., & Johnson, S. (1993). Contraception. In B. J. McElmurry & R. Parker (Eds.), *Annual review of women's health* (Vol. 1, pp. 95–122). New York: National League for Nursing.

McElmurry, B. J., & Huddleston, D. (1991). Self-care and menopause: Critical review of research. *Health Care for Women International, 12,* 15–26.

McElmurry, B. J., & Parker, R. (Eds.). (1993). *Annual review of women's health* (Vol. 1). New York: National League for Nursing Press.

McElmurry, B. J., & Parker, R. (Eds.). (1995). *Annual review of women's health* (Vol. 2). New York: Jones & Bartlett.

McElmurry, B. J., & Parker, R. (Eds.). (1997). *Annual review of women's health* (Vol. 3). New York: Jones & Bartlett.

McElmurry, B., & Zabrocki, E. (1988). Health of older women. In C. Leppa (Ed.), *Women's health perspectives: An annual review* (pp. 161–180). Phoenix, AZ: Oryx.

Meleis, A., Norbeck, J. S., & Laffrey, S. C. (1989). Role integration and health among female clerical workers. *Research in Nursing and Health, 12,* 335–364.

Mercer, R. T. (1986). *First-time motherhood: Experiences from teens to forties.* New York: Springer Publishing Co.

Miaskowski, C. (1997). Pain management in women. In B. J. McElmurry & R. Parker (Eds.), *Annual review of women's health* (Vol. 3). New York: Jones & Bartlett.

Mitchell, E. S. (1990). Multiple triangulation: A methodology for nursing science. *Advances in Nursing Science, 8,* 18–26.

Mitchell, E. S., Woods, N. F., & Lentz, M. J. (1991). Recognizing PMS when your see it: Criteria for PMS sample selection. In D. Taylor & N. Woods (Eds.), *Menstruation, health and illness* (pp. 89–102). Washington, DC: Hemisphere.

Morse, J. M., & Kieren, D. (1993). The Adolescent Menstrual Attitude Questionnaire: Normative scores, part 2. *Health Care for Women International, 14,* 63–76.

Morse, J. M., Kieren, D., & Bottorff, J. (1993). The Adolescent Menstrual Attitude Questionnaire: Scale construction, part 1. *Health Care for Women International, 14,* 39–62.

Muecke, M. (1983). In search of healers: Southeast Asian refugees in the American health care system [Special issue: Crosscultural Medicine]. *Western Journal of Medicine, 139,* 31–36.

Nelson, M. A. (1994). Economic impoverishment as a health risk: Methodological and conceptual issues. *Advances in Nursing Science, 16*(3), 1–12.

Nightingale, F. (1969). *Notes on nursing: What it is and what it is not.* London: Dover. (Original work published 1959)

Nightingale, F. (1979). *Cassandra: An essay.* Old Westbury, CT: Feminist Press.

Nyamathi, A. M., & Lewis, C. E. (1991). Coping of African-American women at risk from AIDS. *Women's Health Inventory, 1*(2), 53–62.

Nyamathi, A. M., Lewis, C., Leake, B., Raskerud, J., & Bennett, C. (1995). Barriers to condom use and needle cleaning among impoverished minority female injection drug users and partners of drug users. *Public Health Reports, 110,* 166–172.

Oakley, L. D. (1986). Marital status, gender role attitude, and Black women's report of depression. *Journal of the National Black Nurses Association, 1,* 41–51.

O'Brien, M. (1982). Pragmatic survivalism: Behavior patterns affecting low-level wellness among minority group members. *Advances in Nursing Science, 4*(3), 13–26.

Olesen, V., Taylor, D., Ruzek, S., & Clarke, A. (1997). Strengths and strongholds in women's health research. In S. Ruzek, V. Olesen, & A. Clarke (Eds.), *Women's health: Complexities and differences* (pp. 580–606). Columbus, OH: Ohio State University Press.

Olshansky, E. F. (1987a). Identity of self as infertile: An example of theory-generating research. *Advances in Nursing Science, 9*(2), 54–63.

Olshansky, E. F. (1987b). Infertility and its influence on women's career identities. *Health Care for Women International, 8*(2,3), 185–196.

Olshansky, E. F. (1998). Responses to high technology infertility treatment. *Image: Journal of Nursing Scholarship, 20*(3), 128–131.

Olshansky, E. (1999). Infertility. In A. Hinshaw, S. Feetham, & J. Shaver (Eds.), *Handbook of clinical nursing research* (pp. 509–516). Thousand Oaks, CA: Sage.

Olson, A. (1989). Osteoporosis. In C. Leppa (Ed.), *Women's health perspectives: An annual review* (Vol. 2, pp. 175–206). Phoenix, AZ: Oryx.

Parker, B., & Mc Farlane, J. (1991). Feminist theory and nursing: An empowerment model for research. *Advances in Nursing Science, 13*(3), 59–67.

Pender, N. J. (1986). Health promotion: Implementing strategies. In B. Logan & C. Dawkins (Eds.), *Family-centered nursing in the community.* Menlo Park, CA: Addison-Wesley.

Pender, N. J. (1987). *Health promotion in nursing practice.* Norwalk, CT: Appleton, Century, Crofts.

Pender, N. J. (1990). Expressing health through lifestyle patterns. *Nursing Science Quarterly, 3*(3), 115–122.

Phillips, L., & Ayres, M. (1999). Supportive and nonsupportive care environments for the eldcrly. In A. Hinshaw, S. Feetham, & J. Shaver (Eds.), *Handbook of clinical nursing research* (pp. 599–628). Thousand Oaks, CA: Sage.

Powers, B. (1982). The use of orthodox and Black American folk medicine. *Advances in Nursing Science, 4*(3), 49–64.

Reinharz, S. (1983). Experiential analysis: A contribution to feminist research. In G. Bowles & R. Klein (Eds.), *Theories of women's studies*. Boston: Routledge & Kegan Paul.

Roberts, B. (1999). Activities of daily living: Factors related to independence. In A. Hinshaw, S. Feetham, & J. Shaver (Eds.), *Handbook of clinical nursing research* (pp. 563–578). Thousand Oaks, CA: Sage.

Rose, J. F. (1990). Psychologic health of women: A phenomenologic study of women's inner strength. *Advances in Nursing Science, 12*(2), 56–70.

Ross, J. (1997). Sexual harassment. In B. J. McElmurry & R. Parker (Eds.), *Annual review of women's health* (Vol. 3). New York: Jones & Bartlett.

Sandelowski, M., & Jones, L. (1986). Social exchanges of infertile women. *Issues in Mental Health Nursing, 8*(3), 173–189.

Sandelowski, M., & Pollock, C. (1986). Women's experiences of infertility. *Image: The Journal of Nursing Scholarship, 18*(4), 140–144.

Shaver, J. (1985). A biopsychosocial view of health. *Nursing Outlook, 33*(4), 186–191.

Smith, B., & MacVicar, M. (1999). Management of mobility and altered physical activity. In A. Hinshaw, S. Feetham, & J. Shaver (Eds.), *Handbook of clinical nursing research* (pp. 363–378). Thousand Oaks, CA: Sage.

Spangler, Z. (1992). Transcultural care values and nursing practices of Philippine-American nurses. *Journal of Transcultural Nursing, 3*(2), 28–37.

Steen, M. (1991). Historical perspectives on women and mental illness and prevention of depression in women, using a feminist framework. *Issues in Mental Health Nursing, 12*, 359–374.

Stevens, P. E., Hall, J. M., & Meleis, A. I. (1992). Examining vulnerability of women clerical workers from five ethnic/racial groups. *Western Journal of Nursing Research, 14*, 754–774.

Stevenson, J. S. (1977). Women's health research. Why, what and so what? *CMR Voice* (Ohio State University School of Nursing), *21*, 1–2.

Stevenson, J. S., & Woods, N. (1986). Nursing science and contemporary science: Emerging paradigms. In O. Sorenson (Ed.), *Setting the agenda for the year 2000*. Kansas City, MO: American Academy of Nursing.

Suarez, L. (1994). Pap smear and mammogram screening in Mexican-American women: The effects of acculturation. *American Journal of Public Health, 84*, 742–746.

Swanson, K. (2000). Predicting depressive symptoms after miscarriage: A path analysis based on the Lazarus paradigm. *Journal of Women's Health Research, 9*, 191–206.

Taylor, D. (1990). Time-series analysis: use of autocorrelation as an analytic strategy for describing pattern and change. *Western Journal of Nursing Research, 12*, 254–261.

Taylor, D. (1999). Effectiveness of professional-peer group treatment: Symptom management for women with PMS. *Research in Nursing and Health, 22,* 496–511.

Taylor, D. (2000). More than personal change: Effective elements of symptom management. *NP Forum, 11*(2), 1–10.

Taylor, D., Woods, N., Lentz, M., Mitchell, E., & Lee, K. (1991). Perimenstrual symptoms: An explanatory model. In D. Taylor & N. F. Woods (Eds.), *Menstruation, health and illness.* Washington, DC: Hemisphere.

Taylor, D., & Woods, N. F. (1996). Changing women's health, changing nursing practice. *Journal of Obstetrical, Gynecological & Neonatal Nurses, 25,* 791–802.

Taylor, D., & Dower, K. (1997). Toward a women-centered health care system: Women's experiences, women's voices, women's needs. *Health Care for Women International, 18,* 407–422.

United States Public Health Service, National Institutes of Health. (1992). *Opportunities for research on women's health.* Bethesda, MD: National Institutes of Health.

Verbrugge, L. (1980). Sex differences in complaints and diagnoses. *Journal of Behavioral Medicine, 3,* 327–355.

Walcott-McQuigg, J. A. (1994). Worksite stress: Gender and cultural diversity issues. *American Association of Occupational Health Nursing Journal, 42,* 528–533.

Warren, B. J. (1994). Depression in African-American women. *Journal of Psychosocial Nursing, 32*(3), 29–33.

Watts, R. I. (1982). Sexual functioning, health beliefs, and compliance with high blood pressure medications. *Nursing Research, 31,* 278–283.

Webster, D. (1988). Women and mental health. In C. Leppa (Ed.), *Women's health perspectives: An annual review* (pp. 14–33). Phoenix, AZ: Oryx.

Webster, D. (1989). Women and mental health. In C. Leppa (Ed.), *Women's health perspectives: An annual review* (pp. 1–18). Phoenix, AZ: Oryx.

Webster, D. (1993). Women and mental health. In B. J. McElmurry & R. Parker (Eds.), *Annual review of women's health* (Vol. 1, pp. 9–28). New York: National League for Nursing, Jones.

White, J. H. (1991). Feminism, eating and mental health. *Advances in Nursing Science, 13*(3), 68–80.

White, M. J., Rintala, D. H., Hart, K., & Fuhrer, M. I. (1994). A comparison of the sexual concerns of men and women with spinal cord injuries. *Rehabilitation Nursing Research, 3*(2), 55–61.

Whitley, N. (1978). The first coital experience of one hundred women. *Journal of Obstetric, Gynecologic and Neonatal Nursing, 7*(4), 41–45.

Williams, D. M. (1989). Political theory and individualistic health promotion. *Advances in Nursing Science, 12*(1), 14–25.

Woods, N. F. (1985). New models of women's health care. *Health Care for Women International, 6,* 193–208.

Woods, N. F. (1988). Women's health. In J. J. Fitzpatrick, R. L. Taunton, & J. Q. Benoliel (Eds.), *Annual review of nursing research* (Vol. 6, pp. 209–236). New York: Springer Publishing Co.

Woods, N. (1994). The United States women's health research agenda; analysis and critique. *Western Journal of Nursing Research, 16,* 467–479.

Woods, N. F. (1995). Women and their health. In C. Fogel & N. F. Woods (Eds.), *Women's health care*. Thousand Oaks, CA: Sage.

Woods, N. F., & Hulka, B. (1979). Symptom reports and illness behavior among employed women and homemakers. *Journal of Community Health, 5*(1), 36–45.

Woods, N. F., Lentz, M., Mitchell, E., & Oakley, L. D. (1994). Depressed mood and self-esteem in young Asian, Black, and White women in America. *Health Care for Women International, 15*(3), 243–262.

Woods, N. F., & Mitchell, E. (1996). Midlife depression: Patterns of depressed mood in midlife women: Observations from the Seattle Midlife Women's Health Study. *Research in Nursing and Health, 19,* 111–123.

Woods, N. F., & Mitchell, E. (1997). Pathways to depressed mood in midlife women: Observations from the Seattle Midlife Women's Health Study. *Research in Nursing and Health, 20,* 119–129.

Woods, N. F., & Mitchell, E. (1999). Anticipating menopause: Observations from Seattle Midlife Women's Health Study. *Menopause, 6*(1).

Woods, N. F., Mitchell, E., & Taylor, D. (1999). From menarche to menopause: Contributions from nursing research and recommendations for practice. In A. Hinshaw, S. Feetham, & J. Shaver (Eds.), *Handbook of clinical nursing research* (pp. 459–484). Thousand Oaks, CA: Sage.

Writing Group of the UCSF Center for Symptom Management Research. (1995). A model for symptom management. *IMAGE: Journal of Nursing Scholarship, 26,* 272–276.

Writing Group of the Expert Panel on Women's Health. (1997). Women's health and women's health care: Recommendations for transformative changes in health care services, nursing education and practice. *Nursing Outlook, 45*(1), 7–15.

Zabrocki, E., & McElmurry, B. (1990). Health of older women. In C. Leppa (Ed.), *Women's health perspectives: An annual review* (pp. 143–174). Phoenix, AZ: Oryx.

Zambrana, R. (1987). A research agenda on issues affecting poor and minority women: A model for understanding their health needs. *Women & Health, 12*(3/4), 137–160.

Chapter 2

Conceptual Models for Women's Health Research: Reclaiming Menopause As an Exemplar of Nursing's Contributions to Feminist Scholarship

Linda C. Andrist and Kathleen I. MacPherson

ABSTRACT

An examination of women's transition through menopause provides a remarkable example of nursing's contributions to feminist scholarship. The predominant biomedical model perpetuates the idea that menopause is a deficiency disease, whereas feminist and nurse scholars have deconstructed this paradigm and have reclaimed menopause as a part of midlife women's developmental stage. We begin this chapter with a review of the birth of women's health scholarship as it is the foundation for theory that undergirds feminist nursing research. We then discuss the tenets of feminist scholarship. The historical context of menopause is reviewed briefly to highlight the ways in which menopause was transformed from a normal physiological event to a disease. Using this as a backdrop, we reviewed nursing studies in two emerging bodies of knowledge. We reviewed 10 studies in the area of "women reclaiming menopause" and found that over all women believe the menopausal transition is a normal developmental stage. The second area of new research looks at "menopause across cultures." The studies of Korean, Indian, and Thai women reviewed demonstrate that similar to other health issues, the experience of Western women cannot be universalized, and most important, researchers must take into consideration the social, political, economic, and cultural forces that impact women's experience of the menopause transition.

Key words: feminist nursing research, menopause, menopause and culture, women's health scholarship

29

Women's transition through menopause is a remarkable example of nursing's contributions to feminist scholarship. At this point in history, menopause is among the most medicalized issue in women's health. Studies published in the medical literature over the past two decades have concentrated on how hormones can be used to prevent diseases of old age, how to help women make decisions about taking hormones, and why women do not comply with therapy. This biomedical model perpetuates the idea that the decline of estrogen levels is a deficiency disease, much like diabetes, and therefore requires medication.

Feminist scholars have deconstructed the biomedical paradigm and nurse scholars are reclaiming menopause as a part of midlife women's developmental stage. Nurses began to ask different questions—what do women know about menopause? What are their sources of information? What is their experience of the transition? How do they make decisions about hormones, given how biomedicine has painted the picture of life after menopause? These kinds of questions arise from a feminist paradigm in which women's lived experience is the critical starting point for all efforts in research. Women's health scholarship, now over 20 years old, has a rich tradition in women's studies, feminist theories, and nursing.

This chapter is slightly different than previous reviews of menopause (Huddleston, 1996; Voda & George, 1986; Woods & Mitchell, 1995) in that we are not reviewing all of the extant literature, but rather nursing literature that has contributed to reclaiming menopause—feminist scholarship. We begin with a brief history of women's health nursing, then discuss characteristics of feminist scholarship. The historical context of menopause is reviewed briefly to underscore the ways in which menopause was transformed from a normal physiological event to a disease and provides the backdrop for our review. Our definition of feminist scholarship is quite broad and includes many scholarly approaches.

THE BIRTH OF WOMEN'S HEALTH SCHOLARSHIP

The women's health movement was grounded in the second wave of feminism in the United States (Nichols, 2000; Rosen, 2000). Women activists in the late 1960s and early 1970s challenged professional authority and the prevailing medical paradigm. Women began meeting and discussing the ways in which the "medical care system" treated them and their health care needs. They advocated for more participation in health care and even lay control over routine health care, and started to dismantle long held beliefs about women's bodies (Geary, 1985; Marieskind, 1975; Ruzek, 1978). In 1969, women activists in Boston held a conference on "Women and their Bodies," which evolved into The Boston Women's Health Book Collective. The first edition of *Our Bodies, Ourselves* was published in 1970 (Boston Women's Health Book Collective, 1971).

Although the profession of nursing was largely silent during the first decade of the women's movement, nurses working in obstetrics and gynecology witnessed the mistreatment of women and related to the groundbreaking work of Gena Corea in her exposé of the medical profession, *The Hidden Malpractice* (1977). Feminist nurses felt caught in a system that perpetuated the oppression of women and many joined forces with lay activists and the nascent field of women's studies. Women's health nursing was probably the strongest link between nursing and the feminist movement in the 1970s and 1980s (Mulligan, 1983). The publication of Leonide Martin's *Health Care of Women* in 1978 was one of the first advanced nursing practice texts that discussed how the women's health movement impacts health care for women. Other texts appeared soon after, included the critique of women as consumers and providers of health care (Hawkins & Higgins, 1981), and embraced a feminist framework that examined health issues across the life cycle, not exclusively obstetrics and gynecology (Fogel & Woods, 1981).

THEORETICAL FRAMEWORKS

Women's health scholarship embodies feminist theories and is a distinct area of women's studies. Nurses began to explicate a women's health theoretical framework in 1981 with the McBrides' classic article, "Theoretical underpinnings for women's health." The McBrides laid out seven issues that frame the specialty of women's health and provide the basis for a theoretical framework. These include: (1) including women as subjects in research; (2) investigating socio-cultural factors that impact health and illness; (3) attending to the ways women are treated in the medical care system, such as unnecessary surgical interventions, excluding women in decision making about treatment choices, and, medicating women without sufficient research; (4) not assuming that male behavior is the norm; (5) asserting that women's health concerns are worthy of serious investigation; (6) investigating overall health rather than solely reproductive issues; (7) appreciating women's life transitions as the norm rather than as disease situations. The framework that addresses these issues has as its core *women's lived experience* as the starting point for health efforts as well as scholarly inquiry.

MacPherson's article, "Menopause as disease: The social construction of a metaphor" (1981), extended the theoretical framework by uncovering the medicalization of menopause and challenging nurses to dismantle the meta-phor. She further encouraged nurses to join forces with activists in the women's health movement and to form self-help groups in which women could become menopause experts. The idea of nurses as activists for social and medical reform was a radical notion at the time and lead to the concept that women's health cannot be divorced from the social, political, and economic forces in society that impact health (Lempert, 1986). The health of women is inevitably connected with the status of women and their place in society. Sherwin noted that the health care system is not the single agent that contributes to women's health; the entire political agenda—local, national, and global—must be ad-dressed (Sherwin, 1987).

The Chicago School of Thought in Women's Health produced a concept paper on nursing practice that incorporated constructs of nursing theory into the women's health framework (1986). They organized the criteria for defining women's health practice according to assumptions, structural issues, process issues, content issues, and outcome issues. Assumptions about women and their health reflected the nursing metaparadigm. Structural issues included comprehensive care across the life span and a relationship between patients and providers that respects each other's strengths. Process issues promoted self-care while content issues encompassed the wholeness of women. Outcome issues proposed the advancement of women taking control over their health and health care.

Shaver (1985) advanced the concept of a biopsychosocial view of human health. She asserted that a human or social ecological model, in which environ-ment, body, and mind interact to determine health, is more in keeping with nursing's concern about the diagnosis and treatment of human responses to actual or potential health problems. Her paper explored fields of inquiry, such as neurochemistry and the stress response, that promote an integrative science of nursing.

Walker and Tinkle (1996) advocated for an integrative science of wom-en's health that incorporates all of the sciences that study women's health in order for women to be viewed holistically and not solely as reproductive beings. While both of these papers are important frameworks for women's health scholarship, Taylor pointed out the importance of the physical and social environment as determinants in women's health (Olesen, Taylor, Ru-zek, & Clarke, 1997).

McBride (1993) embraced this concern when she expanded her earlier work to describe the shift from gynecology to GYN-ecology, noting the relationship between the woman and her environment and the influence on health and health care. In the lead chapter in Dan's book, *Reframing Women's Health* (1994), McBride discussed new theoretical concepts. The concept of difference requires us to acknowledge the differences in women based on a multitude of factors, such as age, race, cultural background, education, sexual preference, and work experience. She further noted a turning point in women's health scholarship, moving from critique of the patriarchal paradigm to assertion, a positive statement of values. McBride stated, "the move to assertion, by contrast, takes the stance that criticizing the extent to which women have been 'constituted' selves must now give way to their becoming 'constituting' selves, persons who define their own experience" (p. 8).

APPLICATION OF THE FRAMEWORK

Nancy Fugate Woods (1985) opened the First International Congress on Women's Health Issues in 1984 with a keynote address on new models of women's health care. These models incorporated the women's health theoretical frame work, addressed the morbidity and mortality of women across the life span, and included comprehensive health promotion, disease prevention, and illness care. Holistic health endeavors and a participatory model of provider–patient interaction were considered central.

The theoretical framework that underpins women's health has been applied to new models of health care for women that guide nursing education (Andrist, 1988; Andrist, 1997a; Andrist, 1998; Cohen, Mitchell, Olesen, Olshansky, & Taylor, 1994; Lewis & Bernstein, 1996; Taylor, 1992), practice (Andrist, 1997b; Taylor, 1995a; Taylor 1995b; Taylor 1995c; Taylor, 1999; Taylor, 2000; Trippet & Bryson, 1995), policy (Maraldo, 1988; Taylor, 1997; Taylor & Woods, 1996; Woods, 1994), and research, which will be discussed in the following section.

The Expert Panel on Women's Health of the American Academy of Nursing wrote a position paper outlining transformative change for women's health care (Writing Group, 1997), setting the stage for the new millennium. Taylor and Woods explored new models of practice based in the theoretical framework—asserting that a changing health care environment and changing health care practices demand that nurses develop new models of care—and placed the profession at the forefront of transforming health care to women (1996).

At the dawn of a new millennium, nurses have developed a definition of women's health that is grounded in the women's health framework: Women's health is defined as health promotion, maintenance, and restoration across the life span. Understanding women and their health is viewed within the context of women's lives and the intersection of economic, social, political, and environmental circumstances (AAN Writing Group, 1997).

FEMINIST RESEARCH

MacPherson's groundbreaking article, "Feminist methods: A new paradigm for nursing research," (1983) laid the foundation for feminist research in nursing. Using a sociology of knowledge approach, in which the influence of existing social structures and institutions are exposed, she further developed scholarly inquiry methods on the lived experience of women.

Duffy's (1985) critique of research on women exposed the impact of male bias on research and the political ramifications of the conventional paradigm. She advocated a feminist critique of research as a method of challenging the dominant scientific discourse and transforming research that is *for* women. MacPherson and Duffy guided the way for feminist scholarship in women's health nursing research.

The nursing literature on feminist perspectives in nursing scholarship has steadily grown since Chinn (1995) wrote her review of feminism and nursing in *The Annual Review of Nursing Research*. Taylor's review of women's health research and knowledge development discussed the variety of ways that nurse scholars have contributed to nursing science. Notably her review was published in an interdisciplinary work, another sign that nurses are making important contributions in feminist scholarship (Olesen, Taylor, Ruzek, & Clarke, 1997).

Nurse scholars are using a rich variety of epistemological frameworks in their work in women's health. Feminist perspectives are embedded in explicitly feminist research (Caroline & Bernhard, 1994; Lauver, 2000; Montgomery, 1994), ecofeminism (McGuire, 1998), participatory research (Maeve, 1999; Predeger, 1996; Taylor & Dower, 1997), narrative stories (Meleis, Arruda, Lane, & Bernal, 1994), Black feminist and womanist epistemology (Banks-Wallace, 2000; Barbee, 1994; Taylor, 1998), critical theory (Henderson, 1995), and critical hermeneutics (Ruangjiratain & Kendall, 1998).

Although each theoretical approach might differ in its world view, we have delineated four characteristics that are common: (1) feminist research is grounded in women's lived experience; (2) the researcher is *in-relation* to those being studied; (3) the researcher's ability to be reflexive is a source of insight; and (4) research findings should be useful to women, thereby contributing to social transformation (Andrist, 1993). These are discussed briefly as they guide our critique of research.

Feminist scholarship includes a critical analysis of women's position in society and of interlocking social relations that impact a woman's particular experience. Patricia Collins (1990) noted that, instead of using additive models of oppression, interlocking models create new paradigms. Rather than an either/or model (race/class), one can conceptualize either/and models of oppression that beg to include other categories of oppression, such as age, sexual orientation, and ability. To this end, feminist research has evolved from a position in which there was debate about a unique "method" (Harding, 1987) to the understanding that there are multiple methods and perspectives that comprise feminist inquiry (Fonow & Cook, 1991; Jayaratne & Stewart; Lorde, 1984; Reinharz, 1992; Stanley, 1990; Stanley & Wise, 1983).

Women's Lived Experience

Beginning with women's lived experience as a resource for analysis implies that the researcher does not outline the agenda but encourages women to talk about their experience, or tell their stories. Women are then able to share what is relevant to them, and in the classic grounded theory approach, the data lead the researcher—which means the focus of the study may change.

By using women's concrete experiences as "situated knowers" (Collins, 1990, p. 17), as well as their place in the social fabric, we can come to understand other women's realities. This approach also reveals that women are not a monolithic group, but differ by many variables that are drawn into our awareness as we compare and contrast difference among and between women across class, race, age, culture, and all the other variables that impact experience. For example, Black feminist scholars have developed theoretical discourses that, while situated in the everyday lives of African American women, also link these experiences to larger structural constraints. They support privileging "lay knowledge" and "everyday theorizing" by African American women and pivoting the center away from Eurocentric, White, middle-class men and women as the normative experience of all peoples (Taylor, 1998).

Researcher In-Relation

Fonow and Cook (1991) stated that attuning oneself to the affective component is one of the fundamental epistemological themes in feminist research. Feminists refuse to ignore the emotional or affective elements in conducting research and in producing social knowledge. We attend to human relations as a source of insight but also as an attempt to create a non-hierarchical relationship with those participating in our research. This approach acknowledges the subjectivity of participants by preserving the "presence of subjects as knowers and actors" (Harding, 1987, p. 105). Grounded in the sociology of knowledge, this concept presumes that reality is socially constructed in the actors' daily and moment-to-moment interpretation of life. It is subjective, to the extent that our individual experience molds our interpretation of the everyday world (Berger & Luckman, 1966).

Recognizing the subjectivity of participants also implies that researchers are not objective, independent knowers. Feminist paradigms see the relationship of the researcher to the subject as being "involved, a sense of commitment, participation and sharing of fate" (Reinharz, 1985).

A researcher in-relation would manage a non-hierarchical relationship by being reciprocal and attempting to maintain parity and using non-oppressive ways of gathering data. Taylor describes "participatory witnessing" in which the researcher (witness) is "less an observer than a teller—that is, one who translates what s/he sees and hears for an audience" (Gordon, 1995, as cited in Taylor, 1998). By bearing witness, the distance between researcher and participant decreases, as the researcher listens in a way that facilitates self-representation and accurate "other-representation."

Reflexivity As a Source of Insight

Reflexivity as a source of insight (Cook & Fanow, 1986) is a major feature of feminist research. It has been described by many scholars as the way in which the researcher describes the experience of being a researcher as well as the effects of the project on the participants. It is the reflection on the experience, the critical examination, and analytical exploration of the nature of the research process (Fonow & Cook, 1991; Stanley, 1990). Reflexivity merges the public and the private, giving voice to how the experience affected the researcher. Zola stated "we must look at that experience—the anxieties, fears, delights, repulsions—as part of the very situation we are trying to understand" (1991, p. 9). Rather than contaminating a project's objectivity, in feminist research reflexivity is critical in restoring the project's pseudo-objectivity (Reinharz, 1992).

Feminist research takes reflexivity one step further to gain insight into the assumptions about gendered relations underlying the study. Consciousness raising, as one of the main tools, exposes previously hidden, taken for granted assumptions, such as power relations. These contradictions lead to emotional catharsis, academic insight, or increased politicization and activism (Fanow & Cook, 1991). The second feature of consciousness raising is examining the effects of the research on the participants. Reflexivity is the concrete analysis of many of the affective components in feminist research; consciousness raising reduces distance between researcher and participants and encourages reciprocity. Central to participatory research, consciousness raising:

> is the meeting ground of theory and practice; it is both the method of achieving a goal and the goal itself. The research process becomes a consciousness-raising experience in which researched and researchers engage

in critical dialogue. This act leads to new understandings of self and new understandings of each other and to the creation of new theories to explain phenomena. (Henderson, 1995, p. 67)

Social Transformation

Feminist scholarship is action research because it is *for* women. MacPherson (1983) reiterated the difference between nursing research *on* women and research *for* women:

> Although nurse researchers increasingly focus on women's issues, this research may or may not be feminist. In the sense that it generally describes the status quo, nursing research uses the old paradigm and tends to be positivistic. While generating useful information, it can simultaneously function to provide rationalizations for existing power distributions, since the paradigm is devoid of any analysis of the inferior status and oppression of women. (p. 18)

Furthermore, the goal of research *for* women provides an explanation of social phenomena that women want and need, rather than for established social systems, such as the medical care community (Harding, 1987). To this end, it is our responsibility to see that lay women have access to our scholarship, be that through offering workshops, writing and speaking in our communities, or having a visible presence in the media.

Because the central theme of feminism is emancipation, social change is the heart of feminist research. There is a continuous dialectic between explicating women's lived experience and exposing inherent contradictions in power relations.

HISTORICAL CONTEXT: FROM HUMORS TO DEFICIENCY DISEASE

Probably the earliest reference to menopause is found in the Old Testament. When Abraham's wife, Sarah, overheard a messenger inform her husband that she would have a child, she laughed and said that she was past the time during which women can bear children (Formanek, 1990). In Galen's time and until sex hormones were discovered in the 1920s, descriptions and explanations of menstruation and menopause were influenced by the theory of "humors." John Friend, an English scholar, was an exception. His book, published in 1729, differentiated menopause from the suppression of menstruation (amenorrhea). He asserted that menopause preserves older women's health—it was not a disease.

The heroic age of sex endocrinology (1918–1941) set the stage for the medicalization of menopause. Dodds, an English researcher, created the first synthetic estrogen, diethystilbesterol (DES), in 1938. Clinical studies were started to test if synthetic estrogen could replace natural estrogen that had already been marketed for the treatment of menopause by some physicians (Bell, 1987). In the 1930s, physicians debated the relative merits of various menopausal treatments. By assuming that menopause could be treated, however, 20th-century medicine defined it as a disease, in contrast to 19th-century medicine when it was believed to be cause of disease (MacPherson, 1981). In the 1960s, the term "estrogen deficiency" was coined to explain menopause as a disease. Dr. Rubin Clay, a San Francisco gynecologist, stated that menopause is a deficiency disease, like diabetes. He prescribed estrogen for virtually all menopausal women for an indefinite period (Clay, as cited in MacPherson, 1981, p. 109).

Robert Wilson's (1966) best-selling book promised that he could prevent and cure menopause with estrogen. In 1975 when a series of studies established that estrogen therapy increased the risk of endometrial cancer, six million women were taking estrogen. The cancer scare of the mid-1970s was overcome by the addition of progestin, a synthetic progesterone, to the estrogen regimen (HRT). From 1980, the promise of protection from chronic diseases of aging, such as osteoporosis and cardiovascular disease (CVD), have made Premarin one of the most often prescribed drugs in the United States. The ubiquitous biomedical paradigm continues to be favored by scientists, physician researchers, and some nurses for menopausal research (MacPherson, 1995).

During the 1990s, studies were tentatively suggesting a link between estrogen and improvement in memory, decreased incidence of Alzheimer's disease, decreased risk of colorectal cancer, and the improvement in collagen content of skin (Andrist, 1998). Hormone replacement therapy was widely recommended by American physicians for disease prevention (Bush, 1992). In 1992, The American College of Physicians issued guidelines recommending that all women should consider preventive hormone therapy. The guidelines said that women with CHD or at risk for CHD are likely to benefit from HRT, and the benefits may outweigh the risks of breast cancer (American College of Physicians, 1992). It is critical to note, however, that there were no long-term data to support this recommendation, and in fact, the College included a caveat in its recommendation—the guidelines may change after results of clinical trials are reported (Woods & Mitchell, 1995). The Women's Health Initiative (WHI), the largest prevention study of midlife women's health in the United States, was designed to investigate these questions. Conclusive data will not be available until 2007. Moreover, at that point in time there seemed to be a consensus that using HRT for five or more years slightly increased the risk of breast cancer, with decreased risk once it was stopped (Andrist, 1998).

Studies appearing in 1998 through spring 2000 began to cast doubt on HRT's ability to protect women from coronary heart disease (CHD). Researchers in the Heart and Estrogen/Progestin Replacement Study (HERS) reported in August 1998 that HRT did not reduce the overall rate of CHD events in postmenopausal women with heart disease (Hulley et al., 1998). In May 2000, the HERS group reported postmenopausal women with CHD on HRT were at increased risk for venous thromboembolic disease (Grady et al., 2000). As of this writing, HRT is not considered appropriate therapy for secondary prevention of CHD in postmenopausal women.

Meanwhile, the dawn of the new millennium brought seemingly bad news about the HRT and breast cancer risk. In January, researchers from the National Cancer Institute (NCI) found that breast cancer risk increased 8% a year for women on HRT as opposed to 1% for women on estrogen alone (Schairer, Lubin, Troisi, Sturgeon, Brinton, & Hoover, 2000). These data, suggesting combined estrogen and progestin increases breast cancer risk more than estrogen alone, were supported by another study published in February (Ross, Hill, Wan, & Pike, 2000). Both studies were criticized, however, as flawed, leaving no direct evidence of the connection between HRT use and breast cancer.

The debate in the research community rages onward, entrenched in the biomedical paradigm. Bear witness to the above commentary—the major questions are how hormones can prevent *diseases* related to menopause. This is hardly science using a women's health framework. What do we know about women's attitudes, given how biomedicine has painted this transition? What do we know about their lived experience? Nurse researchers have led the way in understanding menopause from women's perspectives.

METHOD OF RETRIEVAL

Articles were chosen that had been published after Voda and George's review of menopause for the 1986 issue of *The Annual Review of Nursing Research*. A search of the nursing literature was conducted using CINAHL and MEDLINE from 1985 through April 2000. MacPherson, a long-time member of the Society for Menstrual Cycle Research (SMCR), knows personally several of the feminist scholars who have been studying menopause and publishing their findings. Andrist is conducting a qualitative longitudinal study of the transition through menopause (Andrist, 1998) and is also a member of SMCR.

Studies that used concepts from the women's health theoretical framework and characteristics of feminist research were included for review. In most cases it was difficult to judge whether all characteristics were used, particularly researcher-in-relationship and reflexivity; however, if the study concentrated on women's experiences and noted how the results contribute to change in the health care for women, it was included for review. Because of the explosion of writings on the menopause transition, and two reviews of the hormone therapy debate since 1986 (Huddleston, 1996; Woods & Mitchell, 1995), we chose to concentrate on two emerging bodies of knowledge: Women Reclaiming Menopause and Menopause Across Cultures.

WOMEN RECLAIMING MENOPAUSE

Ten studies were reviewed from 1985 through 1999. Unless otherwise stated, all included convenience samples of EuroAmerican women who were well-educated and in middle- and upper-middle income groups. The results indicate that women believe the menopausal transition is a normal developmental stage, most of the changes they expect or experience are normal, albeit frustrating, and most of the changes can be managed with self-care strategies. Women discuss changes with health care providers, friends, and family, but find that many providers, physicians in particular, are not well versed in menopause beyond the benefits of taking hormones for short- and long-term prevention of disease. Some women experience symptoms that are probably not related to falling estrogen levels (such as joint pain), however, researchers believe women should know about the various symptoms other women experience to avoid anxiety and fear of the unknown. Depressed mood does not appear to be related to menopausal changes or vasomotor symptoms; the most influential factor to depressed mood appears to be life stresses.

Napholz (1985) used an exploratory, descriptive design to examine working women's knowledge of various issues in midlife and the relationship between a woman's knowledge and her age, education, and marital status. The average participant was White, had a high school education, was married, employed full time in an industrial setting, and was 40 years old. The 67 women in this study were knowledgeable about midlife and able to separate issues of midlife with menopause. Half of the sample did not find midlife mysterious and the one-third of the group that felt it was mysterious said they needed more information. Three quarters of the women felt they have had or will have experiences similar to other women. Almost two-thirds had discussed midlife health concerns—one-third had talked to a physician, one-third with friends and one-third with family. The participants who had not talked about menopause had no concerns yet or had not thought about or experienced menopause so far. Half of the respondents were involved in health promotion activities and half rated themselves as above average health or very healthy. A statistically significant correlation was found between present level of health and present level of health when compared with other women.

Engel (1987) assessed the relationship of menopausal stage, current life changes, and degree of acceptance of traditional role orientation to perceived health status in 249 women. Ages of participants ranged from 40 to 55 with a mean of 47 years. Engel stated that the ages spread across the menopause continuum, representing a proportionate sample in each phase (perimenopausal, menopausal, postmenopausal). Contrary to what Engel hypothesized, perceived health status did not improve in cross-sectional groups representing the progression through menopause. Engel commented that this may have been a problem with the definition of perceived health status, or menopause may signify aging in a culture that does not value aging. Current life stress had an inverse relationship to perceived health status, suggesting that negative life changes impact one's perceptions of health. Women clustered toward the modern definition of women's roles, as defined by the Index of Sex Role Orientation—women who "value themselves as individuals more than they value their family role" (Dreyer, Woods, & James, 1981, as cited in Engel, 1987). Engel suggested a qualitative approach to understanding the meanings of menopause.

Bernhard and Sheppard (1993) conducted a descriptive cross-sectional study to determine the relationship among perceived health, menopausal symptoms, and self-care responses in perimenopausal and postmenopausal women. In women with partners, they also looked at dyadic adjustment. In their sample of 99 women who responded to cycle phase, 27 considered themselves perimenopausal and 72 postmenopausal. Most of the women considered themselves in good health. When given the Menopause Symptom Checklist, which is a 28-item scale (Neugarten & Kraines, 1965), the average number of symptoms was 13 and the mean number of worrisome symptoms was 2.49; notably 20 women marked no symptoms as worrisome. The most frequent symptoms were being tired (91%), hot flashes (87%), and irritability or nervousness (76%). The most frequent worrisome symptoms were weight gain (28%) and hot flashes, being tired, and trouble sleeping, at 22% each. Regarding self-care measures in response to symptoms, women said "accepting changes in my body" (97%), "have faith" (94%), and "throw myself into work" (93%). The researchers stated that this reflects a healthy perspective towards menopause and that this sample of healthy women believed they could manage menopause themselves. In contrast to Engels' study, more women in this study were postmenopausal which may have given them perspective.

Quinn's (1991) investigation of the perimenopausal process revealed a substantive theory of "Integrating a Changing Me." This grounded theory study included 12 participants who were all perimenopausal. Five categories comprised the theory: "Tuning into Me," "My Body and Moods," "Facing a Paradox of Feelings," "Contrasting Impressions" and "Making Adjustments." Quinn found that the process of "Integrating a Changing Me" includes merging and overlapping of categories as women integrate a changing self. Beginning with an awareness of changing physical and emotional changes, the paradox of thoughts, perceptions, and feelings related to changes, assimilating information and formulating personal meaning, women adjusted to the process of menopause. Two important results of this study reinforce that women need to be educated about what to expect during the menopause transition. First, women viewed menopause as a normal transition in which they required knowledge about what to expect; they had positive and negative reactions, but were able to adjust to this period in their lives. Second, all of them had negative perceptions about what to expect, based on information from the media, other women, and things that they read; they rarely discussed menopause with husbands, mothers, or friends.

Mansfield and Voda (1997) presented data collected in 1990 from the Midlife Women's Health Survey in which participants reported changes in their menses (80%), physical condition (66%), sexual response (49%), and emotional state (46%). Forty-eight percent reported new premenstrual symptoms; only 8 women out of 351 reported none of the listed symptoms associated with menopause. Mansfield and Voda concluded "that change is a normal part of middle age and should be characterized as such to women whose response to change might be otherwise fear and anxiety."

Women were asked to report common symptoms experienced during midlife, based on Cobb's (1993) book, which lists more than 40 "ailments" associated with menopause. Four of the most common symptoms included weight gain (58%), fatigue (56%), joint pain (52%), and food cravings (51%). Mansfield and Voda acknowledge that these symptoms may have existed prior to midlife or may be more related to aging than to menopause. Nonetheless, they believe it is valuable for women to know how common a variety of ailments are among healthy midlife women, whether or not they are connected to falling estrogen levels. Notably, women also rated themselves positively on overall physical and emotional health, with mean scores of 4.3 and 4.2, respectively (out of a 5-point Likert scale).

In a second Mansfield and Voda survey conducted in 1993, women reported a variety of menstrual cycle changes, from becoming farther apart (30.8%), closer together (33.6%), lasting longer (20.9%), lasting fewer days (36.0%), bleeding more heavily (39.1%) or more lightly (49.7%), passing more clots (25.7%), and different color/texture/odor (19.4%). Respondents in the survey depicted what life is like at midlife. Twenty per cent reported financial problems, 21% experienced the death of a spouse, friend, or relative, 23% had relationship problems, 30% had job problems, 34% reported personal health problems, and 46% reported health problems of a relative or friend (Mansfield & Voda, 1997).

Woods and Mitchell published results from the Seattle Midlife Women's Health Study in 1996 and 1997. They were the only researchers thus far who included women of color. In both studies, their sample included EuroAmerican, African American, and Asian women in the approximate racial/ethnic proportions in the Seattle area. In the first study, they differentiated women who perceived depressed mood as related to menopausal changes and to factors unrelated to menopause in a sample of 347 women. Three patterns of depressed mood, consistent depressed mood (CDM), emerging (EDM), and resolving depressed mood (RDM) were distinguished from women without depressed mood, or absent depressed mood (ADM). Their findings indicated that women with EDM had poorer reported health status, negative socialization about midlife, a history of premenstrual syndrome (PMS), fewer family resources (including a partnered relationship, adequate income, and number of children), and less social support than did women without depressed mood. Women with CDM had more stress, and history of postpartum blues and PMS, than ADM women. Women with CDM also had a history of postpartum blues and PMS, less positive socialization about midlife, and more severe vasomotor symptoms than did women with resolving depressed mood. Women with resolving depressed mood had more stress, fewer family resources, and poorer health status than ADM women. Interestingly, menopausal changes and vasomotor symptoms were absent from most of the models, leading the researchers to state that we must look beyond menopause for explanations of depressed mood in midlife women.

The second study reported pathways to depressed mood for midlife women. Using the Seattle sample of 337 women, Woods and Mitchell tested three models: menopausal transition, stressful life context, and health status. Their findings indicated that the most influential pathway was stressful life context; again, menopausal changes had little explanatory power. Taken together, these two studies demonstrate that depressed mood in midlife women must be examined in light of the women's health framework, not just the medical model.

Aber, Arathuzik, and Righter (1998) reported results of women's perceptions and concerns about menopause. They conducted a nonrandom survey of 320 women between 46 and 55 years; questionnaires were mailed to women in the United States, the United Kingdom, and France. Respondents had attended women's health workshops on hormone therapy, health at midlife, or preventive health.

Participants reported slightly more satisfaction with care received from nurse practitioners (88.2%) than from gynecologists (81%); however, it is difficult to tell whether or not this was statistically significant. Seventeen percent did not think anyone was providing menopausal care for them. Women talked with friends and health care providers less than with family members, yet many woman felt that physicians needed to be "updated on the topic of menopause" (p. 235). Unfortunately, the investigators did not compare the data by nationality, which might have shed some light on any cultural differences among women from different European countries and the United States.

Kittel, Mansfield, and Voda (1998) recruited 61 women from the Midlife Women's Health Study (see Mansfield and Voda above) who self-reported changes in their menstrual cycles. Data were gathered through phone interviews. "Keeping up appearances" was the basic social process discovered. Two key components included ways in which women concealed what were potentially embarrassing or disruptive changes and how women controlled changes. If a woman experienced embarrassing or disruptive changes that she perceived were uncontrollable, she became frustrated and sought help from health care providers. If changes brought little or no threat of social disclosure or loss of control, women generally felt secure or undisturbed. When changes were perceived as uncontrollable but posed no threat of embarrassment, women remained silent or detached. The researchers offer explanations for their results, two of which are particularly important for this review. Women view menstrual cycle changes as potentially disruptive yet manageable with self-care activities. Second, the concealment of cycle changes is potentially isolating because women do not feel comfortable sharing their experiences with one another.

More data from the Seattle Midlife Women's Health Study corroborates women's expectations that menopause is a normal developmental stage and not a medical problem. Woods and Mitchell (1999) reported findings from their cohort (described above) of 508 premenopausal women who were asked to define their images of menopause and expectations of their own experiences. Women expressed 10 different definitions of menopause, however, the most common definitions were: end of menstrual periods (78.7% of the total responses), end of reproductive capacity (37.4%), hormonal changes (20.1%), change of life, and life stage (18.5%). Only 4.1% cited disease risk, and 2.8% said medical care needs. More women were uncertain about what to expect from menopause (24.2%) or expected nothing (22.1%). Most anticipated their experiences would be a mix of positive, neutral, and negative experiences. This study suggests that women anticipate menopause very differently from health care providers and that women need information about what to expect.

MENOPAUSE ACROSS CULTURES

Anthropologists were the first to identify ethnicity and culture as important variables for predicting women's responses to menopause (Beyene, 1986; Flint, 1975; Griffin, 1977; Davis, 1983; Kaufert, 1988; Locke, 1986). The idea of diversity among different races, ethnic groups, and cultures has been slowly taken into account by menopause researchers for two reasons. First, it is not an easy task. Margaret Mead noted that people living in non-industrial societies practiced explicit ceremonial and ritual patterns for transitions like menses and menopause. In contrast, she believed it is more difficult to study people living in industrial societies that practice invisible patterns of behavior (1975). In the modern world, rituals for life transitions are almost nonexistent (Griffin, 1977). Second, our large world and diverse women's experiences of menopause defy simple explanations. People within the United States and from other regions of the world have differences including social classes, incomes, gender relationships, and rural and urban communities. Each region has particular circumstances that cannot be melded together into one generic picture (Rousseau & McCool, 1997).

There has been a trend for American researchers to focus on one or two attributes of White menopausal women, such as age at the time of menopause or the quantity of hot flashes, and then compare these attributes with those of women belonging to a racial or ethnic group. This reductionist approach ignores the total menopausal experience. It does not recognize that culture, ethnicity, race, class, and gender are central to a woman's identity and destiny (Gould, 1989). This void of holism in menopausal research is being partially filled by nurse scholars. Nursing's contributions to the cultural aspects of women's health, including menopause, were promoted by Madeline Leininger's *Journal of Transcultural Nursing* in 1989. The journal, while not directly related to women's health, provided a forum for many research-based reports on the cultural diversities of women's health and illness (Olesen, Taylor, Ruzek, & Clarke, 1997).

Berg and Taylor's research with Filipino American midlife women stresses the influence of cultural perspectives on women's menopausal experiences—research must move beyond the "estrogen-related menopause symptoms" experience. These Filapinas clearly have adopted the Western biomedical position on health care yet continued to believe that menopause was a natural process and reported less distressing symptoms, including common menopause symptoms (Berg & Taylor, 1999a; 1999b). Other examples of culturally sensitive studies that focus on Asian women follow.

KOREAN WOMEN'S MENOPAUSAL EXPERIENCE

Theory

Afaf I. Meleis and colleagues have created a research trajectory on the concept of transitions in women's lives. In 1975, Meleis identified transition as a concept central to nurses; in 1986, Chick and Meleis further refined the concept of transition using content analysis. Schumacher and Meleis defined a transition as "a process that humans undergo when faced with changes in their lives or environment" (1994, p. 193). They also developed a model describing the types of transitions that nurses deal with: properties that characterize transitions, conditions that determine the nature of responses, indicators of healthy transitions, and nursing therapeutics most appropriate for people experiencing transition. In 1999, Im and Meleis applied situation-specific theory to Korean immigrant women's menopausal transition.

We selected Im and Meleis' study (1999) for review. The purpose of the study was to extend the previous model of transitions by including the menopausal experiences of low-income Korean immigrant women in the United States. Findings from the study were used as a main source for modification of the conceptual properties of transitions, conditions shaping the transitions, and indicators of healthy transitions. Quantitative analysis was based on data from 119 first-generation Korean immigrant women who engaged in low-status or low-income work outside their homes; qualitative study using theoretical sampling method included 21 women. Analyses included descriptive and inferential statistics and thematic analysis. Integrative conceptual analysis using deductive and inductive reasoning was conducted to determine modifications in theory based on the descriptions on menopausal transition of Korean immigrant women.

Three main themes were identified: (a) the women gave their menopausal transition far less attention than they did to their immigrant and work transition; (b) menopause was a hidden experience in cultural background; and, (c) the women "normalized," ignored, and endured symptoms. The findings added the following concepts: (a) number, seriousness, and priority of transitions; (b) socioeconomic status; (c) gender; (d) context; (e) attitudes toward health and illness; (f) interrelationships among all conditions, shaping transitions; and (g) symptom management. The proposed situation-specific model is limited in scope; however, it provides understanding of the menopausal transition of Korean immigrant women in context and is a guide for nursing interventions for immigrant women experiencing transition.

Research

Im, Meleis, and Park's (1999) feminist critique of research on menopausal experience of Korean women represents the increasing number of studies on the menopausal experiences of Asian women. Under the strong influence of Western medicine, research is expanding in Asian countries including Thailand (Chompootweep, Tankeyoon, Yanarat, Poomsuwan, 1993; Sukwatana, Meekhangvan, Tamrongrerakul, Tanapat, Asavarait, & Boonjitrpimon, 1991); Hong Kong (Haines, Chung, & Leung, 1994); Malaysia (Ismael, 1994); Singapore (McCarthy, 1994); Philippines (Ramoso-Jalbuena, 1994); Indonesia (Samil, & Wishnuwardhani, 1994); China (Tang, 1994); and, Karachi, Pakistan (Wasti, Robimson, Akhtar, Khan, & Badaruddin, 1994). It is of interest that all these studies were published from 1991 to 1994. Seven were published in 1994 and all appeared in *Maturitas*, the official journal of The International Menopause Society. This organization has been known to promote the disease model of menopause, to work closely with the pharmaceutical companies, and to support educating doctors from underdeveloped countries. The medical education includes hormones as the primary treatment for estrogen deficiency. It is not surprising that the studies listed above have focused on disease-oriented research. Despite the increasing number of studies, the focus has been on simple comparisons of Asian women's symptoms with Western women's and other disease-oriented research topics.

To propose directions for future research on menopause, Im, Meleis, and Park reviewed, analyzed, and critiqued from a feminist perspective 158 studies from 1980 to 1998 on Korean women's experiences of menopause. Data were retrieved through a search of computerized databases in the United States and South Korea. One hundred and one (64%) of the studies were conducted by male researchers, 81 of whom were physicians. Forty (25%) were conducted by nurses. One hundred and twenty five (79%) researchers used a biomedical framework and 44 (28%) of the studies were clinical trials that focused on the effects of hormone therapy on women's menopausal symptoms. Only five qualitative studies by nurse scholars had research questions that were women-centered (Kim, 1996; Kim & Yoo, 1997; Lee, 1994; Lee, 1997; Lee & Chang, 1992). A lack of conceptualizing the menopausal experience presents a void where the cultural, economic, political, and patriarchal backgrounds are ignored.

Im and colleagues noted a lack of rigor in the research. Drawing upon criteria from feminist critique, they found problems with conceptualization, including ethnocentric views of menopause, biomedical perspectives, and language difficulties. Research methods, such as inadequate instruments, passive relations between researchers and research participants, culturally inappropriate communication styles, inadequate study designs, and homogeneous research participants were problematic, as were interpretation and communication of study findings. These issues undermine the conclusions drawn in the majority of the studies about the nature of the menopausal experience of Korean women.

Indian and Thai Women's Experiences of Menopause

Information on women's experiences of menopause in non-Western, non-English speaking, and non-industrialized countries is limited. The data that have been collected show that women's experience of menopause in these countries does not correspond with many of the aspects of American women's experience. The following two studies address new concepts in menopausal research: Midlife women's identity-continuity theory and Western post-colonialism.

The first article explored the attitudes and experiences of menopause among middle-aged fish sellers in a fishing village on the southwest coast of the Indian state of Kerala (George, 1996). The researcher used a triangulation design, employing participant observation, intensive interviewing, and symptom and attitude checklists. Challenges for the researcher included the limitations of surveys and questionnaires based on Western medical literature and assumptions about menopause. Her unfamiliarity with the women's dialect was another obstacle for collecting reliable data. This obstacle was overcome by finding a sociologist from the village to assist in fieldwork and data collection and to communicate with the fish sellers in their own dialect.

The convenience sample of 190 women ranged in age from 35 to 69. They were literate and could perform the addition and subtraction necessary for their daily sales and purchases. The sample was divided into premenopausal (age 49 and younger with $N = 120$) and postmenopausal groups (age 50 and older with $N = 70$).

Findings focused on menopausal symptoms and the fish sellers' attitudes toward menopause. The symptom checklist included symptoms mentioned in menopausal literature. The most frequently reported symptom, other than menstrual irregularities, was weight gain. Seventy percent of the premenopausal women and 40% of the postmenopausal women believed that weight gain accompanied menopause. Only 12% of the premenopausal women and 14% of the postmenopausal women said that they had hot flashes, but none complained of their severity. Five per cent of the premenopausal women and 13% of the postmenopausal women reported vaginal dryness. Fatigue and insomnia had high scores, and cold sweats and depression were mentioned, but in no case did women associate any of the symptoms with menopause per se.

Data indicated that menopause held no negative connotations for village fish-selling women. Women in the sample not only had a positive attitude toward menopause but also expected to feel better after their menstrual years were over because it would be easier to pursue their work as fish sellers. These women saw menopause as one of several milestones in their life cycle as a blessing from God. They clearly differentiated between the biological event of menopause and the problems of physiological aging.

Identity-continuity theory, first proposed by Atchley (1971), provides a fresh explanation of why these women do not rest on being wives or mothers. They see themselves primarily as fish sellers, as their mothers and grandmothers before them. While the women experience several transitory family duties, selling fish is a role that continues throughout their lives. According to Atchley's theory, a firmly based, continuing conviction enables people to remain productive and comfortable with aging.

The researcher's attempt to place the women fish sellers in the sociocultural milieu they experience during midlife and menopause is a strength of this study. Limitations of the study include a need to expand on the research design and methodology. For example, the author did not disclose the name of the symptom checklist.

The second paper (Punyahotra & Street, 1998) offers the concept of postcolonization for theorizing the effect of Western medicine and the international pharmaceutical companies on women's health in developing countries. Menopausal discourse in Thailand is a prime example.

Thailand has been spared physical colonization by a Western country. Although an elected government has replaced the monarchy, two previous monarchs and the present king have successfully fostered a deliberate strategy to introduce and popularize Western medicine, especially from the United States. This has been accomplished in two ways: by sending Thai citizens overseas to study medicine and by incorporating Western medical practices and drug therapies into Thai culture (Punyahotra & Street, 1998).

Thailand has a population of 59.6 million 79% of whom live in rural areas. The average age at menopause is 49.5 years with a life expectation of 20–25 years more. It is common to see rural women of all ages working in the fields. A physically active lifestyle combined with a healthy diet of fruit and vegetables without dairy products and without much saturated fats and rarely drinking alcohol lends to a satisfactory body mass index. Many rural Thai women live in relative poverty and are kept so busy dealing with economic problems, adverse living conditions, and caring for family members that they rarely seek health services if they are accessible. Urban women's lifestyles are quite different due to higher education levels, more sedentary professional occupations, and more interest in their health (Health, 1996). The Ministry of Public Health conducted a major national study of midlife Thai women's menopausal experiences in 1995. The common health complaints reported were skeletal, urinary, and general malaise symptoms associated with aging rather than with menopause.

Two competing discourses dominate thinking about menopause in Thailand. On the one hand, Thai women view cessation of menses as a private matter that is little remarked upon or linked to a cluster of symptoms. On the other hand, Western medicine has constructed the definition and treatment for menopause. Punyahotra and Street (1998) explored these discourses in a qualitative, integrated, exploratory study. They included several important concepts: the Western view of menopause as a deficiency disease requiring hormone treatment for symptoms; the strong alliances between medicine and the drug companies; the sociocultural construction of the healthy mid-life woman needing interventions to fulfil her social and sexual obligations; and, the essentialist contention that all women share the same global experience of menopause.

The authors identified four traditional discourses framing complexities in midlife Thai women's lives. First, Buddhist Thai women believe in reincarnation and creating harmony in relationships and community; therefore, women are more interested in gaining merit for embracing these values than for adopting Western values of individualistic interests in personal health and welfare. Second, Buddhist concepts place menopause in a religious explanatory framework that includes the notion that harmony is desired between the four elements of nature: earth, water, wind, and fire. As in many countries, menopause is also perceived as "the change." Thai women believe that when menstrual blood ceases, women may experience a time of unstable or erratic physical or emotional changes related to the body being out of harmony. This reflects the relationship of the body to the elements. The discourse focuses on integration and well-being rather than individual pathology and symptoms. Third, many Thai women see "the change" as "the golden age." There are several benefits including more freedom and respect without pressure on rural women to maintain youth and beauty (Whittaker, 1996). Fourth, Thai women silence their bodies' experiences that are considered private and not appropriate for social discussion. Silence means that women tolerate health problems; many women wait until they feel ill to seek medical care.

The authors identified several ways in which Western medicine is able to influence women's health care. First, because gynecologists are trained in the West, they are developing Western-style clinics that stress HRT. Women then have contact with health care personnel who have been sensitized to the discourse of menopause as a disease. Overlaying this, is the tendency for Thai people to believe the claims of Western scientific experts and physicians. The fact that the Thai media depicts middle-aged women as needing HRT to retain health and youth plus the alarming information that is being provided by the Western pharmaceutical corporations creates a situation where women are enticed to also view menopause as a disease that needs treatment.

The authors concluded that a focus on health promotion for Thai women could build on positive aspects of the aging experience while providing health education and the benefits of Western medical advances in a culturally appropriate manner. Caution will be necessary to prevent post-colonizing discourses of Western medicine and of drug companies that would marginalize the positive discourses of Thai women on aging or to relegate mid-life women's health to hormonal deficiency problems.

This research review of Asian women's experiences of the menopause transition generally report that, although there are variations, menopause is not the pressing factor responsible for physical and psychological health alterations at midlife. There are indications, however, that the more Western medicine and international pharmaceutical corporations market their therapy and hormones, the more women, especially urban women, will forego their traditional view of menopause as normal and the gateway to aging. Thai women are at risk to further colonization by Western medical discourses even when those discourses have been challenged by critical postmodern arguments in their own Western countries.

In sum, based on research reviewed in this chapter, we have noted that weight gain and fatigue are seen as problems during the menopausal transition for EuroAmerican (Bernard & Shepard, 1993; Mansfield & Voda, 1997) and for Indian fish sellers (George, 1996). Korean and Thai women tend to view menopause as a private matter; menopausal changes as well as symptoms that could be related to illnesses are normalized. In terms of theory, Im and Meleis offer their situation-specific theory, and the Indian and Thai articles open new areas for feminist research and scholarship—the concept of identity—continuity theory and the emphasis on multiple discourses including the influence of post-colonization and pharmaceutical companies.

CHARTING A COURSE FOR THE FUTURE

It is heartening to look back at Voda and George's review of the menopause literature in 1986. They recommended the need for closer linkages between feminist and nursing critique and thinking and the adoption of feminist research methods in nursing. They predicted that feminist scholars studying menopause would place women at the center of the investigation, and women would be viewed as a coherent group, not "floating in a man's world" (Voda & George, 1986, p. 72). They further stated that the normalcy of menopause has not been documented and challenged scholars of the next decade to develop a theory of menopause from a humanistic perspective.

Our chapter bears witness to the substantive gains made by feminist nurse researchers in this area. When women are put at the center of the investigation, we find very different thoughts about menopause than the biomedical paradigm tells us. We have discovered the normalcy of the menopause transition and how women are reclaiming it as part of their midlife development.

There are more challenges ahead. We cannot universalize this transition to all women. The evidence so far seems to be from educated EuroAmerican women. Clearly, much more research needs to be done with women of different ethnic and racial groups; that said, we have noticed an increase in published studies in the past few years.

Research methods need to be focused on rural and poor women in all countries—including Western countries that share these populations. Nurse scholars need to gather data on how these women perceive and adapt to the menopausal transition. They are often devoid of educational and economic resources as exemplified by rural Thai women who keep silent about menopause and are also silent about symptoms of serious illness.

The literature we reviewed about Asian women raises important theoretical issues. Meleis and colleagues' ongoing research on the concept of transition sets an example of creating a feminist, research-based, mid-level theory. Their situation-specific theory, although limited in scope, provides knowledge of the menopausal transition and is a guide for nursing interventions for immigrant women experiencing transition. Meleis and her colleagues believe some of the properties and concepts proposed could enhance understanding of the menopausal transitions of other immigrant women as well. They propose that future theorists focus on situation-specific theories through targeted research with diverse groups of clients who are experiencing transitions. This theoretical approach helps to avoid a major flaw of menopausal research in the past that women are one-dimensional.

As we discussed at the beginning of the chapter, women's health, including menopause, cannot be divorced from social, political, economic, and cultural forces that impact women's health. There is much to gain by exploring and using theories from other disciplines. We could do well to follow feminist academic scholarship on menopause that has emerged from various disciplines, including philosophy, anthropology, sociology, history, psychology, psychiatry, and English. One representative anthology focused on historical, medical, and clinical perspectives on menopause (Formanek, 1990). Another contests the medicalization of menopause by uncovering patriarchal constructs that shape the image and treatment of menopausal women-gendered science and medicine, pharmaceutical companies, and the media (Callahan, 1993).

Another challenge is to move beyond menopause and investigate midlife adult women's development. Nancy Fugate Woods commented in her review in 1993 that "the concept of midlife [is] a complex time for women with personal and social changes having health effects that are as important, if not more important, than the biological changes of menopause" (Woods, 1993,

p. 173). There are published data that, for example, compare health and symptom experiences across the midlife period (Lee & Taylor, 1996) and social and psychological well-being in midlife women (Jacobson, 1993; Miller, Wilbur, Montgomery, & Chandler, 1998).

Biological changes should not be ignored, however. Nursing research investigating biobehavioral and physiologic changes, such as neuroendocrine regulation, must continue (Reame, 2000). The research reviewed above on mood and midlife women documented that depression is not necessarily connected to decreased hormone levels. And, although we did not review studies on women's decisions to take hormones, this is another area that is important to study, as are alternatives to taking hormones. One example is Cohen and colleagues who are studying acupuncture as a treatment for symptoms of menopause (Cohen, Rousseau, & Carey, 1998).

More generally, it is critical for researchers to identify multiple variables that prevent women from caring for their own health. These are universal data that must be uncovered and made a public discourse by feminist researchers. There is evidence that global and essentialist experience of menopause is under attack. Some anthropologists and other social scientists have concluded that the problems associated with menopause are influenced by women's social and cultural environment (Kaufert, 1996).

The 21st century brings promise that women are becoming "constituting selves" and defining their own experience. Nurse scholars can enrich the study of women's health through feminist research that will transform women's health and women's place in the fabric of society the world over. This is the legacy of the "first" wave of women's health nursing scholarship.

REFERENCES

Aber, C. S., Arathuzik, D., & Righter, A. R. (1998). Women's perceptions and concerns about menopause. *Clinical Excellence for Nurse Practitioners, 2*, 232–238.

American College of Physicians. (1992). American College of Physicians guidelines for counseling postmenopausal women about preventive hormone therapy. *Annals of Internal Medicine, 117*, 1038–1041.

Andrist, L. C. (1988). A feminist framework for graduate education in women's health. *Journal of Nursing Education, 27*, 66–70.

Andrist, L. C. (1993). *A model of women-centered practice: Shared decision making between breast cancer surgeons and patients* [CD-ROM]. Abstract from ProQuest File: Dissertation Abstracts Item: 9322337.

Andrist, L. C. (1997a). Integrating feminist theory and women's studies into the women's health nursing curriculum. *Women's Health Issues, 7*(2), 76–83.

Andrist, L. (1997b). A feminist model for women's health care. *Nursing Inquiry,* *4,* 268–274.

Andrist, L. C. (1998). Women's health care: Where are nurse practitioner programs headed? *Clinical Excellence for Nurse Practitioners, 2,* 286–292.

Andrist, L. C. (1998). The impact of media attention, family history, politics, and maturation on women's decisions regarding hormone replacement therapy. *Health Care for Women International, 19,* 243–260.

Atchley, R. C. (1971). Retirement and leisure participation. Continuity or crisis? *Gerontologist, 11,* 13–17.

Banks-Wallace, J. (2000). Womanist ways of knowing: Theoretical considerations for research with African American women. *Advances in Nursing Science, 22*(3), 33–45.

Barbee, E. L. (1994). A Black feminist approach to nursing research. *Western Journal of Nursing Research, 16,* 495–506.

Bell, S. (1987). Changing ideas: The medicalization of menopause. *Social Science and Medicine, 24,* 535–542.

Berg, J., & Taylor, D. (1999a). Symptom experience of Filipino American midlife women. *Menopause, 6,* 115–121.

Berg, J., & Taylor, D. (1999b). Symptom responses of midlife Filipina Americans. *Menopause, 6,* 115–121.

Berger, P. L., & Luckman, T. (1966). *The social construction of reality.* New York: Anchor Books.

Bernhard, L. A., & Sheppard, L. (1993). Health, symptoms, self-care, and dyadic adjustment in menopausal women. *Journal of Obstetric Gynecologic and Neonatal Nursing, 22,* 456–461.

Beyene, Y. (1989). *From menarche to menopause: Reproductive lives of peasant women in two cultures.* Albany, NY: State University of New York.

Boston Women's Health Book Collective. (1971). *Our bodies, ourselves.* New York: Simon and Schuster.

Bush, T. L. (1992). Feminine forever revisited: Menopausal hormone replacement in the 1990s. *Journal of Women's Health, 1*(1), 1–4.

Callahan, J. C. (1993). *Menopause: A midlife passage.* Indianapolis, IN: Indiana University Press.

Caroline, H. A., & Bernhard, L. A. (1994). Health care dilemmas for women with serious mental illness. *Advances in Nursing Science, 16,* 78–88.

Chicago School of Thought in Women's Health. (1986). Nursing practice in women's health—Concept paper [Letter]. *Nursing Research, 35,* 143.

Chick, N. L., & Meleis, A. I. (1986). Transitions: A nursing concern. In P. I. Chinn (Ed.), *Nursing research methodology: Issues and implementation* (pp. 237–257). Rockville, MD: Aspen.

Chinn, P. L. (1995). Feminism and nursing. In J. J. Fitzpatrick & J. Stevenson, S. (Eds.), *Annual review of nursing research* (Vol. 13, pp. 267–289). New York: Springer Publishing Co.

Chompootweep, S., Tankeyoon, M., Yamarat, K., Poomsuwan, P., & Dusitsin, N. (1993). The menopausal age and climacteric complaints in Thai women in Bangkok. *Maturitas, 17,* 64–71.

Cobb, J. (1993). *Understanding menopause: Answers and advice for women in the prime of life.* New York: Plume.

Cohen, S. M., Mitchell, E. O., Olesen, V., Olshansky, E., & Taylor, D. L. (1995). From female disease to women's health: New educational paradigms. In A. J. Dan (Ed.), *Reframing women's health: Multidisciplinary research and practice* (pp. 50–55). Thousands Oaks, CA: Sage.

Cohen, S. M., Rousseau, M. E., & Carey, B. (1998). Menopausal symptoms management with acupuncture. *Menopause: The Journal of the North American Menopause Society, 98,* 257.

Collins, P. H. (1990). *Black feminist thought.* Boston: Unwin Hyman.

Cook, J. A., & Fonow, M. M. (1986). Knowledge and women's interests: Issues of epistemology and methodology in feminist sociological research. *Sociological Inquiry, 56,* 2–29.

Corea, G. (1977). *The hidden malpractice.* New York: Jove/HBJ.

Davis, D. L. (1983). *Nerves and blood: An ethnographic focus on menopause.* St. John, Newfoundland: St. John's Memorial University of Newfoundland Press.

Duffy, M. E. (1985). A critique of research: A feminist perspective. *Health Care for Women International, 6,* 341–352.

Engel, N. S. (1987). Menopausal stage, current life change, attitude towards women's roles, and perceived health status. *Nursing Research, 36,* 353 357.

Flint, M. (1974). Menarche and menopause and Rajput women. *Unpublished Doctoral Dissertation,* City College of New York, New York.

Fogel, C. I., & Woods, N. F. (1981). *Health care of women: A nursing perspective.* St. Louis: C. V. Mosby.

Fonow, M. M., & Cook, J. A. (1991). Back to the future: A look at the second wave of feminist epistemology and methodology. In M. M. Fonow & J. A. Cook (Eds.), *Beyond methodology: Feminist scholarship as lived research* (pp. 1–15). Bloomington, IN: University of Indiana Press.

Formanek, R. (1990). *The meanings of menopause: Historical, medical and clinical perspectives.* Hillsdale, NJ: Analytic Press.

Friend, J. (1729). Emmenologia (T. Dale, trans.). London: Cox.

Geary, M. A. S. (1995). An analysis of the women's health movement and its impact on the delivery of health care within the United States. *Nurse Practitioner, 20*(11), 24–35.

George, T. (1996). Women in a South Indian fishing village: Role identity, continuity, and the experience of menopause. *Health Care for Women International, 17,* 271–279.

Gould, K. H. (1989). A minority feminist perspective on women and aging. In J. D. Garner & S. O. Mercer (Eds.), *Woman as they age: Challenges, opportunity, triumph* (pp. 305–316). Binghamton, NY: Hayworth Press.

Grady, D., Wenger, N. K., Herrington, D., Khan, S., Furberg, C., Hunninghake, D., Vittinghoff, E., & Hulley, S. (2000). Postmenopausal hormone therapy increases risk for venous thromboembolic disease. The Heart and Estrogen/Progestin Replacement Study. *Annals of Internal Medicine, 132,* 689–696.

Griffin, J. (1982). Cultural Models for Coping with Menopause. In A.M. Voda, M. Dinnerstein, & S. R. O'Donnell (Eds.), *Changing perspectives on menopause* (pp. 248–262). Austin, TX: University of Texas Press.

Haines, C. J., Chung, T. K. H., & Leung, D. H. Y. (1994). A prospective study of the frequency of acute menopausal symptoms in Hong Kong Chinese women. *Maturitas, 18*, 175–181.

Harding, S. (Ed.). (1987). *Feminism and methodology*. Bloomington, IN: Indiana University Press.

Hawkins, J. W., & Higgins, L. P. (1981). *Maternity and gynecological nursing: Women's health care*. Philadelphia: J. B. Lippincott.

Health, T. (1996). The national study of pre- and postmenopausal Thai women. Bangkok: The Ministry of Public Health.

Henderson, D. J. (1995). Consciousness raising in participatory research: Method and methodology for emancipatory research. *Advances in Nursing Science, 17*(3), 58–69.

Huddleston, D. S. (1996). Menopause: The hormonal replacement therapy decision. In B. J. McElmurray & R. S. Parker (Eds.), *Annual review of women's health* (Vol. III, pp. 33–45). New York: National League for Nursing.

Hulley, S., Grady, D., Bush, T., Furberg, C., Herrington, D., Riggs, B., & Vittinghoff, E. (1998). Randomized trial of estrogen plus progestin for secondary prevention of coronary heart disease in postmenopausal women. Heart and Estrogen/Progestin Replacement Study (HERS) Research Group. *Journal of the American Medical Association, 19*, 605–613.

Im, E-O., & Meleis, A. I. (1999). A situation-specific theory of Korean immigrant women's menopausal transition. *Image: Journal of Nursing Scholarship, 331*, 333–338.

Im, E-O., Meleis, A. I., & Park, Y. S. (1999). A feminist critique of research on menopausal experience of Korean women. *Research in Nursing & Health, 22*, 410–420.

Ismael, N. N. (1994). A study on the menopause in Malaysia. *Maturitas, 19*, 205–209.

Jacobson, J. M. (1993). Midlife baby boom women compared with their older counterparts in midlife. *Health Care for Women International, 14*, 427–436.

Jayaratne, T. E., & Stewart, A. J. (1991). Quantitative and qualitative methods in the social sciences: Current feminist issues and practical strategies. In M. M. Fonow & J. A. Cook (Eds.), *Beyond methodology: Feminist scholarship as lived research* (pp. 85–106). Bloomington, IN: University of Indiana Press.

Kaufert, P.A. (1996). The social and cultural context of menopause. *Maturitas, 23*, 169–180.

Kaufert, P., Gilbert, P., & Hassard, T. (1988). Researching the symptoms of menopause: An exercise in methodology. *Maturitas, 10*, 117–131.

Kim, A. K. (1996). A phenomenological study on women's menopausal experience. Master's thesis, Hanyang Universty, Seoul. The Republic of Korea.

Kim, A. K., & Yoo, F. K. (1997). The meaning of menopause experience by women. *Journal of Korean Women's Health Nursing, 3*, 75–76.

Kittell, L. A., Mansfield, P. K., & Voda, A. M. (1998). Keeping up appearances: The basic social process of the menopausal transition. *Qualitative Health Research, 8*, 618–633.

Lauver, D. (2000). Commonalities in women's spirituality and women's health. *Advances in Nursing Science, 22*(3), 76–88.

Lee, K. H. (1997). Korean urban women's experience of menopause: New life. *Health Care for Women International, 18,* 139–148.

Lee, K. H., & Chang. (1992). Korean urban women's experience of menopause: New life. *The Korean Journal of Maternal and Child Health Nursing, 2,* 70–86.

Lee, K., & Taylor, D. (1996). Is there a generic midlife woman? Health status and symptom experience in midlife working women. *Menopause, 3,* 154–164.

Lee, M. (1994). Adaptation process to menopause. *Korean Journal of Nurses Academic Society, 24,* 623–633.

Lempert, L. B. (1986). Women's health from a woman's point of view: A review of the literature. *Health Care for Women International, 7,* 255–275.

Lewis, J. A., & Bernstein, J. (1996). *Women's health: A relational perspective across the life cycle.* Boston: Jones and Bartlett.

Locke, M. (1986). Ambiguities of aging: Japanese experience and perceptions of menopause. *Culture, Medicine and Psychiatry, 10,* 23–27.

Lorde, A. (1984). *Sister outsider.* Trumansberg, NY: The Crossing Press.

MacPherson, K. I. (1981). Menopause as disease: The social construction of a metaphor. *Advances in Nursing Science, 3,* 95–113.

MacPherson, K. I. (1983). Feminist methods: A new paradigm for nursing research. *Advances in Nursing Science, 6*(2), 17–25.

MacPherson, K. I. (1995). Going to the source: Women reclaim menopause [Review Essay]. *Feminist Studies, 21,* 347–357.

Maeve, M. K. (1999). The social construction of love and sexuality in a women's prison. *Advances in Nursing Science, 21*(3), 46–65.

Mansfield, P. K., & Voda, A. M. (1997). Woman-centered information on menopause for health care providers: Findings from the midlife women's health survey. *Health Care for Women International, 18,* 55–72.

Maraldo, P. (1988). The economics of women's health. *Nursing Economics, 6*(3), 128–131.

Marieskind, H. (1975). The women's health movement. *International Journal of Health Services, 5*(2), 217–223.

Martin, L. L. (1978). *Health care of women.* Philadelphia: J. B. Lippincott.

McBride, A. B. (1993). From gynecology to gyn-ecology: Developing a practice-research agenda for women's health. *Health Care for Women International, 14,* 315–325.

McBride, A. B., & McBride, W. L. (1981). Theoretical underpinnings for women's health. *Women and Health, 6*(1/2), 37–55.

McBride, A. B., & McBride, W. L. (1994). Women's health scholarship: From critique to assertion. In A. J. Dan (Ed.), *Reframing women's health: Multidisciplinary research and practice* (pp. 3–12). Thousand Oaks, CA: Sage.

McCarthy, T. (1994). The prevalence of symptoms in menopausal women in the Far East: Singapore segment. *Maturatas, 19,* 199–204.

McGuire, S. (1998). Global migration and health: Ecofeminist perspectives. *Advances in Nursing Science, 21*(2), 1–16.

Mead, M. (1975). *Blackberry winter: My earlier years.* New York: Pocket Books.

Meleis, A. I. (1975). Role insufficiency and role supplementation: A conceptual framework. *Nursing Research, 24,* 246–271.

Meleis, A. I., Arruda, E. N., Lane, S., & Bernal, P. (1994). Veiled, voluminous, and devalued: Narrative stories about low-income women from Brazil, Egypt, and Colombia. *Advances in Nursing Science, 17*(2), 1–15.

Mitchell, A. M., Wilbur, J., Montgomery, A. C., & Chandler, P. (1998). Social role quality and psychological well being in employed Black and White midlife women. *American Association of Occupational Health Nurses Journal, 46,* 371–378.

Montgomery, C. (1994). Swimming upstream: The strengths of women who survive homelessness. *Advances in Nursing Science, 16*(3), 34–45.

Mulligan, J. E. (1983). Some effects of the women's health movement. *Advances in Nursing Science,* 1–9.

Napholz, L. (1985). A descriptive study on working women's knowledge about midlife menopause and health care practices. *Occupational Health Nursing, 33,* 510–512.

Neugarten, B. L., & Kraines, R. J. (1965). 'Menopause symptoms' in women of various ages. *Psychosomatic Medicine, 27,* 266–273.

Nichols, F. H. (2000). History of the women's health movement in the 20th century. *Journal of Obstetrics, Gynecological and Neonatal Nursing, 29*(1), 56–64.

Olesen, V. L., Taylor, D., Ruzek, S. B., & Clarke, A. E. (1997). Strengths and strongholds in women's health research. In S. B. Ruzek, V. L. Olesen, & A. E. Clarke (Eds.), *Women's health: Complexities and differences* (pp. 580–606). Columbus, OH: University of Ohio Press.

Predeger, E. (1996). Womanspirit: A journey into healing through art in breast cancer. *Advances in Nursing Science, 18*(3), 48–58.

Punyahotra, S., & Street, A. (1998). Exploring the discursive construction of menopause for Thai women. *Nursing Inquiry, 5,* 96–103.

Quinn, A. A. (1991). A theoretical model of the perimenopausal process. *Journal of Nurse Midwifery, 36*(1), 25–29.

Ramosso-Jalbuena, J. (1994). Climacteric Filipino women: A preliminary survey in the Philippines. *Maturitas, 19,* 183–190.

Reame, N. E. (2000). Neuroendocrine regulation of the perimenopause transition. In R. Lobo, J. Kelsey, & R. Marcus (Eds.), *Menopause: Biology and pathology* (pp. 95–110). San Diego: Academic Press.

Reinharz, S. (1985). Feminist distrust: Problems of context and content in sociological work. In D. Berg & K. Smith (Eds.), *Exploring clinical methods for social research* (pp. 153–172). Beverly Hills: Sage.

Reinharz, S. (1992). *Feminist methods in social research.* New York: Oxford University Press.

Rosen, R. (2000). *The world split open: How the modern women's movement changed America.* New York: Viking Penguin.

Ross, R. K., Paganini-Hill, A., Wan, P. C., & Pike, M. C. (2000). Effect of hormone replacement therapy on breast cancer risk: Estrogen versus estrogen plus progestin. *Journal of the National Cancer Institute, 92,* 328–332.

Rousseau, M. E., & McCool, W. F. (1997). The menopausal experience of African American women: Overview and suggestions for research. *Health Care for Women International, 18,* 233–250.

Ruangjiratain, S., & Kendall, J. (1998). Understanding women's risk of HIV infection in Thailand through critical hermeneutics. *Advances in Nursing Science, 21*(2), 42–51.

Ruzek, S. B. (1978). *The women's health movement: Feminist alternatives to medical control.* New York: Praeger.

Samil, R. S., & Wishnuwardhani, S. D. (1994). Health of Indonesian women city-dwellers of perimenopausal age. *Maturitas, 19,* 191–197.

Schairer, C., Lubin, J., Troisi, R., Sturgeon, S., Brinton, L., & Hoover, R. (2000). Menopausal estrogen and estrogen-progestin replacement therapy and breast cancer risk. *Journal of the American Medical Association, 283,* 485–491.

Schumacher, K. L., & Meleis, A. I. (1994). Transitions: A central concept in nursing. *Journal of Nursing Scholarship, 26,* 119–127.

Shaver, J. F. (1985). A biopsychosocial view of human health. *Nursing Outlook, 33,* 186–191.

Sherwin, S. (1987). Concluding remarks: A feminist perspective. *Health Care for Women International, 8,* 293–304.

Stanley, L. (1990). *Feminist praxis: Research, theory, and epistemology in feminist sociology.* London: Routledge.

Stanley, L., & Wise, S. (1983). *Breaking out: Feminist consciousness and feminist research.* London: Routledge and Kegan Paul.

Sukwatana, P., Meekhangvan, J., Tamrongterakul, T., Tanapat, Y., Asavarait, S., & Boonjitrpimon, P. (1991). Menopause symptoms among Thai women in Bangkok. *Maturitas, 13,* 217–228.

Tang, G. W. (1994). The climacteric of Chinese factory workers. *Maturitas, 19,* 177–182.

Taylor, D. (1992). The nurse specialist in women's health: A model for graduate education. *NAACOG's Women's Health Nursing Scan, 6*(6), 1–2.

Taylor, D. (1995a). Perimenstrual symptoms and disorders. In W. Star, L. Lommel, & M. Shannon (Eds.), *Women's primary care: Protocols for practice.* Washington, DC: American Nurses' Association.

Taylor, D. (1995b). Midlife women's health. In W. Star, L. Lommel, & M. Shannon (Eds.), *Women's primary care: Protocols for practice.* Washington, DC: American Nurses' Association.

Taylor, D. (1995c). Perimenopausal transition. In W. Star, L. Lommel, & M. Shannon (Eds.), *Women's primary care: Protocols for practice.* Washington, DC: American Nurses' Association.

Taylor, D. (1997). Improving women's health. *National Women's Studies Association Journal, 9*(1), 89–98.

Taylor, D. (1999). Effectiveness of professional-peer group treatment: Symptom management for women with PMS. *Research in Nursing and Health Care, 22,* 496–511.

Taylor, D. (2000). More than personal change: Effective clements of symptom management. *NP Forum, 11*, 1–10.

Taylor, D., & Dower, C. (1997). Toward a women-centered health care system: Women's experiences, women's voices, women's needs. *Health Care for Women International, 18*, 407–422.

Taylor, D. L., & Woods, N. F. (1996). Changing women's health, changing nursing practice. *Journal of Obstetrics, Gynecological, and Neonatal Nursing, 25*, 791–802.

Taylor, J. Y. (1998). Womanism: A methodologic framework for African American women. *Advances in Nursing Science, 21*(1), 53–64.

Timmerman, G. M. (1999). Using a women's health perspective to guide decisions made in quantitative research. *Journal of Advanced Nursing, 30*(3), 640–645.

Trippet, S. E., & Bryson, M. R. (1995). A model of women's health nursing. *Health Care for Women International, 16*, 31–41.

Voda, A. M., & George, T. (1986). Menopause. In H. Werley (Ed.), *Annual review of nursing research* (Vol. 4, pp. 55–75). New York: Springer Publishing Co.

Walker, L. O., & Tinkle, M. B. (1996). Toward an integrative science of women's health. *Journal of Obstetrics, Gynecologic, and Neonatal Nursing, 25*, 379–382.

Wasti, S., Robinson, S. C., Akhtar, Y., Khan., S., & Badaruddin, N. (1993). Characteristics of menopause in three socioeconomic urban groups in Karachi, Pakistan. *Maturitas, 16*, 61–69.

Whittaker, A. (1996). Quality of care for women in northeast Thailand: Intersections of class, gender, and ethnicity. *Health Care for Women International, 17*, 435–447.

Wilson, R. A. (1966). *Feminine forever.* New York: M. Evans.

Woods, N. F. (1985). New models of women's health care. *Health Care for Women International, 6*, 193–208.

Woods, N. F. (1994). The United States women's health research agenda analysis and critique. *Western Journal of Nursing Research, 16*, 467–479.

Woods, N. F., & Mitchell, E. S. (1995). Midlife women: Decisions about using hormone therapy for preventing disease in old age. In B. J. McElmurray & R. S. Parker (Eds.), *Annual review of women's health* (pp. 11–39). New York: NLN.

Woods, N. F., & Mitchell, E. S. (1996). Patterns of depressed mood in midlife women: Observations from the Seattle Midlife Women's Health Study. *Research in Nursing & Health, 19*, 111–123.

Woods, N. F., & Mitchell, E. S. (1997). Pathways to depressed mood for midlife women: Observations from the Seattle midlife women's health study. *Research in Nursing and Health, 20*, 119–129.

Woods, N. F., & Mitchell, E. S. (1999). Anticipating menopause: Observations from the Seattle midlife women's health study. *Menopause: The Journal of the American Menopause Society, 6*, 167–173.

Writing Group of the 1996 AAN Expert Panel on Women's Health. (1997). Women's health and women's health care: Recommendations of the 1996 AAN Expert Panel on Women's Health. *Nursing Outlook, 45*(1), 7–15.

Zola, I. K. (1991). Bringing our bodies and ourselves back in: Reflections on a past, present, and future "medical sociology." *Journal of Health and Social Behavior, 32*(1), 1–16.

PART II

Research on Women's Social Roles and Health

Chapter 3

Women As Mothers and Grandmothers

ANGELA BARRON MCBRIDE AND CHERYL PROHASKA SHORE

ABSTRACT

This chapter analyzes the literature on women as mothers; research reports published between January 1985 and December 1999 were reviewed. As in the past, almost all of the extant studies analyzed the experience of mothers in their children's first year of life. Although therapeutic suggestions were made in many studies, relatively few interventions have been implemented and evaluated. More studies are needed that go beyond traditional family forms and that explore mothers' role development over the full course of their children's growth and development. Additional longitudinal research that views maternal role development as a process is indicated.

Key words: maternal role, women—parents

Until the latest round of the women's movement, inaugurated in the United States with the publication of Betty Friedan's *The Feminine Mystique* (1963), the principal conceptualization of women as mothers was prescriptively on what they should do for the sake of their children rather than on the growth and development experienced by mothers in this role (McBride, 1973). The literature on parenthood as a developmental crisis dates back decades (LeMasters, 1957), but the focus of that literature historically has been on the successful attachment/bonding of the mother so that the child's subsequent development might be ensured (Bowlby, 1969). When the first author last reviewed the topic of women as mothers (McBride, 1984), the majority of research reports

63

were found to focus on the adjustment of first-time mothers in the first few months postpartum, and the overwhelming majority of studies were descriptive, based on relatively small samples ($n < 40$). The parenting experience, beyond the child's first year of life, was almost completely unaddressed, although nonnurse researchers were beginning to write about the various stages of parenting over the life cycle (Galinsky, 1981).

Nursing research has long been concerned with these matters because the profession has believed itself to be responsible for strengthening the mother-infant bond. The work of Rubin (1967a, 1967b) on maternal role attainment has profoundly shaped research and practice in this area. Her naturalistic case recordings gave rise to Mercer's (1981) theoretical framework for studying a range of factors that impact on the maternal role, which, in turn, led to considerable research on maternal identity (Mercer, 1995). This chapter explores the research, largely set in motion by these nurse pioneers, in the last 15 years.

METHODS OF REVIEW

Computer-assisted searches were conducted using the data bases CINAHL and PsycInfo. Keywords "maternal role" and "women, parents" were used to locate articles, books, and book chapters published between January 1985 and December 1999. A subsequent search of "maternal health" and "mothers, health" was conducted in order to track the link between social role and maternal well-being. Hand searches also were conducted in various journals that focus on family and parenting. Seemingly relevant literature, cited by other authors, was also reviewed (the ancestry approach). Reports were included if they were research based (using either quantitative or qualitative methods), pertained to the mothering role, and were published in English journals or books. Since the focus was on mothering as a psychosocial role, research reports that focused primarily on pregnancy, labor and delivery, and/or breastfeeding were not included. Reports were also not included that largely addressed the developmental trajectory of the child, although it was frequently difficult to make judgments about the latter because most of the literature remains focused on how the experience of the mother affects the child. Whenever possible, information is provided about the diversity of the populations sampled because previous research tended not to include minority participants.

MATERNAL ROLE

Mercer (1985, p. 198) defined maternal role attainment "as a process in which the mother achieves competence in the role and integrates the mother behaviors into her established role set, so that she is comfortable with her identity as a mother." Most of the studies conducted on this subject in recent years have been undertaken by nurses who have asked a range of questions about maternal role attainment: Does it vary by the age of the mother? Does maternal competency vary over the course of the first year? Do primiparas and multiparas have a different experience?

Maternal Role Attainment

Making use of role theory and symbolic interactionism for her theoretical underpinnings, Mercer (1985, 1986) explored role attainment over the first year of motherhood in three age groups (15–19, 20–29, and 30–42 years). Maternal role attainment was assessed in this sample of 242 in terms of four measures—Feelings About the Baby, Gratification in the Mothering Role, Maternal Behaviors, and Ways of Handling Irritating Child Behaviors. Women in the different age groups began with different levels of proficiency, with nonteenagers being more psychosocially advantaged, but there were no significant differences by maternal age in self-image or role strain, and the infant's temperament and health status did not predict maternal role attainment.

Positive self-concept was *the* major variable accounting for successful role attainment. All women felt more positive about their babies and more competent at 4 months than they did either at 1 month or later (8 and 12 months). Indeed, most women (64%) had internalized the role by 4 months. The challenge most frequently mentioned by all mothers was lack of personal time. The finding that may be of most importance to future research, however, is that role attainment behaviors did not show a positive linear increase over the year. For example, mothers generally felt less competent at 8 months than they did at 4 months. From a methodological point of view, there was some evidence that the instruments may have not had the same cultural relevance to minority participants (38% of the sample).

Primiparous (*n* = 64) and multiparous (*n* = 60) women were interviewed 1–3 days postdelivery and again 4–6 weeks later by Walker and her associates (Walker, Crain, & Thompson, 1986a, 1986) with regard to Self-Confidence, Myself as Mother, and My Baby. Not surprising, multiparas saw themselves more positively as mothers than primiparas. Over time, mothers' attitudes toward themselves became more positive, even as they came to view their babies somewhat less positively. Self-confidence was important to maternal identity and maternal feeding behavior, but less so for multiparas than for primiparas. This mostly White sample was restudied when the child was 9-years old to see if earlier maternal role attainment predicted subsequent competence or behavior problems in the children (Walker & Montgomery, 1994). Over 60% of the original sample participated in this follow-up. Only an affective subset of maternal identity correlated modestly with children's adjustment, thus providing relatively little evidence of the predictive power of maternal role attainment in shaping children's subsequent behavior.

In another study by Walker (1989) involving 173 mothers of infants, work status and a difficult infant were associated with perceived stress, but a health-promoting lifestyle contributed additively to perceptions of less stress and maternal identity. Following that lead and other pilot work (Walker & Preski, 1995), Preski and Walker (1997) studied two cohorts of mothers who were either 6 or 12 months postpartum at recruitment, then assessed them again at two time periods when their children were 12–18 months and 30–36 months ($n = 122$, 99% White). Maternal identity was assessed at recruitment; maternal lifestyle was measured at all three time periods; child behavior problems were assessed at the end. Maternal identity was not related to child adjustment, but there was an inverse relationship between mothers with health-promoting lifestyles and their children's behavior problems. The authors consequently suggest that a healthy maternal lifestyle may be an important marker in family assessment, although it is important to point out that mothers assessed both their own behavior and that of their children, so those judgments were not independent assessments.

Majewski (1986, 1987) studied the extent to which Transition to the Maternal Role and Role Conflict were influenced by Employment Role Attitude and Marital Satisfaction in 86 first-time mothers (8% minority). Data were collected at some point 5 to 18 months after the birth of the child. Unemployed mothers did not experience less role conflict than employed mothers; however, mothers with careers ($n = 30$) experienced more role conflict than mothers with jobs ($n = 15$), and role conflict was associated with difficulty in making the transition. Transition to the maternal role was correlated with marital satisfaction. This research is flawed when viewed in light of Mercer's aforementioned research because the mothers' experience was assessed any time over a 14-month span, so the experience of the respondents was not the same. For example, the mother with a 5-month-old and the mother with an 18-month-old have children at different developmental stages and are consequently likely to think differently about transition to the maternal role.

Virden (1988) evaluated maternal anxiety and mother-infant mutuality as measures of maternal role adjustment in primiparous women ($n = 60$, 40% minority). At 1 month postpartum, 33 were breastfeeding, 13 were bottle-feeding, and 14 were using a combination approach. Those women who breastfed had less anxiety and more mutuality than bottle-feeding women, but there is no way of knowing whether those with less anxiety were originally more inclined toward breastfeeding.

Maternal–fetal attachment has been of concern to health professionals because it is presumed to shape consequent postpartum attachment (Cranley, 1981); antenatal attachment has been found to moderate postpartum depression (Priel & Besser, 1999). Koniak-Griffin (1988) found that prenatal attachment was best predicted in one group of adolescents ($n = 90$) by a planned pregnancy, intent to keep the infant, and presence of a support network. Davis and Akridge (1987) wondered if a prenatal intervention aimed at directing first-time mothers' attention to their fetuses would promote post-delivery attachment. There were no differences between experimental ($n = 10$) and control ($n = 12$) groups. Gottesman (1992) found that the older the woman was, the more likely she was to interact with her fetus. Sorenson and Schuelke (1999) suggested that routine assessment of prenatal fantasies may be helpful in understanding women's expectations.

Kemp and colleagues (Kemp, Sibley, & Pond, 1990) compared adolescent and adult low-income, first-time mothers ($n = 52$, 85% minority) on factors affecting maternal role attainment. Participants were assessed for Prenatal Attachment, then videotaped the first day or two postpartum with their babies during feeding, after which they described their Maternal-Infant Adaptation. There were no significant differences in the two groups on either tool. Fowles (1996, 1998) recruited a sample of 136 primiparous women (8% minority) from prenatal classes and assessed the relationships among prenatal attachment, maternal role attainment, and postnatal depression 9–14 weeks after birth. Prenatal attachment was positively related to maternal role attainment; postpartum depression was negatively related to maternal role attainment. Only 49% of her respondents had internalized the maternal role by two months postpartum.

Pridham and her associates (1991) found that experienced mothers evaluated their parenting more positively than inexperienced mothers, although the more educated were more negative in their self-evaluations, perhaps because of higher expectations ($n = 140$, 61% multiparae). In another study, Pridham (1987) found that the meaning attached to having an infant had more to do with sense of self in multiparous women than it did in primiparous women ($n = 83$). From the first week to three-months postpartum, the most satisfying factor of mothering did not change—the baby's growth and development, including personality expression—but what was most difficult did change, from getting up at night to feed the baby to not having enough time for oneself.

Brouse (1988) and Flagler (1988) both conducted intervention studies aimed at teaching primiparous women about their babies (30–45 minutes and 15–20 minutes, respectively) in the hope of easing the transition to the maternal role. Brouse measured maternal anxiety and maternal lifestyle adjustment at 3 days and 3 weeks postpartum ($n = 31$). Flagler measured maternal role competence early postpartum and 4–6 weeks later ($n = 61$). Both interventions did not result in demonstrable changes. Merely providing information may be no guarantee that the mother knows how to use that information. The instruments used may not have been sensitive to the changes occasioned by the interventions. Is it even reasonable to believe that mother's anxiety related to child rearing will be significantly affected by one interaction that took place weeks ago?

Mercer and Ferketich (1994) studied 121 high-risk women (HRW) and 182 low-risk women (LRW), about 30% minority, at 1, 4, and 8 months postpartum to see if HRW report lower maternal competence than LRW and if there is a relationship between maternal competence and maternal attachment over time. Maternal competence was significantly related to maternal attachment, but no differences were found between groups in maternal competence over time. Self-esteem and mastery were consistent predictors of maternal competence.

Mercer and Ferketich (1995) re-analyzed essentially the same sample in terms of the differences between primiparous and multiparous women. The two groups did not differ in their sense of maternal competence over time. Inexperienced women's competence was higher at 4 and 8 months than earlier, but did not change much over time for experienced women. Brouse (1985) also studied self-concept in 52 primiparous and 21 multiparous women over time (in the third trimester, 2–3 weeks postpartum, and 4–6 weeks postpartum). There were no differences in self-concept by parity, and level of self-concept was not significantly related to level of perceived comfort in the mothering role.

Bullock and Pridham (1988) interviewed mothers of healthy newborns at 30 and 90 days after birth to ascertain sources of confidence and uncertainty ($n = 49$). On the whole, mothers perceived themselves to be relatively competent, however, properties of the infant were the only sources significantly related to perceived problem-solving competence, raising questions about what means mothers use to form judgments about their performance. Grace (1993) explored changes in perceptions of What Being the Parent of a New Baby Is Like at 1, 3, 4 1/2, and 6 months. Individual differences were relatively stable over time ($n = 76$). Mothers who were increasingly pleased with their role performance also demonstrated increasing mastery in the maternal role, even though the baby was less central to their thoughts over time. This study also suggested that all multiparas do not have the same experience, with mothers of three or more being more pleased with their role performance than mothers of two, although mothers with larger-than-average families may be a self-selected group, already inclined in that direction before the experience.

There is some evidence that first-time mothers experience more fatigue and less vitality at one month postpartum than multiparous women (Waters & Lee, 1996), and this has been attributed to the challenges of maternal role attainment. Flagler (1989, 1989) also urged that more attention be paid to fatigue during the initial postpartum weeks. She found that mothers ($n = 20$) who used negative descriptors to indicate how they felt physically also experienced more anxiety and less mutuality with their infants. Rutledge and Pridham (1987) found that amount of perceived rest was associated with perceptions of competence in infant care and feeding for breastfeeding mothers ($n = 140$, 6% minority).

Pridham and her colleagues (1986) also studied the stressors and supports mothers experienced in the first 90 days with a new baby ($n = 38$ primiparas, 24 multiparas). As their infants grew older, the mothers' perceptions of stressors decreased. Multiparous women were more likely to report activities and plans as stressors. Interestingly enough, lack of time was the reason given by the majority of women who refused to participate in the study. Parks and colleagues (1999) have studied the consequences of persistent maternal fatigue over the first 18 months after birth ($n = 229$, 100% White). More than half of the sample (52%) was persistently fatigued (Milligan et al., 1997), and 6% of the variance in infant development was accounted for by that variable. Persistent fatigue was related to perceived maternal health, but not to infant health. It should also be noted that Gross and Semprevivo (1989) identified low energy as an issue in mentally ill mothers' care of their young children.

These research reports, taken as a whole, indicate that nurse researchers have explored various aspects of maternal role attainment. The sample sizes in these studies were comparatively larger than those reported in the past (McBride, 1984) and generally demonstrated at least some concern for including minorities, but the focus continued to be on the experience of the first-time mother. Although most studies also remained concerned with the mother's experience in the first year of parenthood, more studies are now going beyond that time frame. Just about all of the studies ended with some statement that the findings are relevant to practice, but exactly how is far from obvious. There are consistent findings that positive self-concept (self-esteem and/or a sense of mastery) is associated with maternal role attainment, but how to strengthen positive self-concept in women is not clear because a sense of self does not seem likely to be influenced by a one-time psychoeducational interaction. The good news in the research is that most women eventually internalize the maternal role, although this does not necessarily happen in the first weeks postpartum, as had been implied in earlier theoretical statements.

The research of Mercer and her associates (Mercer, 1985, 1986; Mercer & Ferketich, 1994, 1995) has most changed the field because it has demonstrated that maternal role attainment, including development of corresponding senses of competence and/or satisfaction, is neither a static nor a linear process. Until this work, there was more of a sense that maternal role attainment was either present or absent, rather than fluctuating with changing circumstances. Koniak-Griffin (1993) made the important methodological point that measurement of maternal role attainment is prone to a lack of correspondence between attitudinal and behavioral assessments, particularly as the mothering role evolves. For example, the woman may be asked to rate herself globally as a mother, but then her competence in a specific area is monitored, with modest correlation between the two estimates because they are not measuring the same phenomenon. Looked at this way, it is not surprising that there was little relationship in the Walker and Montgomery (1994) study between maternal identity and adjustment in 9-year-olds.

Both the anecdotal and the research literature have long pointed out that mothers of young children are pressed for time and persistently fatigued. That phenomenon was underscored in several studies, pointing to the likelihood that mothering may be more shaped by physiological considerations than behavioral scientists typically credit. The findings that a health-promoting lifestyle can have positive consequences on maternal well-being and child adjustment suggest that this line of inquiry is beginning to move away from merely documenting negative associations between fatigue and competence to suggesting a means by which mothers' self-care behaviors can have positive consequences. What accounts for the observed differences remains unexplained. Do mothers with health-promoting lifestyles begin with advantages (and so do their infants), or does exercise contribute to positive mood which then has consequences for how positively the mother then rates her own performance and that of her child?

Maternal Role Attainment in Special Circumstances

Though the previously discussed research contained some studies of the experience of teenagers, nurses have been particularly concerned with this age group. Koniak-Griffin and Verzemnieks (1991) studied a sample of 20 primiparous adolescents (95% minority) to see if four 1 1/2-hour classes would improve maternal role attainment. There was a significant increase in maternal–fetal attachment scores over time for those in the experimental group ($n = 9$), but no difference in actual mothering behaviors. As with other studies, there was a positive correlation between affective perceptions of self and of baby at each testing period. Because participants were all living in a large residential maternity home, the possibility of across-group contamination needs to be considered, particularly since those in the control group subsequently asked to also receive classes.

With a similar population, they (Koniak-Griffin, Verzemnieks, & Cahill, 1992) videotaped structured teaching tasks at 1 and 2 months postpartum. Mothers in the experimental group reviewed the 1-month tape and received feedback that reinforced positive behaviors and encouraged desired mother-child interactions. At 2 months, these adolescent mothers ($n = 15$) scored higher than the control group ($n = 16$) on the growth fostering and responsiveness subscales of the Nursing Child Assessment Teaching Scale.

Patterson (1997) analyzed the experience of 32 adolescent mothers, their 1-year-old children (22% minority), and the children's involved maternal grandmothers. Using the Strange Situation laboratory procedure for assessing the availability of attachment figures, it was found that 44% of children were securely attached to their mothers, but 72% were securely attached to their grandmothers. Of the 11 children insecurely attached to their mothers, 82% were securely attached to their grandmothers. Awake time with grandmothers was strongly associated with secure attachment, but awake time with mothers was not. Only three children were neither attached to mother nor grandmother. Flaherty (1988; Flaherty, Facteau, & Garver, 1987) analyzed the functions of Black grandmothers in adolescent mothering at three time periods (immediately postpartum, two weeks later, and 3 months postpartum) and found that the adolescent mothers served as primary caregivers, while the grandmothers served as important "back-up persons."

Lesser and colleagues (Lesser, Anderson, & Koniak-Griffin, 1998) used qualitative methods to categorize adolescents' responses ($n = 36$, 100% minority) to preparation-for-motherhood classes. Three major themes emerged from the data regarding the maternal role: responsibility, respect, and reparation. These same researchers (Lesser, Koniak-Griffin, & Anderson, 1999) followed a sub-sample ($n = 15$) who were depressed perinatally and interviewed them 24 months postpartum. The findings suggest that the experience of motherhood can be positive in previously self-destructive adolescents, serving as an opportunity to change and prove themselves. Higginson (1998) found that the competitive nature of the teen culture can be used to advantage when teen parents are urged to compete with one another to be the best mother.

There are several important studies that demonstrate the effects of early intervention and home visitation by nurses on vulnerable, largely adolescent, mothers (Kitzman et al., 1997; Koniak-Griffin et al., 1999; Olds & Korfmacher, 1997; Olds et al., 1998; O'Sullivan & Jacobsen, 1992; Williams-Burgess, Vines, & Ditulio, 1995). Though interventions are aimed at facilitating the maternal role, outcomes are described more often in terms of physical and social benefits (e.g., decreased premature birthrate, decreased antisocial behavior) than in terms of maternal role identity or competence per se, though the latter is assumed to be responsible for the former. For example, Kitzman and colleagues (1997) described the intervention ($n = 1139$, 92% African American) as, on average, seven home visits during pregnancy and 26 visits from birth to the child's second birthday, with the emphasis being on setting and meeting small, achievable objectives between visits. The protocols were based on theories of "human ecology, human attachment, and self-efficacy" (p. 646). These studies have collectively demonstrated the effectiveness of home visitation by nurses, but the deciding features that make these interactions so successful have not been adequately described. What is in the "black box" of nursing care that is the causative agent of change? Are there aspects of these over-time interactions that are essential and that are not essential to the therapeutic process? To what extent should home visitation by nurses be modified depending upon community need, or is there a tried-and-true intervention protocol that works in most communities?

Maternal response to a high-risk infant was also previously considered, but deserves special consideration. Zabielski (1994) queried first-time mothers with full-term and pre-term babies ($n = 42$, 19% minority) one year after their child's birth. There were no significant differences between groups on How I Feel About My Baby, Myself As A Mother, and maternal role satisfaction, though mothers with full-term babies recalled first feeling like a mother sooner than those with pre-term babies. Having a pre-term infant can have continuing consequences for the mother's health (Brooten et al., 1988; Gennaro, 1988). Gennaro and Krouse (1996) followed 68 mothers of infants born before 37 weeks of gestation over the first 6 months postpartum. The majority of these mothers (65%) reported having to alter their normal activities because of ill health. By the half-year point, 19% of the mothers continued to rate their health as fair to very poor. Substantial morbidity has also been reported five years following the birth of a premature low-birthweight infant by non-nurse investigators (Haas & McCormick, 1997).

Miles and her associates (1999) have examined maternal role attainment when the child is medically fragile ($n = 67$, 46% minority). Data were collected at enrollment and hospital discharge, and at 6, 12, and 16 months after birth. Findings indicated that such mothers experience both distress and growth as a consequence of their child's condition. Distress was mostly shaped by maternal characteristics (e.g., less education, lower perceived control), hospital environmental stress, and worry about the child's health. Growth was influenced by some of the same variables (e.g., hospital environmental stress, worry about the child's health) but also by maternal role attainment. Maternal role attainment had no impact on depressive symptoms, but being involved with the child and maternal identity had an impact on maternal growth.

Raines (1999) interviewed seven mothers whose infants had a genetic anomaly only identified at birth. Respondents described a sense of diminished maternal role and the problem of "false protection" whereby staff are not straightforward in their communications. Miles and Holditch-Davis (1995) analyzed mothers' recollections of the birth of their preterm infants in light of their parenting of these children at three years of age ($n - 27$, majority African American). These mothers evidenced a compensatory parenting style whereby the children were viewed as both normal *and* special. The authors recommended further study of the advantages and disadvantages of such a parenting style. Parents of multiple birth infants (Holditch-Davis, Roberts, & Sandelowski, 1999) also comment on the specialness of these children and managing their care is a major concern. Holditch-Davis, Sandelowski, and Harris (1998) studied 70 couples to see if a history of infertility problems altered early parent-infant interactions in infertile couples who subsequently become parents through adoption or pregnancy, only to find no negative consequences.

Findings regarding maternal role attainment in special circumstances provide some reasons to be optimistic: young children may be securely attached to grandmothers even if they are not attached to their mothers (Patterson, 1997); home visitation by nurses to vulnerable mothers is effective short-term *and* long-term (Kitzman et al., 1997; Olds et al., 1998); the experience of motherhood can serve as an opportunity for self-destructive adolescents to change (Lesser, Koniak-Griffin, & Anderson, 1999); and mothering a medically fragile infant can be a growth experience (Miles et al., 1999). The link between maternal vitality and maternal role success deserves further investigation, given findings regarding maternal morbidity long after the birth of a premature low-birthweight infant (Haas & McCormick, 1997).

The Maternal Role: Cultural Considerations

There is a growing body of literature on the maternal role from a cross-cultural perspective. Taking the lead in this line of inquiry, Meleis and colleagues (1990) have studied the experience of low-income women in multiple cultures. A Brazilian sample of clerical employees ($n = 60$) responded to the Women's Roles Interview Protocol translated into Portuguese. The 33 who were mothers described their maternal role as child care-taking and general upbringing, including care when children are ill. The mothers liked the intimacy, the caring, and the energizing parts of the role. They disliked having limited time with their children and the fact that caring can be fatiguing. Stressful aspects included worries, lack of resources, and role overload. The most important resource used to support their maternal role was child care help (e.g., day-care centers, extended family, partner support, and job flexibility). The authors speculated that the more satisfied mothers are with child care help and job flexibility, the less stress they are likely to describe in their role as mothers. This study did not describe the ages of the children, so it is not clear how the findings apply by stage of motherhood.

Stevens and Meleis (1991) used the same Women's Roles Interview Protocol to study maternal role experience in a U.S. sample of 87 clerical workers (76% minority). Like their Brazilian counterparts, these women experienced satisfaction in their children's growth and development; they were stressed by the worries they had in raising their children. They coped with the stresses of motherhood using a range of strategies—acceptance, problem-solving, talking with their children, seeking time for themselves, etc. These women depended on tangible aid from partners, extended family, and friends, although 25 of the 54 women living with spouses complained that their partners were unresponsive to their requests for help with domestic responsibilities.

Also using qualitative content analysis to understand the role experience of women, another study (Messias, Hall, & Meleis, 1996) focused on impoverished Brazilian women employed in the domestic service sector. In this sample of 75, 93% were mothers of at least one child. These mothers experienced similar satisfactions in the role (e.g., witnessing the child's growth, closeness) and stresses (e.g., time constraints, worries), but they also were concerned, more than the women in the two previous studies, with meeting basic needs. Fatigue and health concerns were prominent in their descriptions of their experience. In the face of heavy role demands, they relied for support on religion and their own inner resources.

A Colombian sample of "por dia" domestic workers (n = 60) included 46 respondents with at least one child (Bernal & Meleis, 1995). Children's companionship and pleasure in their growth were major satisfactions in these women's lives; poverty and the children's behavior/illnesses were major stressors. The mothers responded to stress physiologically (e.g., crying, loss of appetite) or by isolating themselves; others talked with friends, and 5% of this sample used drugs.

Low-income Mexican women (n = 41), 85% of whom were mothers with children up to five years of age, were also given the Women's Roles Interview Protocol to elicit their satisfactions, stressors, and coping strategies (Meleis et al., 1996). "Giving to child" was described as the greatest role satisfaction in 68% of responses. These mothers worried about their children's health and their limited resources, including not having enough time to spend with their children. These mothers coped by "juggling priorities," taking advantage of the extended family, being well-organized, and problem solving. Like many other mothers, these respondents described considerable role overload.

Siantz (1990) analyzed maternal acceptance and rejection in Mexican-American migrant farmworker mothers with children 3–5 years old (n = 100).

As with the previously reported study by Meleis and her colleagues (1996), the family was a source of strength. Total social support available accounted for 75% of the variance in mothers' acceptance/rejection of their children. In living with the problems of being a migrant farmworker parent, a mother's access to a variety of supportive persons may be a key factor in shaping her response to her children.

Hattar-Pollara and Meleis (1995) studied the experience of Jordanian immigrant mothers of adolescents living in California ($n = 30$). Content analysis was used to identify key themes in their parenting. One issue shaping maternal behavior was maintaining a Jordanian identity (avoiding loss of honor and a bad reputation). The second issue, somewhat at odds with the first, was helping their children become socially integrated and well adjusted. To realize these mandates, the mothers engaged in a number of behaviors: nurturing the child and encouraging cultural identification; disciplining to promote cultural adherence; advocating for the teen and mediating between spouse and child; and vigilant parenting.

These studies, sensitive to cultural considerations, are similar to other research in this area, which found time constraints and fatigue to be important in understanding maternal role experience. But this line of research, taken as a whole, is much more mindful of issues surrounding the person-environment fit. Repeatedly, the support of others functioned as a strength in shouldering maternal responsibilities. These studies raise significant questions about whether maternal attachment and competence can be fully understood removed from issues of environmental supports and stressors, including the presence or absence of partner's investment in the child, child care availability, extended family, and job flexibility.

Beyond the First Year of Mothering

All of the cross-cultural studies investigated maternal role beyond the child's first year of life, and more research is moving in that direction. Koniak-Griffin and Verzemnieks (1995) studied the perceptions parents had of their 24 month olds and found that there was a strong correlation between the perceptions of working mothers and fathers, but not between unemployed mothers and their husbands. Employed mothers tended to identify fewer child behaviors as problematic than did unemployed mothers.

Gross and Rocissano (1988) have studied maternal confidence in parenting toddlers ($n = 50$), and found that mothers of boys want to know different information than mothers of daughters. For example, mothers of girls (42%) were more interested in knowing what to do when the child has a temper tantrum than those with boys (22%), but mothers of sons (41%) were more interested in managing the child's aggressiveness with other children than those with daughters (21%). This study noted that mothers are simultaneously becoming more confident and less confident about their children's progress because the child is changing, thus requiring the mother to change, too. Sullivan and McGrath (1999) studied 184 mothers (11% minority) and their 4-year-old children in order to explore mothers' tendencies to be supportive or controlling of their children's autonomy. An optimal style was associated with maternal responsivity and involvement, as well as higher educational level and being older.

McBride (1987) found that the very nature of parenting changes when children are in their second decade: "Where once the emphasis was on cuddling, safeguarding, instructing, admonishing, improving, and caring for, now encouraging the child to come into her own takes precedence over making her your own" (p. 149). Ohashi (1992) used Locke's expectancy theory to describe the experience of 102 mothers of teens (8% minority). Encountering at least one positive surprise in parenting was associated with maternal role satisfaction. Out of 21 items, mothers' experience was generally more positive than expected on 8 items, but it was more negative than expected on 13 items. The three areas that mothers rated most negatively had to do with teens' smoking/drug use, setting limits, and balancing the child's independence with parental authority. On average, these mothers felt competent; they rated their behavior only one scale step below the ideal they aimed to be. Mays (1992) noted that value attainment was a more useful predictor of satisfaction in this study than the discrepancies between experience and expectation.

Thomas (1995) has been interested in how being a mother influences her health in midlife. In a secondary analysis of 238 middle-aged women, the least healthy women reported more child-rearing concerns than did the most healthy women. The differences between the two groups was greatest in worrying about their children's well-being. The least healthy were unsure of themselves and prized being needed by their children and being helped by them. Thomas (1997) wondered whether these mothers' expectations for both their children and themselves might not be unrealistic.

Mercer, Nichols, and Doyle (1988) took an even broader perspective and compared life histories of 50 mothers with 30 non-mothers (aged 60 or older, 4% minority). The women were asked about turning points in their lives. Mothers described a greater number of transitions in their lives, and 30% of them reported reaching adult status at 15 years or younger, compared to only 3% of non-mothers. On the whole, mothers described a less stable career trajectory than did non-mothers. Findings, however, were shaped not only by personal experience but also by historical events, e.g., age at the time of the 1929 Depression.

Nurses are becoming interested in research on grandmother caregivers (Dowdell & Sherwen, 1998). For example, Musil (1998) studied 90 grandmothers (75% African American) with and without primary responsibility for raising their grandchildren. Those grandmothers most invested in caring for their grandchildren experienced greater overall parenting stress and comparatively little social support. Caliandro and Hughes (1998) interviewed 10 grandmothers (100% minority) who have primary responsibility for their HIV-positive grandchildren. The themes that emerged included: upholding the family; being a strong woman; living in the child-centered present; and living with a constricting environment. Using a similar interview-oriented methodology, Reese and Murray (1996) queried 16 women (50% African American) about their experience as great-grandmothers. Finding opportunities to influence their great-grandchildren—through being wise, religion, telling stories, and/or transmitting values—provided meaning to their lives.

These studies demonstrate that nurse scientists are beginning to expand their investigations of maternal role beyond the transition to parenthood, but there is a paucity of research on how mothers handle their children's transitions to the school years, the teenage years, and through the adult years (McCubbin, 1999). In the first author's experience, "parenting teenagers" is a phrase more likely to be interpreted in American society as referring to teen parents than as referring to parents' facilitation of their teenage children because there is more interest in the beginnings of the mothering role than in the course of women's experience as mothers. It is interesting to note the growing focus on the grandmother role but that literature tends to ignore or discount what the woman is doing as mother to the child's mother. In doing so, there is a danger that grandmother will be understood (and valued) only in terms of her interactions with the young and not for what she does to affirm the parenting of the adult child, an important area in need of further research.

Emerging research tends to be qualitative in approach rather than quantitative, in large measure because the focus is on getting the questions right rather than on finding answers. What is more, instruments with established psychometric properties may not exist. This situation is more likely to be the case in research beyond the first year of mothering because so little has been done to study women's experience in those years. To the extent that nurses play a role in facilitating a variety of normative family transitions beyond the postpartum period, then they must develop a better understanding of the full range of maternal worries and concerns and how they can be addressed to promote maximal functioning, for there is existing evidence that mothers who are worried are at risk themselves.

SUMMARY AND RESEARCH RECOMMENDATIONS

The start of the 21st century is an interesting period in the mothering literature. Concern post World War II about the consequences of maternal deprivation, with its conclusions about the importance of early bonding and subsequent greater understanding of the nascent capacities of newborns, led to decades of emphasis on the importance of the mother's role in the child's beginnings. More recent information about the extent of genetic determination has, however, brought to the fore countervailing arguments that "it's all in the wiring," so mothers may not be all that important in shaping the child's behavior. Add to those shifting paradigms, a greater interest in the mother's own growth and development as she lives out that role (summed up in the notion that if "mamma's happy, then everybody is happy"), and it is clear that the nature-nurture debates of old must be revisited with a fresh sense of the complexities involved.

A greater appreciation of the complexities involved is beginning to be visible in the nursing research reviewed for this chapter. For example, one is left with the impression that maternal attachment can no longer be described as simply present or absent postpartum, for maternal competence and satisfaction change with the circumstances. Positive self-concept is associated with maternal role attainment, but that perception of self may have less to do with specific competencies than with whether the mother has developed an overall sense of mastery. Yet that overall sense of mastery may, in turn, be affected by how she performs in new situations.

Self-concept may be psychosocially shaped because being older, more educated, experienced, and supported by others generally make a positive difference. But positive self-concept also seems to be shaped by physiological and affective states—healthy lifestyle and not being depressed. It would, therefore, seem that woman as mother can only be fully understood from a biopsychosocial perspective, but that has not been the orientation of most research in the area.

Mercer (1985) pointed the way to what must be *the* major research recommendation when she defined maternal role attainment as "a process," but the nursing research in this area has infrequently used the over-time methods necessary to the study of process. A process analysis would, for example, be not only concerned with the relationship between maternal role satisfaction and child outcomes, but with mother-child interaction as a mediating factor (Lerner & Galambos, 1985, 1986). A mother may conclude that a child is difficult, particularly if she is tired and/or depressed, which may set in motion another round of problem behavior in the child, compounded perhaps by the pressure of new developmental or environmental requirements. Sprey

(2000) has argued that one must be mindful of the direction of process away from beginnings to some point in the future and the problem of ordered states changing to disorder over time, thus explaining why "there are far more ways to be unhappy than happy in a close relationship."

All of these points make clear the need for additional longitudinal studies in order to assess the extent to which any correlation between parenting and child's behavior "is not due *solely* to the effect of children on parenting behavior" (Collins et al., 2000) or due solely to the effect of mother on child behavior. Such an approach is also likely to provide some evidence of differentiated patterning in sub-populations of mothers, rather than confirming heretofore monolithic notions of good vs. bad mothers. Or to put it another way, we must find out if there are different ways to be happy and unhappy in the mother-child relationship, so interventions can be tailored to that patterning. And does that patterning vary if one is a single mother, an adoptive mother, a stepmother, or a grandmother raising a child on her own—types of mothers not usually studied?

The literature is impressive in documenting that home visitation by nurses can make a major difference in the lives of vulnerable mothers and their children, but more attention to process issues would also clarify what there is in these interactions that is so effective. Kitzman and colleagues (1997) summarized their approach as working with mothers to set and meet small, achievable objectives between visits, and that seems to be an approach likely to facilitate the mastery so linked to maternal competence and satisfaction, but more needs to be understood about how these desirable outcomes come to pass. Indeed, more needs to be understood about how positive self-concept in a mother fits with the burgeoning general literature on self-concept and mastery. Finally, it would seem that "maternal role attainment" is itself a phrase that needs to be retired, for it implies a static situation rather than a fluctuating process, and that way of thinking, with its implication that comfort with the mothering role can be *achieved*, has precluded taking a needed lifespan approach to the mothering role.

REFERENCES

Bernal, P., & Meleis, A. I. (1995). Being a mother and a *por dia* domestic worker. Companionship and deprivation. *Western Journal of Nursing Research, 17*, 365–382.

Bowlby, J. (1969). *Attachment* (Vol. 1). Attachment and loss series. New York: Basic Books.

Brooten, D., Gennaro, S., Brown, L., Butts, P., Gibbons, A., Bakewell-Sachs, S., & Kumar, S. (1988). Anxiety, depression, and hostility in mothers of preterm infants. *Nursing Research, 37*, 213–216.

Brouse, A. J. (1988). Easing the transition to the maternal role. *Journal of Advanced Nursing, 13*, 167–172.

Brouse, S. H. (1985). Effect of gender role identity on patterns of feminine and self-concept scores from late pregnancy to early postpartum. *Advances in Nursing Science, 7*(3), 32–48.

Bullock, C. B., & Pridham, K. F. (1988). Sources of maternal confidence and uncertainty and perceptions of problem-solving competence. *Journal of Advanced Nursing, 13*, 321–329.

Caliandro, G., & Hughes, C. (1998). The experience of being a grandmother who is the primary caregiver for her HIV-positive grandchild. *Nursing Research, 47*, 107–113.

Collins, W. A., Maccoby, E. E., Steinberg, L., Hetherington, E. M., & Bornstein, M. H. (2000). Contemporary research on parenting. The case for nature and nurture. *American Psychologist, 55*, 218–232.

Cranley, M. S. (1981). Development of a tool for the measure of maternal attachment during pregnancy. *Nursing Research, 30*, 281–284.

Davis, M. S., & Akridge, K. M. (1987). The effect of promoting intrauterine attachment in primiparas on postdelivery attachment. *Journal of Obstetric, Gynecologic, and Neonatal Nursing, 16*, 430–437.

Dowdell, E. B. (1998). Grandmothers who raise grandchildren: A cross generational challenge to caregivers. *Journal of Gerontological Nursing, 24*(5), 8–13.

Flagler, S. (1988). Maternal role competence. *Western Journal of Nursing Research, 10*, 274–290.

Flagler, S. (1989a). Relationships between stated feelings and measures of maternal adjustment. *Journal of Obstetric, Gynecologic, and Neonatal Nursing, 19*, 411–416.

Flagler, S. (1989b). Semantic differentials and the process of developing one to measure maternal role competence. *Journal of Advanced Nursing, 14*, 190–197.

Flaherty, M. J. (1988). Seven caring functions of Black grandmothers in adolescent mothering. *Maternal-Child Nursing Journal, 17*, 191–207.

Flaherty, M. J., Facteau, L., & Garver, P. (1987). Grandmother function in multigenerational families: An exploratory study of Black adolescent mothers and their infants. *Maternal-Child Nursing Journal, 16*, 61–73.

Fowles, E. R. (1996). Relationships among prenatal maternal attachment, presence of postnatal depressive symptoms, and maternal role attainment. *Journal of Society of Pediatric Nurses, 1*, 75–82.

Fowles, E. R. (1998). The relationship between maternal role attainment and postpartum depression. *Health Care for Women International, 19*, 83–94.

Friedan, B. (1963). *The feminine mystique.* New York: Dell.

Galinsky, E. (1981). *Between generations: The six stages of parenthood.* New York: Times Books.

Gennaro, S. (1988). Postpartal anxiety and depression in mothers of term and preterm infants. *Nursing Research, 37*, 82–85.

Gennaro, S., & Krouse, A. (1996). Patterns of postpartum health in mothers of low birth weight infants. *Health Care for Women International, 17*, 35–45.

Gottesman, M. M. (1992). Maternal adaptation during pregnancy among adult early, middle, and late childbearers: Similarities and differences. *Maternal-Child Nursing Journal, 20*, 93–110.

Grace, J. T. (1993). Mothers' self-reports of parenthood across the first 6 months postpartum. *Research in Nursing and Health, 16*, 431–439.

Gross, D., & Rocissano, L. (1988). Maternal confidence in toddlerhood: Its measurement for clinical practice and research. *Nurse Practitioner, 13*(3), 19–20, 22, 25, 27, 29.

Gross, D., & Semprevivo, D. (1989). Mentally ill mothers of young children. *Journal of Child and Adolescent Psychiatric Nursing, 2*, 105–109.

Haas, J. S., & McCormick, M. C. (1997). Hospital use and health status of women during the 5 years following the birth of a premature, low-birthweight infant, *American Journal of Public Health, 87*, 1151–1155.

Hattar-Pollara, M., & Meleis, A. I. (1995). Parenting their adolescents: The experiences of Jordanian immigrant women in California. *Health Care for Women International, 16*, 195–211.

Higginson, J. G. (1998). Competitive parenting: The culture of teen mothers. *Journal of Marriage and the Family, 60*, 135–149.

Holditch-Davis, D., Roberts, D., & Sandclowski, M. (1999). Early parental interactions with and perceptions of multiple birth infants. *Journal of Advanced Nursing, 30*, 200–210.

Holditch-Davis, D., Sandelowski, M., & Harris, B. G. (1998). Infertility and early parent-child interactions. *Journal of Advanced Nursing, 27*, 992–1001.

Kemp, V. H., Sibley, D. E., & Pond, E. F. (1990). A comparison of adolescent and adult mothers on factors affecting maternal role attachment. *Maternal-Child Nursing Journal, 19*(1), 63–75.

Kitzman, H., Olds, D. L., Henderson, C. R., Jr., Hanks, C., Cole, R., Tatelbaum, R., McConnochie, K. M., Sidora, K., Luckey, D. W., Shaver, D., Engelhardt, K., James, D., & Barnard, K. (1997). Effect of prenatal and infancy home visitation by nurses on pregnancy outcomes, childhood injuries, and repeated childbearing: A randomized controlled trial. *Journal of the American Medical Association, 278*, 644–658.

Koniak-Griffin, D. (1988). The relationship between social support, self-esteem, and maternal-fetal attachment in adolescents. *Research in Nursing and Health, 11*, 269–278.

Koniak-Griffin, D. (1993). Maternal role attainment. *IMAGE: Journal of Nursing Scholarship, 25*, 257–262.

Koniak-Griffin, D., Mathenge, C., Anderson, N. L. R., & Verzemnieks, I. (1999). An early intervention program for adolescent mothers: A nursing demonstration project. *Journal of Obstetric, Gynecologic, and Neonatal Nursing, 28*(1), 51–59.

Koniak-Griffin, D., & Verzemnieks, I. (1991). Effects of nursing intervention on adolescents' maternal role attainment. *Issues in Comprehensive Pediatric Nursing, 14*, 121–138.

Koniak-Griffin, D., & Verzemnieks, I. (1995). The relationship between parental ratings of child behaviors, interaction, and the home environment. *Maternal-Child Nursing Journal, 23*, 44–56.

Koniak-Griffin, D., Verzemnieks, I., & Cahill, D. (1992). Using videotape instruction and feedback to improve adolescents' mothering behaviors. *Journal of Adolescent Health, 13*, 570–575.

LeMasters, E. E. (1957). Parenthood in crisis. *Marriage and Family Living, 19*, 352–355.

Lerner, J. V., & Galambos, N. L. (1985). Maternal role satisfaction, mother-child interaction, and child temperament: A process model. *Developmental Psychology, 21*, 1157–1164.

Lerner, J. V., & Galambos, N. L. (1986). Child development and family change: The influences of maternal employment on infants and toddlers. *Advances in Infancy Research, 4*, 39–86.

Lesser, J., Anderson, N. L. R., & Koniak-Griffin, D. (1998). "Sometimes you don't feel ready to be an adult or a mom:" The experience of adolescent pregnancy. *Journal of Child and Adolescent Psychiatric Nursing, 1*(1), 7–16.

Lesser, J., Koniak-Griffin, D., & Anderson, N. L. R. (1999). Depressed adolescent mothers' perceptions of their own maternal role. *Issues in Mental Health Nursing, 20*, 131–149.

Majewski, J. L. (1986). Conflicts, satisfactions, and attitudes during transition to the maternal role. *Nursing Research, 35*, 10–14.

Majewski, J. (1987). Social support and the transition to the maternal role. *Health Care for Women International, 8*, 397–407.

Mays, R. M. (1992). Response to "Maternal role satisfaction: A new approach to assessing parenting." *Scholarly Inquiry for Nursing Practice an International Journal, 6*, 151–154.

McBride, A. B. (1973). *The growth and development of mothers*. New York: Harper & Row.

McBride, A. B. (1984). The experience of being a parent. In H. H. Werley & J. J. Fitzpatrick (Eds.), *Annual review of nursing research* (Vol. 2, pp. 63–81). New York: Springer Publishing Co.

McBride, A. B. (1987). *The secret of a good life with your teenager*. New York: Times Books.

McCubbin, M. (1999). Normative family transitions and health outcomes. In A. S. Hinshaw, S. L. Feetham, & J. L. F. Shaver (Eds.), *Handbook of clinical nursing research* (pp. 201–230). Thousand Oaks, CA: Sage.

Meleis, A. I., Douglas, M. K., Eribes, C., Shih, F., & Messias, D. K. (1986). Employed Mexican women as mothers and partners: Valued, empowered and overloaded. *Journal of Advanced Nursing, 23*(1), 82–90.

Meleis, A. I., Kulig, J., Arruda, E. N., & Beckman, A. (1990). Maternal role of women in clerical jobs in southern Brazil: Stress and satisfaction. *Health Care for Women International, 11*, 369–382.

Mercer, R. T. (1981). A theoretical framework for studying the factors that impact on the maternal role. *Nursing Research, 30,* 73–77.

Mercer, R. T. (1985). The process of maternal role attainment over the first year. *Nursing Research, 34,* 198–204.

Mercer, R. T. (1986). Predictors of maternal role attainment at one year postbirth. *Western Journal of Nursing Research, 8*(1), 9–32.

Mercer, R. T. (1995). *Becoming a mother. Research on maternal identity from Rubin to the present.* New York: Springer Publishing Co.

Mercer, R. T., & Ferketich, S. L. (1994). Predictors of maternal role competence by risk status. *Nursing Research, 43,* 38–43.

Mercer, R. T., & Ferketich, S. L. (1995). Experienced and inexperienced mothers' maternal competence during infancy. *Research in Nursing and Health, 18,* 333–343.

Mercer, R. T., Nichols, E. G., & Doyle, G. C. (1988). Transitions over the life cycle: a comparison of mothers and nonmothers. *Nursing Research, 37,* 144–151.

Messias, D. K. H., Hall, J. M., & Meleis, A. I. (1996). Voices of impoverished Brazilian women: Health implications of roles and resources. *Women and Health, 24*(1), 1–20.

Miles, M. S., & Holditch-Davis, D. (1995). Compensatory parenting: How mothers describe parenting their 3-year-old, prematurely born children. *Journal of Pediatric Nursing, 10,* 243–253.

Miles, M. S., Holditch-Davis, D., Burchinal, P., & Nelson, D. (1999). Distress and growth outcomes in mothers of medically fragile infants. *Nursing Research, 48,* 129–140.

Milligan, R. A., Parks, P. L., Kitzman, H., & Lenz, E. (1997). Measuring women's fatigue during the postpartum period. *Journal of Nursing Measurement, 5,* 3–16.

Musil, C. M. (1998). Health, stress, coping, and social support in grandmother caregivers. *Health Care for Women International, 19,* 441–455.

Ohashi, J. P. (1992). Maternal role satisfaction: A new approach to assessing parenting. *Scholarly Inquiry for Nursing Practice: An International Journal, 6,* 135–150.

Olds, D., Henderson, C. R., Jr., Cole, R., Eckenrode, J., Kitzman, H., Luckey, D., Pettitt, L., Sidora, K., Morris, P., & Powers, J. (1998). Long-term effects of nurse home visitation on children's criminal and antisocial behavior. 15-year follow-up of a randomized controlled trial. *Journal of the American Medical Association, 280,* 1238–1244.

Olds, D. L., & Korfmacher, J. (1997). The evolution of a program of research on prenatal and early childhood home visitation: Introduction [Special Issue: Home visitation I]. *Journal of Community Psychology, 25,* 1–7.

O'Sullivan, A. L., & Jacobsen, B. S. (1992). A randomized trial of a health care program for first-time adolescent mothers and their infants. *Nursing Research, 41,* 210–215.

Parks, P. L., Lenz, E. R., Milligan, R. A., & Han, H-R. (1999). What happens when fatigue lingers for 18 months after delivery? *Journal of Obstetric, Gynecologic, and Neonatal Nursing, 28,* 87–93.

Patterson, D. L. (1997). Adolescent mothering: Child-grandmother attachment. *Journal of Pediatric Nursing, 12,* 228–237.

Preski, S., & Walker, L. O. (1997). Contributions of maternal identity and lifestyle to young children's adjustment. *Research in Nursing and Health, 20*, 107–117.

Pridham, K. F. (1987). The meaning for mothers of a new infant: Relationship to maternal experience. *Maternal-Child Nursing Journal, 16*, 103–122.

Pridham, K. F., Egan, K. B., Chang, A. S., & Hansen, M. (1986). Life with a new baby: Stressors, supports, and maternal experience. *Public Health Nursing, 3*, 225–239.

Pridham, K. F., Lytton, D., Chang, A. S., & Rutledge, D. (1991). Early postpartum transition: Progress in maternal identity and role attainment. *Research in Nursing and Health, 14*, 21–31.

Priel, B., & Besser, A. (1999). Vulnerability to postpartum depressive symptomatology: Dependency, self-criticism and the moderating role of antenatal attachment. *Journal of Social and Clinical Psychology, 18*, 240–253.

Raines, D. A. (1999). Suspended mothering: Women's experiences mothering an infant with a genetic anomaly identified at birth. *Neonatal Network, 18*(5), 35–39.

Reese, C. G., & Murray, R. B. (1996). Transcendence: The meaning of great-grandmothering. *Archives of Psychiatric Nursing, 10*, 245–251.

Rubin, R. (1967a). Attainment of the maternal role: Part I. Processes. *Nursing Research, 16*, 237–245.

Rubin, R. (1967b). Attainment of the maternal role: Part II. Models and referrants. *Nursing Research, 16*, 342–346.

Rutledge, D. L., & Pridham, K. F. (1987). Postpartum mothers' perceptions of competence for infant care. *Journal of Obstetric, Gynecologic, and Neonatal Nursing, 16*, 185–194.

Siantz, M. L. D. (1990). Maternal acceptance/rejection of Mexican migrant mothers. *Psychology of Women Quarterly, 14*, 245–254.

Sorenson, D. S., & Schuelke, P. (1999). Fantasies of the unborn among pregnant women. *Maternal-Child Nursing Journal, 24*, 92–97.

Sprey, J. (2000). Theorizing in family studies. Discovering process. *Journal of Marriage and the Family, 62*, 18–31.

Stevens, P. E., & Meleis, A. I. (1991). Maternal role of clerical workers: A feminist analysis. *Social Science and Medicine, 32*, 1425–1433.

Sullivan, M. C., & McGrath, M. M. (1999). Proximal and distal correlates of maternal control style. *Western Journal of Nursing Research, 21*, 313–334.

Thomas, S. P. (1995). Psychosocial correlates of women's health in middle adulthood. *Issues in Mental Health Nursing, 16*, 285–314.

Thomas, S. P. (1997). Distressing aspects of women's roles, vicarious stress, and health consequences. *Issues in Mental Health Nursing, 18*, 539–557.

Virden, S. F. (1988). The relationship between infant feeding method and maternal role adjustment. *Journal of Nurse-Midwifery, 33*(1), 31–35.

Walker, L. O. (1989). Stress process among mothers of infants: Preliminary model testing. *Nursing Research, 38*, 10–16.

Walker, L. O., Crain, H., & Thompson, E. (1986a). Maternal role attainment and identity in the postpartum period: Stability and change. *Nursing Research, 35*, 68–71.

Walker, L. O., Crain, H., & Thompson, E. (1986b). Mothering behavior and maternal role attainment during the postpartum period. *Nursing Research, 35*, 352–355.

Walker, L. O., & Montgomery, E. (1994). Maternal identity and role attainment: Long-term relations to children's development. *Nursing Research, 43*, 105–110.

Walker, L. O., & Preski, S. (1995). Are maternal health behaviors related to preschool children's adjustment? A preliminary report. *Journal of Developmental and Behavioral Pediatrics, 16*, 345–349.

Waters, M. A., & Lee, K. A. (1996). Differences between primigravidae and multigravidae mothers in sleep disturbances, fatigue, and functional status. *Journal of Nurse-Midwifery, 41*, 364–367.

Williams-Burgess, C., Vines, S. W., & Ditulio, M. B. (1995). The parent-baby venture program: Prevention of child abuse. *Journal of Child and Adolescent Psychiatric Nursing, 8*(3), 15–23.

Zabielski, M. T. (1994). Recognition of maternal identity in preterm and fullterm mothers. *Maternal-Child Nursing Journal, 22*(1), 2–36.

Chapter 4

Women and Employment: A Decade Review

ABSTRACT

Contemporary women fulfill multiple social roles: wife or partner, parent and caregiver to elders, worker in the labor force. This chapter focuses on women and employment. Nursing research from the past decade on women and their role in the work force, with emphasis on the relationships between paid work and women's other social roles and their health is reviewed. Major categories of nursing research contributions are summarized, including populations studied, methodological approaches, and major findings. Suggestions for emphases in future research are included.

Key words: employment, women's health, work and family

Contemporary women fulfill multiple social roles: wife or partner, parent and caregiver to elders, worker in the labor force. The impact of these social roles, both individually and in combination, on the health of women has been the subject of increasing study in nursing and other disciplines.

This chapter focuses on women and employment. The purpose of the chapter is to review nursing research during the past decade on women and their employment role, with emphasis on the relationships between paid work and women's other social roles and their health. Major categories of nursing research contributions will be summarized including populations studied, methodological approaches, and major findings. Suggestions for emphases in future research are included.

Women work both within and outside the home, in both unpaid and paid labor. Work has been defined as any form of productive activity that contributes to the supply of valued goods and services. Within this definition both paid work and unpaid housework are forms of productive activity, however, the contexts, value, rewards, and costs of these two forms of labor differ (Lombardi & Ulbirch, 1997; Kahn, 1991). The importance of women's unpaid household, caregiving, and volunteer work is vital in society and is significantly understudied and undervalued (Messias et al., 1997; Im, 2000; Schroeder & Ward, 1998). Research on women's unpaid work as mothers and caregivers is reviewed elsewhere in this volume. Therefore this chapter will focus primarily on paid employment; the terms "employment" and "work" will be used interchangeably in this context.

HISTORICAL AND DEMOGRAPHIC PERSPECTIVES ON WOMEN AND EMPLOYMENT

Throughout history, work has been an important dimension of women's lives, however, the widespread entry of women across all socioeconomic groups into the paid labor force has occurred largely since World War II. World War II provided women in the United States with exposure to new job skills, work experience, and rewards (both economic and intrinsic satisfactions). Single and married women, with and without young children, from all socioeconomic groups joined the labor force. At the end of the war, however, many women returned to traditional family roles focusing on unpaid household and family work. In the 1960s, there began a dramatic movement of women into the paid labor force in the United States which continues to the present. By the mid-1990s, women's labor force participation rate rose to 58.8%, with women representing 46% of the total labor force. It has been projected that by 2005 women's labor force participation will reach 63% (Hertz & Wootton, 1996; U.S. Department of Labor Bureau of Labor Statistics, 1995; Costello, Stone, & Dooley, 1994; Costello, Krimgold, & Dooley, 1996; Costello, Miles, & Stone, 1998).

Women's involvement in paid work is likely to span 30 or more years of their adult lives. The majority no longer leave the labor force to bear and rear children as they did in the past; since 1990, women in their childbearing years (i.e., 25 to 44) have had the highest rate of labor force participation of all women, and the proportion of older women (55 to 64) in the labor force exceeds 50%. In 48% of married couples with children, both parents work and women are increasingly likely to be employed as their children get older. The labor force participation rate for women with children under one year

(54.6%) is comparable to that of women with no children; employment rates steadily increase with the age of the youngest child: under 3 years (57.1%), under 6 years (60.3%), 6–17 years (76%). Seventy-one percent of working mothers reported they worked to support the family (Women's Bureau U.S. Department of Labor, 1994). Nearly three-quarters of all women employed in 1992 were working full time, however, women are more likely than men to work part time, representing two-thirds of all part-time workers. Women with children under age 6 are most likely to be employed part-time. When women work part-time, they are more likely than men to do so voluntarily (Herz & Wootton, 1996).

Although the income gap between men and women has been narrowing in the past decade, employed women continue to earn less than men. In 1994, median earnings for women working full-time was 76% of the median for men. The lessening of the income gap may be due, in part, to changes in occupations of women; the greatest increase in female employment in the past decade has been in professional and managerial positions; in 1994 men and women were nearly equally represented in this occupational group (Herz & Wootton, 1996).

Employment patterns and earnings differ for selected groups of women based on age, education, and ethnicity. Older women experience a larger earnings gap with men than do younger women. These differences reflect, to some extent, differences in educational attainment but may also be a reflection of age, racial, or gender discrimination. Among all age, racial, and ethnic groups, women with more education are more likely to have higher earnings; differences in earnings between women of different races within each educational level are small. African American and Hispanic women are more likely to work part-time involuntarily and less likely to hold professional and managerial positions (Herz & Wootton, 1996).

CONCEPTUAL PERSPECTIVES

The research to date examining women, work, and health has focused almost exclusively on how work, *added to* women's other roles and responsibilities, influences their health. This research has derived from two main theoretical perspectives, the role-stress perspective and the role-expansion perspective (Barnett, 1996; Killien, 1999; Frankenhaeuser, Lundberg, & Chesney, 1991; Sorensen & Verbrugge, 1987).

The role-stress perspective proposes that specific social roles occupied by women (e.g., parent, partner, worker) are each sources of unique stressors that may be harmful to an individual's physical and mental well-being. Further, simultaneously maintaining multiple roles compounds health problems through cumulative stress (role overload) and competing demands (role conflict). Research derived from this perspective has focused on the direct effects of workplace stress on health as well as stress associated when employment roles are combined with family roles. Such research employs a scarcity hypothesis that presumes that individual resources of time and energy have an upper limit that can be exhausted by multiple and conflicting role responsibilities (Frankenhaeuser et al., 1991).

The role-expansion perspective emphasizes that social roles provide resources to individuals that directly or indirectly maintain or enhance health. Employment provides access to income, health care benefits, and social support, while also providing an expansion of opportunities for building knowledge, skills, self-esteem and also alternative sources of reward and satisfaction, thereby promoting health. In a classic paper, Verbrugge (1996) ranked women with various role configurations by health status as indicated by incidence of acute illness, illness restricted days, chronic illness limitations, and self-rated health status. Employed, married women, with or without children, were found to have the best health outcomes. In contrast, women with the absence of these roles fared increasingly less well. In the more recent Commonwealth Fund survey, employed women of all ages and racial/ethnic groups were also found to have better health than non-working women; the least healthy women were those who were not employed, but would like to be (Hartmann, Kuriansky, & Owens, 1996).

Difficulties in evaluating these two perspectives regarding the effects of employment on health are related to insufficient understanding or control of several factors. First, healthier people may acquire and maintain employment more easily than those who are less healthy (i.e., the "healthy worker effect"). Second, multiple roles may be incompatible with sick-role behavior and thus decrease sensitivity to symptoms or willingness to respond to symptoms. Third, the interactive effects of work and family roles and individual characteristics have only recently been recognized and studied (Meleis, Norbeck, & Laffrey, 1989).

METHODS OF RETRIEVAL

The literature that formed the basis for this chapter was limited to a review of research published between January 1990 and June 2000. A computer search of MEDLINE AND CINAHL (Cumulative Index to Nursing and Allied Health Literature) covering the period 1990–2000 and using the search terms "employment or work" and "women" and "health" was conducted. To limit the potentially broad scope of literature reviewed, only studies published in nursing journals or those authored by investigators identified as nurses or employed in schools of nursing were included in the analysis. Thus, while significant research on women's work and health has been conducted and published beyond nursing, this review attempts to focus on the contributions to knowledge within the scope of nursing research, as defined previously. All citations meeting the above criteria were reviewed for applicability by reading the title and/or abstract of the study. Additionally, some articles identified in the reference lists of others were added to the review. Articles retained for analysis included only data-based reports of original research in which: a) women participants were the focus of the study; b) work/employment was a major variable in the conceptual framework for the study or in the analysis; c) employment was linked directly or indirectly with physical and/or emotional health; and d) employment was conceptualized as a social role rather than a geographic location. Thus excluded, for example, were studies of worksite programs for women in which work was only mentioned as an intervention site. A recent review of these latter studies was written by Lusk (1997). Only studies published in English and primarily those using U.S. samples were included. Important research has been conducted internationally, however, since access to international journals was more limited and a comprehensive review could not be assured, this review did not include international studies. Undoubtedly, relevant articles were missed, and their omission limits the scope of this review.

THEMES

Between 1990–2000, approximately 120 published reports of research on work and women's health meeting the above criteria were identified. These reports addressed the influence of employment on women's health and well-being during different life phases, the influence of employment on other social roles of women, and balancing of multiple roles.

Influence of Employment on Women's Health and Well-Being

EMPLOYMENT AND WOMEN'S GENERAL HEALTH

The majority of papers published during the past decade focused on general or non-reproductive aspects of women's health and employment. The health variables addressed included psychological distress, anger, stress, life satisfaction, depression, blood pressure, and health practices including exercise. Employment variables studied ranged from employment status (i.e., employed vs. nonemployed) to attributes of employment including job quality, job satisfaction, job stress, work environment, attitudes towards employment, and role conflict. The majority of papers reported on quantitative analysis of questionnaire data although qualitative analysis from interviews and focus groups were also included. Studies included participants from diverse occupational groups, incomes, ages, and ethnic/racial groups. Clerical workers and nurses were the occupational groups most frequently studied.

Employment, Stress, and Well-Being.   Much of the research on employment and women's health focuses on work as a source of stress. Stress in the workplace may be related to physical demands, job design, job tasks or the nature of the work, work environment, or interpersonal relationships as well as role overload or role conflict. Stress has been cited as the primary problem for working women, identified by almost 60% of women (Dear, 1995; Jenkins, Layne, & Kisner, 1992). A number of nurse investigators have examined life contexts of women, including employment and its relationship to health outcomes.

Woods and colleagues (Woods, Lentz, Mitchell, & Oakley, 1994; Woods, Lentz, & Mitchell, 1993) examined personal and social resources, socialization, and social demands and roles (including employment) on self-esteem and depression in a community sample of 461 Asian, Black, and White women ages 18–45 years. Over three-quarters of participants were employed. Different regression models were constructed for each ethnic group. Asian women had the highest rates of employment (93%) and highest self-esteem scores, while Black women had the highest rate of depression (14%). Employment status failed to enter the regression models for depressed mood or self-esteem for any of the three groups, but income was predictive of depressed mood for Asian women and predictive of self-esteem in White women. Napholz (1994) also investigated self-esteem and depression in a sample of 106 mostly White, employed women ages 22–62 years. She specifically examined the relationship of sex role orientation to these indices of psychological well-being and found that women who were undifferentiated in sex role orientation had significantly higher depression scores, lower self-esteem scores, and lower life satisfaction scores than those with clearly defined sex role orientation. Lack of social support was a predictor of psychological distress among Japanese female auto workers (but not Japanese male employees or American male or female employees) at a Japanese-managed automobile plant in the United States (Gage & Takeshita, 1996).

Lee and colleagues (Lee, Lentz, Taylor, Mitchell, & Woods, 1994) examined fatigue as a response to environmental demands in women's lives in a secondary analysis of daily diary data from a sample of 227 women ages 18–45 years in an urban community. They found that depression and anxiety were more significantly related to self-reported fatigue and vitality than employment variables that included income, occupation, and hours of work.

The psychosocial health of women who made the transition from welfare to employment was the focus of a study by Kneipp (2000). The study was a secondary analysis of longitudinal data originally collected to examine personal characteristics most associated with the need for welfare. No differences in psychosocial health (including depression, self-esteem, self-efficacy, and emotional support) were found between women who left welfare for employment and those remaining on welfare. The author suggested that the life circumstances of the women leaving welfare for employment rarely improved and that these difficult life circumstances overwhelmed any benefits to health that employment might have offered.

Clerical workers experience both mental and physical stress in their jobs; stress has been associated with characteristics of the work environment, low pay, and role conflict. Common symptoms for clerical workers include depression, muscular fatigue, visual discomfort, and musculoskeletal disorders. Role experiences of female clerical workers in the U.S. have been described in a series of reports by Meleis and colleagues (Stevens, Hall, & Meleis, 1992; Hall, Stevens, & Meleis, 1992a; Hall, Stevens, & Meleis, 1992b; Meleis & Stevens, 1992; Stevens & Meleis, 1991). Participants in the study included 87 women with children, representing five ethnic groups, who were employed as clerical workers in four organizations in the western U.S. Most (87%) were employed full time, but half reported annual family incomes of less than $25,000 and experienced serious economic difficulties. Data were collected through a structured interview and analyzed using qualitative methods. Vulnerabilities in the work role for these women included being in jobs with limited opportunities for advancement or development, experiencing ethnic/racial tensions at work, inadequacies of economic resources, and interference with their maternal responsibilities and commitments. Women's abilities to integrate their employment, maternal, and spousal roles were related to health outcomes. A separate analysis of 46 women employed as clerical workers in patient care areas of health care organizations further described relative powerlessness, occupational hazards, and stresses in dealing with ill clients as issues for these women (Hall et al., 1992a).

Several investigators have contributed to the depth of our understanding of the work environment for nurses. McCloskey (1990) examined the concepts of autonomy (control over work activities) and social integration (relationships with co-workers) in a sample of nurses in their sixth and twelfth months of employment. Low autonomy and low social integration was associated with low job satisfaction, low work motivation, poor commitment to the organization, and less intent to stay employed. Decker (1997) surveyed 376 hospital-based nurses to identify factors associated with job satisfaction and psychological distress. Positive relationships with co-workers were predictive of job satisfaction but not predictive of psychological distress, while longer tenure on the unit was associated with both outcomes. In a phenomenological study of the experience of work-related anger in female nurses, Smith, Droppleman, and Thomas (1996) identified characteristics of a hostile work environment contributing to nurses' anger that included scapegoating, disrespectful treatment, and lack of support. Schaefer and Moos (1996) examined effects of work stressors and work climate on job morale and functioning among 405 staff in long-term care facilities. Stressors from relationships and workload were associated with lower job satisfaction, job-related distress, depression, and physical symptoms.

Two studies focused on substance use in nurses. In a study of smoking behavior of 307 nurses at a military medical center, Alexander and Beck (1990) found that 22% were current smokers and 23% were former smokers. Current smokers reported significantly more job stress, job dissatisfaction, and less social support than either former smokers or nonsmokers. Trinkoff, Zhou, Storr, and Soeken (2000) examined use of substances including alcohol, marijuana/cocaine, and prescription-type drugs in a sample of 3600 nurses who participated in the Nurses Worklife and Health Study. Nurses were more likely to use these substances when workplace access to substances increased, when their social networks included more drug users, when religiosity decreased, and when role strain (indicated by high job demands and depressive symptoms) increased.

Shift work is another stressor that has been examined. Lee (1992) surveyed 760 registered nurses about their sleep patterns and sleep quality; women working nights and rotating shifts had a higher incidence of sleep disturbances and excessive sleepiness. These findings have particular relevance for the nursing profession, as shown in two studies by non-nurse investigators in which nurses were the participants. The study of 635 nurses by Gold and associates (Gold, Rogacs, Bock, Tosteson, Baum, Speizer, & Czeisler, 1992) found that nurses working either the night shift or rotating shifts had twice the number of accidents or errors compared to nurses working day or evening shifts. In a prospective study of female nurses between 1988 and 1992, Kawachi and associates (Kawachi, Colditz, Stampfer, Willett, Manson, Speizer, & Hennekens, 1995) found an increased relative risk of coronary heart disease among participants who worked rotating shifts as compared to those who never rotated shifts; this risk increased among women who had experienced shift work for over 6 years duration.

Few studies were found which examined the effectiveness of positive elements of the work environment or interventions to reduce stress among workers. Thomas, Riegel, Gross, and Andrea (1992), however, tested differences in job-related stress among emergency department nurses after implementing staff-generated strategies. Sources of stress were identified by staff, and interventions included a problem-focused task force, classes in conflict resolution, assertive communication, and situational leadership. There were no significant post-test differences on staff burnout, but other predictors of burnout (e.g., low social support) were identified for future research. DesCamp and Thomas (1993) focused on the benefits of play at work as a mediator between job stressors and job strain (job dissatisfaction, workload dissatisfaction, and job motivation). A questionnaire was administered to 72 female registered nurses employed in hospitals in three western U.S. states. Three types of play at work were examined: active physical play, gaming, and use of humor. Physical play at work buffered the effects of stressors on job dissatisfaction and workload dissatisfaction but not on job motivation, while humor and gaming were unrelated to job strain.

Employment and Health Practices.   A number of investigators have examined the effect of employment on health practices and health-promoting or health-damaging behaviors. In a qualitative study of 34 low-income women employed in long-term care facilities, Nelson (1997) found that work occupied the central position in most of the women's lives and exerted the greatest influence on their health practices including exercise, rest, and diet. Time, energy constraints, and financial needs presented barriers to desired health practices. Woods, Lentz, and Mitchell (1993) found in telephone interviews that women who were employed were more likely to use alcohol, ate fewer meals, and got less sleep at night. Similarly, Walker and Best (1991) found that employed women with young infants reported less healthy lifestyles than homemakers. Duffy (1997), however, found no relationships between employment characteristics and health promotion behaviors reported by a sample of 397 employed, Mexican American women.

Sedentary behavior has been identified as a major public health problem for women, contributing to obesity and other health problems. Employment status and hours of work per week were not related to physical activity and exercise in surveys conducted by Woods et al. (1993) and Wilbur, Miller, Montgomery, and Chandler (1998). Nies, Vollman, and Cook (1999) used focus groups to explore mid-life African American women's experiences with physical activity. Among other factors identified as contributing to physical activity was the presence of an ability to use exercise facilities at work. Similarly, Pender, Walker, Sechrist, and Frank-Stromborg (1990) reported that enrollment in a workplace health promotion program had positive effects on healthy lifestyles.

Sexual Harassment and Workplace Violence.   Although the legal community seeks to establish as a standard what the "reasonable person" or "reasonable woman" would identify as harassment in the workplace, men and women have been found to differ in their perceptions of what constitutes a hostile and harassing work environment. Large surveys of working women suggest that half of all working women will be harassed at some point during their working lives (Fitzgerald, 1993). Williams (1996) studied the prevalence and impact of workplace sexual harassment and violence experienced by a random sample of 1130 registered nurses. While the response rate of 30% poses potential for bias in the respondents, 57% reported a personal experience with sexual harassment and 26% reported being the victim of a physical assault at work. Patients and clients were the most frequent perpetrators of sexual harassment and physical assault, and physicians were responsible for over half of the sexual assaults. Sexual harassment and physical assault each were significantly associated with job satisfaction.

Rogers and Maurizio (1993) described the experiences of sexual harassment reported by 735 community care workers for the elderly in rural communities. The majority (95%) of the workers were women, and 28% reported experiencing harassment on the job, 15% by their elderly clients. In a study of job stressors among male and female firefighters and paramedics, Murphy, Beaton, Cain, and Pike (1994) found that, while there were few gender differences in either job stressors or symptoms of stress, females were more likely to report job discrimination. Females were also more likely to report conflict with co-workers, while their perception of support at work and at home were similar to their male colleagues. Work-related conflict in this mixed-gender sample was significantly associated with decreased job satisfaction, decreased work morale, and increased symptoms of stress (Beaton, Murphy, Pike, & Corneil, 1997). Spratlen (1994) extended the conceptualization of harassment to include perceived maltreatment as a source of stress in the workplace.

Work-related assaults were studied by Findorff-Dennis, McGovern, Mull, and Hung (1999). Ten randomly selected participants were selected for qualitative interviews from a population of 429 individuals who reported an assault that resulted in a wage loss claim. The impact of the assault was not associated with the severity of the injury, however, health and quality of life 4 years after the assault were significantly affected and resulted in job changes, chronic pain, changes in functional status, and depression. Levin, Hewitt, and Misner

(1998) explored through focus groups the perspectives on assault of nurses working in hospital emergency departments; half of the 22 participants had been assaulted at work. Analyses suggested that personal, workplace, and environmental factors all contribute to assault. While verbal and physical assaults affect nurses' personal and professional lives, only physical assaults are treated.

Homicide is the leading cause of worksite mortality for women (followed by motor vehicle injuries); homicide ranks third as the cause of worksite mortality for men (Lusk, 1992). An analysis of medical examiner and coroner reports by Levin, Hewitt, and Misner (1996) indicated that most of the occupational homicides occurred in the retail trade and were associated with robbery, handguns, and women working alone. An excellent review of research on workplace violence in Canada and the United States was recently published (Hewitt & Levin, 1997).

Occupational Health and Safety.   Hand, arm, and neck symptoms associated with repetitive movements at work have been termed repetitive strain or cumulative trauma disorders. Higher rates of these disorders have been reported in females. Risk factors may include differences in stature, physiology, and the nature of jobs performed by women. For example, tools and work equipment are frequently designed for men and may be inappropriate for women's anatomical characteristics. Occupations in which women may be especially exposed to these disorders include secretarial and clerical positions, assembly line workers, hairdressers, and cleaner/domestics (Lusk, 1997). Strasser, Lusk, Franzblau, and Armstrong (1999) examined the relationship between perceived psychological stress and upper extremity cumulative trauma disorders in a sample of 354 workers in manufacturing. Stress was only weakly associated with these disorders and the authors suggested that the measurement of stress was problematic. Hess (1997) studied the relationship between perceived stress and symptoms of repetitive strain injuries, particularly carpel tunnel syndrome. In this sample, perceived stress was significantly associated with repetitive strain symptoms as was use of a computer for four or more hours daily. Back injuries of nurses were studied by Garrett, Singiser, and Banks (1992) to identify risk factors and potential preventive strategies. Results indicated that those at greatest risk of back injury were female nurses in early phases of assignment on long-term care units, nurses on evening shifts, and nurses who weighed in excess of 200 pounds.

Morris (1999) examined risk factors for injuries among temporary workers in manufacturing settings, using a survey and focus group methodology with employees and employers as participants. Of note was that temporary employees were reluctant to report injuries because they perceived doing so would lead to a loss of work opportunities; furthermore, employers believed that reported injuries were not always legitimate.

Dewar (1996) examined gender differences in the health and safety concerns of farm workers, using data from the 1988 New York Farm Family Survey. Women farm workers' health concerns included physical problems and occupational hazards, whereas men were concerned about counseling related to workplace accidents and skin hazards.

EMPLOYMENT AND WOMEN'S ILLNESS EXPERIENCES

When women experience acute and chronic illnesses, their social roles, including employment, are likely to be affected. Nursing research has addressed the relationships between employment and women's experiences of cardiac disease, cancer, and HIV.

Reviere and Eberstein (1992) used longitudinal data from the U.S. National Health and Nutrition Survey to analyze the effects of family and work roles and role changes on the incidence of coronary heart conditions in a sample of 3097 midlife women. Among the findings was that women who were homemakers (not employed) and those who left the labor force were at higher risk for these conditions than were employed women. Hamilton and Seidman (1993) compared the recovery of men and women after acute myocardial infarction (AMI), focusing on return to employment as one of the dimensions of recovery. While participants reported that nurses gave little or no counseling concerning resumption of return to work, women received less counseling than men. Riegel and Gocka (1995) studied quality of life in a sample of 96 women who had a diagnosis of myocardial infarction. A large proportion (45%) of the variance in quality of life was accounted for by three variables: employment status, social support, and self-esteem. Return to work was predictive of a higher quality of life and may also be associated with the other predictors, social support and self esteem.

Sarna (1994) described physical functional status in a sample of 69 women diagnosed with lung cancer, the third most common cancer for women in the United States. The majority (58.9%) experienced reduced energy, and 28% reported interference with work due to physical limitations. Concerns of 102 women were solicited by questionnaire following diagnosis of breast cancer by Wang, Harris, and Liu (1999). Concerns about work and finances were expressed more frequently by younger women, those who were unmarried, and non–White women. Burman and Weinert (1997) also used questionnaires to obtain data about concerns of 294 rural men and women experiencing cancer. Gender differences in concerns were found, with women less likely than men to feel that their job security was threatened; few felt discriminated against at work. Dow, Ferrell, and Anello (1997) conducted a qualitative study of the demands of long-term cancer surveillance among 34 survivors of thyroid cancer, the majority of whom were women and employed. The physical symptoms related to thyroid hormone withdrawal were severe and debilitating and had a major impact on work capacity and scheduling during periods of hypothyroidism. Carter (1997) also used qualitative analysis of interviews to describe the experiences of 10 women who had lymphedema after breast cancer treatment. While most were able to continue normal lives, they reported impairments of work and social relationships.

Sowell, Seals, Moneyham, Demi, Cohen, and Brake (1997) studied quality of life in a sample of 264 women receiving treatment for HIV/AIDS. Participants were primarily middle-aged, African American women living in poverty conditions. Those working full-time reported an overall better quality of life than those who were unemployed; they had fewer restrictions in functioning, less anxiety, and fewer symptoms. Lee, Portillo, and Miramontes (1999) examined fatigue in a sample of 100 ethnically diverse women with HIV, using questionnaires and noninvasive monitoring of sleep. As a group, these women perceived high levels of fatigue unrelieved by a night of sleep and also showed sleep disturbance. Evening and morning fatigue was compared according to role differences between women; evening fatigue was significantly higher in women who were employed than in women not employed, but there was no difference between the groups in morning fatigue.

The impact of urinary incontinence (UI) on 1113 female university employees was studied by Fitzgerald, Palmer, Berry, and Hart (2000); 21% reported UI at least monthly. The impact on work included fatigue as a result of interrupted sleep, embarrassment, alteration of concentration, and emotional distress.

EMPLOYMENT AND WOMEN'S REPRODUCTIVE HEALTH

Health During Menstruation.   Concern about the ability of women to function in responsible employment positions while menstruating has, in the past, been a basis for gender discrimination in employment. Lee and Rittenhouse (1991) examined the prevalence of perimenstrual symptoms in a cross-section of professionally employed women; these women did not differ from other cross-sections of the population in their reports of symptoms. Lee and Rittenhouse (1992) found that employed women with premenstrual symptoms were less satisfied with their social lives, had less social support, lower psychological well-being, and more physical health problems than nonsymptomatic women.

Health During Pregnancy and Postpartum.   It has been estimated that 85% of the female labor force will become pregnant sometime during their working years (Killien, 1990; Paul, 1994). The literature has documented no direct, negative effects of employment during pregnancy on the health of pregnant women themselves. Intense exercise, however, has been associated with amenorrhea and difficulty conceiving, and other strenuous work including prolonged standing and heavy lifting has been associated with preterm labor (Gabbe & Turner, 1997). In a report of data from a survey of members of the Association of Women's Health, Obstetric, and Neonatal Nurses (AWHONN), Luke, Memelle, Keith, Monuz, et al. (1995) showed that the risk of preterm birth increased for female nurses working more than 36 hours per week, more than 10 hours per shift, and standing for four to six hours per shift. Youngblut and Ahn (1997) used secondary analysis of a dataset from 171 women with high-risk pregnancies to examine their employment patterns and the relationship of prenatal employment to preterm birth. No relationships were found between employment and preterm labor in this sample, however, prescribed bedrest was associated with stopping work prenatally. The majority of women with high risk pregnancies who planned to return to work postpartum did so.

The reproductive outcomes associated with occupational exposure to hazardous substances have been a major focus of research in occupational health. Within nursing, McAbee, Gallucci, and Checkoway (1993) reported on a study of nurses' occupational exposures. Their findings indicate that more attention needs to be paid to radiation exposure and to the potential synergy between exposure to multiple workplace hazards.

Symptom experiences and functional ability during pregnancy and postpartum, particularly that of fatigue, have been a focus of nursing research during the past decade. Several cross-sectional and longitudinal surveys have documented changes in health during this reproductive phase of employed women's lives. A series of studies by Lee and associates have documented sleep and fatigue experiences of employed, childbearing women. Lee and DeJoseph (1992) found no differences in reports of general vitality and fatigue or of feelings of tiredness or energy at work between employed and non-employed groups of pregnant and postpartum women. Lee and Zaffke (1994, 1999) examined how pregnancy and postpartum influenced fatigue and energy among a sample of 42 women, the majority of whom were employed, using questionnaires and biological measures gathered before, during, and after pregnancy. While fatigue levels changed longitudinally with women reporting high levels of fatigue during the first trimester of pregnancy, employment was unrelated to perceptions of fatigue either prior to or throughout pregnancy and postpartum. Gardner (1991) described a decline in self-reported fatigue at 2 days, 2 weeks, and 6 weeks postpartum among 35 healthy women. Parks, Lenz, Milligan, and Han (1999) found, in a secondary analysis of a community hospital sample, that 52% of mothers of full-term infants experienced persistent fatigue that continued for 18 months after delivery; employment status at 3 or 18 months was unrelated to persistent fatigue.

Tulman and associates (Tulman, Fawcett, Groblewski, & Silverman, 1990; Tulman & Fawcett, 1990) gathered questionnaire data from 92 women at 3 and 6 weeks and 3 and 6 months postpartum; 58% were employed by 6 months postpartum. By this time, many still had not returned to their usual level of energy and 60% reported they had not yet fully resumed usual occupational activities. This finding is consistent with that of Mike, McGovern, Kochevar, and Roberts (1994) who surveyed a stratified, random sample of postpartum women who had been employed during pregnancy. Among their small sample of 26 women who were at least six months postpartum, 82% reported one or more work or activity limitations due to feeling tired or unwell. In a study of 1003 women at six weeks postpartum, regular vigorous exercise was associated with greater weight loss, more frequent participation in fun activities, and better postpartum adaptation; employment status was not associated with the level of exercise (Sampselle, Seng, Yeo, Killion, & Oakley, 1999).

Killien and associates (Killien, 1998; Killien, Habermann, & Jarrett, 2000) surveyed 149 employed, married women at five occasions from mid-pregnancy through 12 months postpartum to determine the impact of returning to employment on maternal health. While reports of physical and emotional symptoms declined significantly from pregnancy throughout the postpartum period, mothers' perceptions of their functional ability and their global perception of their health also decreased significantly. Employment characteristics (work environment, job satisfaction, income adequacy, and work/family interference) explained 19% to 34% of the variance in health status at each postpartum occasion. Interference between work and family was the most consistent predictor of health.

Postpartum depression has been a focus of nursing research in the past. The few studies focused on this health problem during the past decade, however, including a meta-analysis by Beck (1996), did not include employment as a major variable in the analysis (Beck, 1996; Hall, Kotch, Browne, & Rayens, 1996; Logsdon, McBride, & Birkimer, 1994).

Interference of work with seeking health care during pregnancy has been explored by several investigators. Johnson, Primas, and Coe (1994) used content analysis of postpartum interview data from 15 low-income Hispanic and non-Hispanic White respondents to determine barriers to seeking prenatal care. Among the 11 barriers identified was that the participants were concerned about missing work in order to seek care. Higgins and Woods (1999) conducted postpartum interviews with 12 urban New Mexican women who had received no prenatal care; the sample was predominantly non-Hispanic White and low-income. Within this sample, missing work and losing wages was again given as a reason for not seeking care during pregnancy.

Employment During Midlife and Menopause.   The health of women in midlife was the focus of the Seattle Midlife Women's Health Study by Woods and Mitchell which includes extensive data gathered through interviews with a population-based sample of 508 women from three racial/ethnic groups (Asian American, African American, and European American) ages 35 to 55 years (Woods & Mitchell, 1996). One of the most notable features of this sample in contrast to prior studies of midlife women from earlier birth cohorts was the centrality of employment and personal achievement in their lives and the challenge of balancing work and family (Woods & Mitchell, 1997a). Similarly, in a study of personal goals of 250 recently divorced women, employment was frequently identified as a primary goal, particularly for older women (Duffy, Mobray, & Hudes, 1990).

Depression is the most common reason for women seeking mental health care. During midlife, endocrine changes that occur during perimenopause have been hypothesized as the source of depression. In reports focusing on depressed mood in midlife women, employment status failed to discriminate women experiencing patterns of depressed mood from those not experiencing depression. Menopausal changes had little explanatory power, but stressful life context was the most influential in accounting for depressed mood (Woods & Mitchell, 1997b).

Lee and Taylor (1996) examined the health and symptom experiences of women ages 40 to 60 years who were employed as nurses at least 32 hours per week. During midlife, job satisfaction was reported as "moderately satisfying" and did not differ by age. Stress, tension, and well-being also did not differ by age. Women in all age groups considered themselves healthy and likely to remain so in the future; the average number of sick days reported was 2–3 days in the past 6 months, with women ages 50 to 55 years having the highest mean of 3.1 days. The majority (60% to 70%) did not experience PMS, fatigue, or depression. Thus, health during the menopausal transition did not appear significantly impact the ability to continue employment.

Influence of Employment on Women's Other Social Roles

EMPLOYMENT AND MOTHERHOOD

Employment Decisions.   While the majority of studies have focused on experiences of ill health or symptoms of employed women during pregnancy, some have focused on the reasons for and benefits of employment during pregnancy and postpartum. Sorenson and Tschetter (1994) surveyed 210 attendees of prenatal classes, most of whom had middle and upper incomes, about their plans for prenatal employment. While the most frequent reason given for planning employment was financial obligations, enjoyment of the job, identity as a career/professional person, and stimulation were also frequently mentioned. The major reasons given for planning non-employment were to have time with children and believing in the importance of full-time mothering. Kelley and Boyle (1995) conducted a qualitative study of pregnant women employed in the service industry. Participants attributed benefits to employment including income, socialization, personal growth opportunities, and social support. They reported coping with the additional demands of pregnancy by adapting home and work schedules but also identified role conflicts between work and home. Similarly, Killien (1993) found that women were motivated to return to work postpartum because of the benefits of employment including income, health care benefits, social support, and personal rewards.

Youngblut and colleagues reported on a series of analyses exploring the employment decisions and attitudes of women with children born preterm and/or at low birth weight (LBW). Employed mothers in two-parent families with 3-month-old, preterm infants held more positive attitudes towards employment but reported less choice and satisfaction with their employment decisions than nonemployed mothers (Youngblut, Loveland Cherry, & Horan, 1990). In a similar study of single mothers of LBW preschoolers, employed mothers held more positive attitudes toward working and were more satisfied with their employment decision than were non-employed mothers. Nonemployed single mothers preferred to be working but were not able to do so, perhaps due to lower education and more children (Youngblut, Singer, Madigan, & Swegart, 1997). In each of these studies, employment decisions were unrelated to health-related characteristics of the child. The stability of mothers' attitudes towards employment, employment status, and consistency between employment attitudes and behaviors over 15 months was examined by Youngblut (1995). Mothers of preterm and full-term infants displayed considerable stability in attitudes, behaviors, and consistency over this period. Availability of child care and financial need influenced attitude/behavior consistency.

Booth and Kelly (1999) explored the impact of having a special needs child on maternal employment decisions in a sample of 166 mothers. Prior to the birth of their children, most mothers were employed full time but, by the child's first birthday, most were employed less than 10 hours per week. The needs of the child affected their work plans for the future as well, especially if the child had chronic health problems or required adaptive equipment. Finding quality and affordable child care was a primary reason influencing the decision to limit employment.

Miller (1996) described the processes by which career-committed women managed their transitions to motherhood and back to the workplace in the first year postpartum. Her qualitative study, using the constant-comparative method, included 70 interviews with 35 middle-class participants from the time of becoming pregnant through reentering the workforce postpartum. In her rich description, she presented an overall process in which women "improvised" an identity that encompassed being women with both babies and careers that served to reduce the conflict between themselves and the people and situations around them.

Changes in the welfare system limits the time a person can receive welfare benefits; this change has particular impact on employment choices for single mothers with young children. Youngblut, Brady, and Brooten (2000) conducted a qualitative study of single mothers' experiences of being unemployed and the barriers to employment for women desiring employment. From focus group interviews with nine women, central themes related to employment emerged. Single mothers expressed a sense of obligation to their children and saw employment as a way to provide for their families, but also believed that no one could raise their children as well as they could and felt that "being there" was important. The primary obstacle to employment was child care, its cost, availability, and quality. The other central obstacle was lacking support (financial and with child care) from the child's father and from other friends and family members to enable them to work or attend school.

Breastfeeding.   The nursing research published in the past decade showed a concentration of studies addressing the influence of women's employment on breastfeeding decisions and practices. The majority focused specifically on how returning to employment in the postpartum period affected the duration of breastfeeding. All nursing research studies reviewed indicated that employment was associated with a shorter duration of breastfeeding. While employment status was not found to be related to the decision to initiate breastfeeding (Visness & Kennedy, 1997), both intentions to return to employment (O'Campo, Faden, Gielen, & Wang, 1992; Kearney & Cronenwett, 1991) and actually returning to employment during the first postpartum year (Visness & Kennedy, 1997) were associated with decreased duration of breastfeeding.

While no differences were found between employed and non-employed women in breastfeeding satisfaction (Kearney & Cronenwett, 1991), women who had intended to combine breastfeeding and employment but did not reported significantly more sadness, depression, and guilt than did those who followed their intended method of infant feeding (Chezem, Montgomery, & Fortman, 1997).

Success in combining breastfeeding and employment was found to be associated with taking a longer postpartum leave from work (Visness & Kennedy, 1997) and working fewer hours, being older, more highly educated, and professionally employed (Hills-Bonczyk, Avery, Savik, Potter, & Duckett, 1993). The duration of breastfeeding was lengthened when employed women were highly committed to breastfeeding and experienced support, including workplace accommodations such as facilities to express and store breastmilk and flexible hours (Hills-Bonczyk et al., 1993; Hills-Boncyzyk, Tromiczak, Avery, Potter, Savik, & Duckett, 1994). Bridges, Frank, and Curtin (1997) found that employers' prior experience with breastfeeding employees and knowledge of other businesses' experiences were predictive of employer support for breastfeeding.

Several interventions to assist working mothers who wish to breastfeed while working have been tested. Cronenwett, Stukel, Kearney, et al. (1992) conducted a prospective experimental study of the effects of planned bottle use during early postpartum on breastfeeding outcomes. Women ($n = 121$) who were committed to breastfeed for at least 6 weeks were randomly assigned to either a group that avoided bottle feeding for the first 6 weeks postpartum or to a group that offered one bottle daily between 2 and 6 weeks postpartum in addition to breast-feeding. Group assignment had no effect on breast-feeding problems, achievement of breastfeeding duration goals, or breastfeeding duration of at least 6 months postpartum. Duckett (1992) described the outcomes of an experimental study in which 50 primiparas who planned to return to work were randomly assigned to either a control group or an experimental group, which received videotaped and one-to-one anticipatory guidance on breastfeeding and working as well as an opportunity to use a breast pump. While not statistically significant, women in the experimental group had a longer breastfeeding duration, on average, than controls. In a clinical trial of the effectiveness of a peer counselor support group for low-income breastfeeding women on breastfeeding duration, the intention to return to work shortened breastfeeding duration by 6–9 weeks (Arolotti, Cottrell, Lee, & Curtin, 1998).

Parenting.   Killien (1998) examined maternal gratification, parenting stress, and maternal separation anxiety in a sample of women returning to work during the first postpartum year. Women completed questionnaires at 1, 4, and 8 months postpartum, and results indicated that parenting experiences improved throughout this time. The length of time the mother remained at home postpartum was unrelated to parenting stress or separation anxiety at 8 months, and only mildly associated with maternal gratification. The number of hours of work per week at 8 months was unrelated to maternal gratification and separation anxiety, and mildly associated with parenting stress. Employed mothers who reported more fatigue and depression were less gratified with parenting, had more parenting stress, and experienced more separation anxiety.

Reports from two combined samples of two-parent families address the impact of maternal employment on fathers' participation in care of preschool children (Darling-Fisher & Tiedje, 1990; Tiedje & Darling-Fisher, 1993). One sample ($n = 214$) included couples in which the wives' employment status varied (housewives, part-time and full-time workers); the other sample ($n = 139$) included couples in which the wives held professional/managerial positions. Fathers' involvement in child care varied by the employment status of their wives, with husbands being more involved when their wives were employed. In couples where the wife was employed in a professional/managerial position, child care was shared more equally than in all other situations, however, women remained the primary caregivers regardless of employment status. Jones and Heermann (1992) similarly reported that in their sample of 351 families of full term infants, mothers provided the majority of infant care although the proportion of fathers increased when mothers were employed.

One parenting concern for women has been the belief that maternal employment is detrimental to children. Several studies in nursing have focused on child outcomes related to maternal employment. Broom (1998) compared parental sensitivity to infants and toddlers in two-parent families in which the mother was either employed or not employed. Employed mothers were more sensitive to their 3 month-old children than were non-employed mothers; at both occasions, parental sensitivity was associated with marital quality. Youngblut, Loveland-Cherry, and Horan (1991, 1993, 1994) investigated the effects of maternal employment on child development and family functioning for families with preterm infants at 3 months, 12 months, and 18 months. Maternal employment at 3 months was unrelated to the child's mental or psychomotor development at all occasions. Mothers' attitude/behavior consistency, however, was positively associated with the child's psychomotor development, and the degree of choice in employment mothers had was positively related to some child development outcomes.

Youngblut, Singer, Madigan, Swegart, and Rodgers (1998) also examined differences in parent-child and family relationships for employed and non-employed single mothers of preschool children. Employed mothers had more positive perceptions of their children and provided more enriching home environments for their preschool children than did non-employed mothers. When sociodemographic factors (income, number of children, mother's education) were statistically controlled, however, employment was not related to any of the mother-child or family variables. Consistency between employment attitudes and employment behavior was related to more positive maternal perceptions of her child. The preschoolers with employed mothers were hospitalized more often than preschoolers with nonemployed mothers, although the number of children with health problems was unrelated to mothers' employment status. The authors speculated that maternal employment might have increased the children's exposures to infectious diseases or that maternal employment might provide health care insurance coverage that influenced hospital admissions.

EMPLOYMENT AND FAMILY CAREGIVING

Employed women are four times more likely to be caregivers to ill and elderly family members than employed men (Stone & Stone, 1990). Krach and Brooks (1995) reported that caregivers of the elderly report a variety of personal health care problems related to caregiver burden and miss an average of eight days of work annually related to caregiving responsibilities. The stress associated with family caregiving may be especially problematic when added to caregiving that is a woman's occupational responsibility as well. Ross, Rideout, and Carson (1994) conducted a qualitative study of 40 nurses employed full-time who also cared for others in their private lives. Analysis of diary and interview data indicated that most participants experienced high levels of stress while also experiencing rewards from dual-caregiving. Similarly, Hawkins (1996) examined the relationship between workforce participation and caregiving stress in a small sample of women caring for frail, elderly parents. Employed caregiving daughters had significantly higher stress scores than unemployed caregiving daughters. Caregiving stress has been found to be associated with physical symptoms, psychological symptoms, and depression (Phillips, Morrison, Steffl, Chae, Cromwell, & Russell, 1995). Although family caregiving responsibilities may increase the stress of working women, employment has been shown to protect women from negative health effects following bereavement. In a study of 157 widows, aged 55 to 75 years, Aber (1992) found that work history and work attitude were statistically significant predictors of women's health two years after the death of a spouse.

Home care for the elderly and chronically ill in need of long-term care is often cited to be less "costly." To challenge that assumption, Ward and Brown (1994) studied 53 primary caregivers for a person with AIDS (PWA). Caregivers reported an average of 8.5 hours daily performing personal care tasks and 5 hours weekly performing household tasks. Using a market valuation method, they calculated the cost of unpaid care for one PWA as in excess of $25,000 annually. Ward's (1990) discussion of valuation methods applied to determining the costs of kin care shows much promise for documenting the cost of women's caregiving, often devalued in policy analyses on the economics of home care. The devaluing of the unpaid caregiving of women was discussed by Angus (1994) as an "ideology of separate spheres" which designates paid activity in the public sphere as work and therefore valued, while unpaid activities pursued in the private sphere of the home are overlooked. Not only is this unpaid work at home a source of stress which interacts with or compounds workplace stress to effect women's health, but also this work is often done to promote the health of others.

EMPLOYMENT AND MARRIAGE AND FAMILY FUNCTIONING

There was considerably less focus in the nursing literature on the impact of women's employment on marital and family functioning. The descriptive studies published during the last decade focused predominantly on marital and family functioning of employed women during the early childbearing years.

Marital quality following birth of a child was studied by Broom (1998) in her longitudinal study of single and dual employed families. Marital quality declined in both groups between 3 and 30 months postpartum, and at the latter occasion, marital quality was lower for couples in which the wife was employed. The influence of maternal employment on family functioning in families of vulnerable children was the subject of a longitudinal investigation by Youngblut, Loveland-Cherry, and Horan (1994). They followed two-parent families with preterm infants from birth through 18 months postpartum and found no differences in family cohesion or adaptability related to employment status or number of hours worked by mothers. Attitude/behavior consistency and the ability of the mother to choose employment or not seemed to be more influential to family functioning than was employment status per se. Gennaro (1996; Generro & Krause, 1996) conducted a prospective study of families of 224 preterm, low birthweight infants to determine the impact of preterm birth on the family. Families were interviewed over the telephone for six months after the infant's hospital discharge. Employed mothers left employment early due to prenatal complications and either failed to return to work, worked fewer hours, or took extended postpartum leaves. Simultaneously, unreimbursed family expenses increased, contributing to increased economic pressures on families.

The clerical workers interviewed by Stevens, Hall, and Meleis (Stevens, Hall, & Meleis, 1992; Meleis & Stevens, 1992) identified several areas of vulnerability related to their partners. Negotiating household responsibilities was a stressor within their marriages and made other role obligations more difficult to meet. Many women also described being monitored and restricted by male spouses, and 14% of the sample reported physical abuse from current or former male partners. As these employed workers attempted to cope with stress in their multiple roles, they frequently reported coping as a solitary effort rather than one supported by their spouses. While employment and income often offers increased power to women in relationships, these investigators documented, that, for women in clerical work, these advantages may not be realized.

Balancing Multiple Roles

Several studies contributed to our understanding of the interaction among multiple roles occupied by employed women. These studies primarily focus on role conflicts and role balance or on the comparison of role benefits and stress among the roles of work, marriage, and parenthood.

Kenney (2000) surveyed 299 women ages 18 to 66 years to identify stressors, personality traits, and health problems by age groups. Young women (18–29) reported the most physical and emotional symptoms of health problems. Midlife women (30–45) had significantly more stressors than other women but fewer health problems, perhaps due to healthy personality traits. Older women (46–66) had fewest symptoms, highest healthy personality traits, and fewest stressors. Juggling multiple responsibilities of spouses, children, aging parents, and work while trying to maintain "inner balance" contributed to the higher stressors of young and midlife women.

Hall (1991, 1992) compared the experiences of men and women in dual-earner families following the birth of their first child. She found that, while each partner's experience was a process of redefining roles, women more than their male partners experienced role strain and placed lower priority on meeting their own needs. Rankin (1993) interviewed 118 mothers of preschoolers who were employed at least 30 hours a week about the stresses and rewards of their experiences. Sixty-two percent reported a high level of stress; major stresses included lack of time, child problems, and guilt. Stevens, Hall, and Meleis (1992) described the juggling of work, marriage, and parenting by the women in their study of clerical workers which included strained relationships, child care concerns, and financial stress.

Thomas (1995) examined psychosocial correlates of women's health in middle adulthood using secondary analysis of data on 238 midlife women with varying constellations of employment, marriage, and parental roles; 76% were employed. Women reporting the best health in midlife had the fewest concerns about their roles as workers, wives, and mothers. Miller, Wilbur, Montgomery, and Chandler (1998) examined relationships among job, partner, and parent role quality and psychological well-being in employed Black and White midlife women. Professionals reported greater well-being than non-professionals. When race, occupational groups, and menopausal status were held constant, partner and parent role quality were related to well-being but job role quality was not.

Gottlieb, Kelloway, and Martin-Mathews (1996) examined work-family conflict, stress, and job satisfaction among 101 nurses who also had responsibility for the care of a child and/or elderly family member. Family support, perceived organizational support for family life, workload size, and involvement in child care were the major factors responsible for the outcomes. Decker (1997) found among hospital nurses that interference of work with non-job activities was associated with both lower job satisfaction and psychological distress; the study did not examine the extent to which family interfered with work.

Despite the numerous studies describing the challenges of employed women attempting to balance multiple roles, very few projects have examined strategies to assist these women. Social support during transitions in and out of employment were the subject of a qualitative, prospective study by Harrison, Neufeld, and Kushner (1995). Women returning to work following an extended absence or retiring from full-time employment were interviewed about access and barriers to social support. These transitions often took as long as two years to complete, and accessing desired support was found to be difficult for some women. Collins, Tiedje, and Stommel (1992) tested the effects of six-session, small group intervention on the well-being of mothers who were returning to work within six months of their infants' births. At one year after delivery, participants in the intervention reported significantly increased levels of marital satisfaction.

SUMMARY

During the past decade a significant number of published research papers have focused on women's employment role. This attention to women's employment is no doubt reflective of a growing awareness of the proportion of women who have added paid employment to the constellation of other social roles they occupy and also awareness of its influence on women's health.

What are the research questions that these studies have addressed? The majority of studies have asked, in some way, how employment influences women's well-being or symptom experience or how employment has affected women's family roles or other family members. While some studies have examined the influence of women's health on their employment, fewer studies have asked how women's family members or family roles affect their employment. This focus may reflect a traditional view of women's gender roles that women's family work is central and that employment is "added on." Thus, for example, investigators are concerned about whether maternal employment is harmful for children but rarely ask how women's caregiving responsibilities are detrimental for employment! The considerable focus on women's employment during pregnancy and early years of childrearing also appears to reflect the cultural tension between women's roles as mothers and members of the labor force. Most samples have also been limited exclusively to women participants. This approach may be a response to the historical exclusion of women in research on employment. As a result of the "gender-segregation" of samples, exploration of gender differences in the influence of employment roles on health has not progressed.

Which women have been the focus of research? Samples are becoming more ethnically, racially, and socioeconomically diverse but the majority of participants remain White, well educated, and middleclass. In samples where diversity is present, race and class were rarely variables included in the analyses, thus the opportunity to more fully understand the influence of these important contexts for women and their employment experiences was lost (General Accounting Office, 2000). Qualitative studies more frequently either focused on historically underrepresented women or included diverse life contexts in the analyses. Women's employment experiences across the lifespan have not been fully represented. The emphasis in the past decade has been on women during childbearing and midlife. As a result, we know little about the employment experiences of young women entering the workforce, single or women without children, or older women approaching retirement.

How has employment been conceptualized and measured? Employment has been treated as a unitary rather than a diverse experience. Clerical work and nursing have been the primary occupations of women studied. When more occupationally diverse samples have been studied, occupational type has not been included as a variable in analysis. While women are more likely than men to be employed part-time or as temporary workers and are increasingly working multiple jobs, employment has usually been treated as a binary variable with study participants categorized as "employed" or "not employed." Occupational health studies have included more complex measurements of employment and other studies could benefit from this broader approach. The limited attention to job type, income, hours of work, and employment conditions has in turn limited the complexity of knowledge that has been generated from research.

What methods of study have been used? Both qualitative and quantitative approaches are represented in the nursing research of the past decade, resulting in descriptions of women's employment experiences and knowledge of associations among employment and other variables. This research has identified variables associated with both health-promoting and health-damaging consequences for employed women, however, studies which incorporate these variables into intervention and outcomes studies are rare. It is in this area that nurse scientists can make major contributions. Many studies have used limited longitudinal designs, spanning the duration of selected life transitions such as recovery from illness or pregnancy. Additionally, several cohort studies have contributed to our knowledge of the influence of employment roles at different points in women's lives.

What emerges from this research, taken as a whole, is that employment per se presents no particular risk to women's health or that of their families. Employment can be a resource that promotes women's health and family well-being, however, certain occupations, work environments, or combination of contextual factors present risks for some or all women exposed to them.

Work environments and conditions that are particularly detrimental for women are those in which the jobs are physically strenuous or involve use of equipment that is not ergonomically correct. Difficult interpersonal relationships with supervisors or coworkers, especially those that involve sexual or racial discrimination, harassment or abuse, contribute to emotional distress, job dissatisfaction, and physical symptoms. Employment can have negative effects on health when women cope with role stress, conflict, and overload through health-damaging behaviors such as smoking, substance abuse, inadequate nutrition, and exercise. But employment settings that have worksite health promotion programs, exercise facilities, lactation support facilities, and supportive colleagues can assist women to engage in health promoting practices.

Women who are employed in jobs with limited income, access to health care and other benefits plus few opportunities for development and advancement do not realize the health advantages associated with employment. Women who experience difficult life circumstances, with limited social support from family and friends, frequently find employment an added burden, not a benefit or resource.

Since most women are employed throughout adulthood, transitions in their lives co-occur with their employment. The workplace, organized on a male model, often fails to acknowledge that workers have personal and family lives. The studies of women's experiences of childbearing and childrearing, personal and family illness, and bereavement suggest that the task of negotiating a balance between multiple role obligations is primarily left to the individual woman. This solitary coping and problem-solving adds to the role burden and stress experienced by women during these life transitions. Data from multiple studies suggest that women manage these situations without harm to children, spouses, family members, or their employment, but perhaps at the expense of their personal health and well-being.

FUTURE DIRECTIONS

This review suggests several directions for future research. It is time to move forward from descriptive studies, especially on employment of mothers with young infants, towards more complex questions. Research to date has typically failed to sufficiently incorporate the complexity of work and family variables in study measures and designs to generate promising interventions for promoting, maintaining, or restoring health to employed women. There is a paucity of research to guide interventions to improve the health of employed women at the individual, group, worksite, or policy level. The unique perspective of nurse scientists, with their focus on developing clinical therapeutics to promote human health, is likely to place nursing research at the forefront of this endeavor. Nurse scientists are especially well prepared to link the perspectives and findings of occupational health research, women's health research, and family health research.

Projected future changes in the female workforce will also influence important areas for consideration by nurse scientists. Women will continue to enter the labor force and gender segregation of occupations will likely disappear, especially in those occupations traditionally dominated by men. The workforce of the future will exhibit more age and ethnic diversity. As mandatory retirement policies evaporate, economic needs increase, and the population ages, there will be an increased age of workers. These changes will have implications for common health concerns of women in the workplace. Research on women's employment transitions as they age and experience changes in their family contexts, including retirement, has not been included in the portfolios of nursing research.

Existing research clearly illustrates that neither a health-risk nor a health-benefits perspective has been adequate in answering questions related to women and work. Future research needs to be guided by more complex and holistic frameworks that account for the full complexity of women's lives.

Research is needed which continues to focus on groups of women who have been underrepresented or unidentified in the past, especially minority women, older women, and women with fewer socioeconomic resources. In addition to studying special health issues for occupational groups in which the largest numbers of women are represented, it will be important to identify areas of concern in occupations in which women were previously underrepresented. Various units of analysis will need to be employed in the future. Most research to date on women, work, and health considers the individual as the principal unit of analysis. Yet family and organizational outcomes are equally important to consider in the future. Individual health outcomes such as physical and emotional symptoms continue to be important outcomes for study. The focus on women's reproductive health, however, must be extended to other areas of concern for women's health including cardiovascular health, cancer, and emotional well-being. In addition, indicators of the impact of health on the ability to function in work and family roles should be considered. Family outcomes to be considered include indicators of family relationship quality such as marital and parenting quality. Organizational outcomes might include measures of productivity and cost/benefit analysis of workplace policies and programs.

Consideration needs to be given to the interpretation and dissemination of results. A critical challenge will be the framing and interpretation of research results in a way to effectively inform policy makers and women themselves.

ACKNOWLEDGMENT

The author gratefully thanks Dr. Mary Salazar for her careful review and comment on this chapter.

REFERENCES

Aber, C. S. (1992). Spousal death, a threat to women's health: Paid work as a "resistance resource." *Image: Journal of Nursing Scholarship, 24,* 95–99.

Alexander, L. L., & Beck, K. (1990). The smoking behaviour of military nurses: the relationship to job stress, job satisfaction and social support. *Journal of Advanced Nursing, 15,* 843–849.

Angus, J. (1994). Women's paid/unpaid work and health: Exploring the social context of everyday life. *Canadian Journal of Nursing Research, 26,* 23–42.

Arolotti, J. P., Cottrell, B. H., Lee, S. H., & Curtin, J. J. (1998). Breastfeeding among low-income women with and without peer support. *Journal of Community Health Nursing, 15,* 163–178.

Barnett, R. C. (1996). *Toward a review of the work/family literature: Work in progress.* Wellesley, MA: Wellesley Center for Research on Women.

Beaton, R. D., Murphy, S. A., Pike, K., & Corneil, W. (1997). Social support and network conflict in firefighters and paramedics. *Western Journal of Nursing Research, 19,* 297–313.

Beck, C. T. (1996). A meta-analysis of predictors of postpartum depression. *Nursing Research, 45,* 297–303.

Booth, C. L., & Kelly, J. F. (1999). Child care and employment in relation to infants' disabilities and risk factors. *American Journal of Mental Retardation, 104,* 117–130.

Bridges, C. B., Frank, D. I., & Curtin, J. (1997). Employer attitudes toward breastfeeding in the workplace. *Journal of Human Lactation, 13,* 215–219.

Broom, B. L. (1998). Parental sensitivity to infants and toddlers in dual-earner and single-earner families. *Nursing Research, 47,* 162–170.

Burman, M. E., & Weinert, C. (1997). Concerns of rural men and women experiencing cancer. *Oncology Nursing Forum, 24,* 1593–1600.

Carter, B. J. (1997). Women's experiences of lymphedema. *Oncology Nursing Forum, 24,* 875–882.

Chezem, J., Montgomery, P., & Fortman, T. (1997). Maternal feelings after cessation of breastfeeding: Influence of factors related to employment and duration. *Journal of Perinatal and Neonatal Nursing, 11,* 61–70.

Collins, C., Tiedje, L. B., & Stommel, M. (1992). Promoting positive well-being in employed mothers: A pilot study. *Health Care for Women International, 13,* 77–85.

Costello, C., Krimgold, B., & Dooley, B. (1996). *The American woman, 1996–97, Where we stand: Women and work.* New York: W. W. Norton.

Costello, C., Miles, S., & Stone, A. J. (1998). *The American woman, 1999–2000: A century of change—What's next?* New York: W. W. Norton.

Costello, C., Stone, A. J., & Dooley, B. (1994). *The American women: 1994 95, Where we stand, women and health.* New York: W. W. Norton.

Cronenwett, L., Stukel, T., Kearney, M. H., Barrett, J., Covington, C., DelMonte, K., Reinhardt, R., & Rippe, L. (1992). Single daily bottle use in the early weeks postpartum and breastfeeding outcomes. *Pediatrics, 90,* 760–766.

Darling-Fisher, C. S., & Tiedje, L. B. (1990). The impact of maternal employment characteristics on fathers' participation in child care. *Family Relations, 39,* 20–26.

Dear, J. A. (1995). Work stress and health '95. *Vital Speeches of the Day, 62,* 39–42.

Decker, F. H. (1997). Occupational and nonoccupational factors in job satisfaction and psychological distress among nurses. *Research in Nursing & Health, 20,* 453–464.

DesCamp, K. D., & Thomas, C. C. (1993). Buffering nursing stress through play at work. *Western Journal of Nursing Research, 15,* 619–627.

Dewar, D. M. (1996). Farm health and safety issues: Do men and women differ in their perceptions? *American Association of Occupational Health Nursing Journal, 44,* 391–401.

Dow, K. H., Ferrell, B. R., & Anello, C. (1997). Balancing demands of cancer surveillance among survivors of thyroid cancer. *Cancer Practice, 5,* 289–295.

Duckett, L. (1992). Maternal employment and breastfeeding. *NAACOG's Clinical Issues in Perinatal and Women's Health, 3,* 701–712.

Duckett, L., Henly, S., Avery, M., Potter, S., Hills-Bonczyk, S. G., Hulden, R., & Savik, K. (1998). A theory of planned behavior-based structural model for breastfeeding. *Nursing Research, 47,* 325–336.

Duffy, M. (1997). Determinants of reported health promotion behaviors in employed Mexican American women. *Health Care for Women International, 18,* 149–163.

Duffy, M. E., Mobray, C. A., & Hudes, M. (1990). Personal goals of recently divorced women. *Image: Journal of Nursing Scholarship, 22,* 14–17.

Findorff-Dennis, M. J., McGovern, P. M., Bull, M., & Hung, J. (1999). Work related assaults. The impact on victims. *American Association of Occupational Health Nursing Journal, 47,* 456–465.

Fitzgerald, L. F. (1993). Sexual harassment. Violence against women in the workplace. *American Psychologist, 48,* 1070–1076.

Fitzgerald, S. T., Palmer, M. H., Berry, S. J., & Hart, K. (2000). Urinary incontinence: Impact on working women. *American Association of Occupational Health Nursing Journal, 48,* 112–118.

Frankenhaeuser, M., Lundberg, U., & Chesney, M. (1991). *Women, work, and health: Stress and opportunities.* New York: Plenum Press.

Gabbe, S. G., & Turner, L. P. (1997). Reproductive hazards of the American lifestyle: Work during pregnancy. *American Journal of Obstetrics and Gynecology, 176,* 826–832.

Gage, L. W., & Takeshita, Y. J. (1996). Coping with stress in a cross-cultural setting: the case of Japanese and American employees of a Japanese plant in the United States. *American Association of Occupational Health Nursing Journal, 44,* 278–287.

Gardner, D. L. (1991). Fatigue in postpartum women. *Applied Nursing Research, 4,* 57–62.

Garrett, B., Singiser, D., & Banks, S. M. (1992). Back injuries among nursing personnel: the relationship of personal characteristics, risk factors, and nursing practices. *American Association of Occupational Health Nursing Journal, 40,* 510–516.

General Accounting Office. (2000). *Increased research on women's health* (Rep. No. GAO/HEHS-00-96). Washington, DC.

Gennaro, S. (1996). Leave and employment in families of preterm low birthweight infants. *Image: Journal of Nursing Scholarship, 28,* 193–198.

Gennaro, S., & Krouse, A. (1996). Patterns of postpartum health in mothers of low birth weight infants. *Health Care for Women International, 17,* 35–45.

Gold, D., Rogacz, S., Bock, N., Tosteson, T., Baum, T., Speizer, F., & Czeisler, C. (1992). Rotating shift work, sleep, and accidents related to sleepiness in hospital nurses. *American Journal of Public Health, 82,* 1011–1014.

Gottlieb, B. H., Kelloway, E. K., & Martin-Mathews, A. (1996). Predictors of work-family conflict, stress, and job satisfaction among nurses. *Canadian Journal of Nursing Research, 28,* 99–117.

Hall, J. M., Stevens, P. E., & Meleis, A. I. (1992b). Developing the construct of role integration: A narrative analysis of women clerical workers' daily lives. *Research in Nursing & Health, 15,* 447–457.

Hall, J. M., Stevens, P. E., & Meleis, A. I. (1992a). Experiences of women clerical workers in patient care areas. *Journal of Nursing Administration, 22,* 11–17.

Hall, L. A., Kotch, J. B., Browne, D., & Rayens, M. K. (1996). Self-esteem as a mediator of the effects of stressors and social resources on depressive symptoms in postpartum mothers. *Nursing Research, 45,* 231–238.

Hall, W. (1991). The experience of fathers in dual-earner families following the births of their first infants. *Journal of Advanced Nursing, 16,* 423–430.

Hall, W. (1992). Comparison of the experience of women and men in dual-earner families following the birth of their first infant. *Image: Journal of Nursing Scholarship, 24,* 33–37.

Hamilton, G. A., & Seidman, R. N. (1993). A comparison of the recovery period for women and men after an acute myocardial infarction. *Heart and Lung, 22,* 308–315.

Harrison, M. J., Neufeld, A., & Kushner, K. (1995). Women in transition: Access and barriers to social support. *Journal of Advanced Nursing, 21,* 858–864.

Hartmann, H., Kuriansky, J., & Owens, C. (1996). Employment and women's health. In M.Falik & K. Collins (Eds.), *Women's health: The Commonwealth Fund Survey* (pp. 296–323). Baltimore: Johns Hopkins University Press.

Hawkins, B. (1996). Daughters and caregiving: Taking care of our own. *American Association of Occupational Health Nursing Journal, 44,* 433–437.

Herz, D., & Wootton, B. (1996). Women in the workforce: An overview. In C. Costello, B. Krimgold, & B. Dooley (Eds.), *The American woman, 1996–97, Where we stand: Women and work* (pp. 44–78). New York: W. W. Norton.

Hess, D. (1997). Employee perceived stress. Relationship to the development of repetitive strain injury symptoms *American Association of Occupational Health Nursing Journal, 45,* 115–123.

Hewitt, J. B., & Levin, P. F. (1997). Violence in the workplace. *Annual Review of Nursing Research, 15,* 81–99.

Higgins, P. G., & Woods, P. J. (1999). Reasons, health behaviors, and outcomes of no prenatal care: Research that changed practice. *Health Care for Women International, 20,* 127–136.

Hills-Bonczyk, S. G., Avery, M. D., Savik, K., Potter, S., & Duckett, L. J. (1993). Women's experiences with combining breast-feeding and employment. *Journal of Nurse Midwifery, 38,* 257–266.

Hills-Bonczyk, S. G., Tromiczak, K. R., Avery, M. D., Potter, S., Savik, K., & Duckett, L. J. (1994). Women's experiences with breastfeeding longer than 12 months. *BIRTH, 21,* 206–212.

Im, E. O. (2000). A feminist critique of research on women's work and health. *Health Care for Women International, 21,* 105–119.

Jarrett, M., Heitkemper, M., & Shaver, J. (1995). Symptoms and self-care strategies in women with and without dysmenorrhea. *Health Care for Women International, 16,* 167–178.

Jenkins, E. L., Layne, L. A., & Kisner, S. M. (1992). Homicide in the workplace: The U.S. experience, 1980–1988. *American Association of Occupational Health Nursing Journal, 40,* 215–218.

Johnson, J. L., Primas, P. J., & Coe, M. K. (1994). Factors that prevent women of low socioeconomic status from seeking prenatal care. *Journal of American Academy of Nurse Practitioners, 6,* 105–111.

Jones, L. C., & Heermann, J. A. (1992). Parental division of infant care: contextual influences and infant characteristics. *Nursing Research, 41,* 228–234.

Kahn, R. L. (1991). Forms of women's work. In M. Frankenhaeuser, U. Lundberg, & M. Chesney (Eds.), *Women, work, and health: Stress and opportunities* (pp. 65–83). New York: Plenum Press.

Kawachi, I., Colditz, G., Stampfer, M., Willett, W., Manson, J., Speizer, F., & Hennekens, C. (1995). Prospective study of shift work and risk of coronary heart disease in women. *Circulation, 92,* 3178–3182.

Kearney, M. H., & Cronenwett, L. (1991). Breastfeeding and employment. *Journal of Obstetric, Gynecologic and Neonatal Nursing, 20,* 471–480.

Kelley, M. A., & Boyle, J. S. (1995). How much is too much? A study of pregnant women in service industry jobs. *Journal of Obstetric, Gynecologic and Neonatal Nursing, 24,* 269–275.

Kenney, J. W. (2000). Women's 'inner balance': A comparison of stressors, personality traits and health problems by age group. *Journal of Advanced Nursing, 31,* 639–650.

Killien, M. G. (1990). Working during pregnancy: Psychological stressor or asset? *NAACOG'S Clinical Issues in Perinatal and Women's Health, 1,* 325–332.

Killien, M. G. (1993). Returning to work after childbirth: Considerations for health policy. *Nursing Outlook, 41,* 73–78.

Killien, M. G. (1998). Postpartum return to work: Mothering stress, anxiety, and gratification. *Canadian Journal of Nursing Research, 30,* 53–66.

Killien, M. G. (1999). Women's work, women's health. In A. S. Hinshaw, S. Feetham, & J. Shaver (Eds.), *Handbook of clinical nursing research* (pp. 457–481). Thousand Oaks, CA: Sage.

Killien, M. G., Habermann, B., & Jarrett, M. (in press). Influence of employment characteristics on postpartum mothers' health. *Health Care for Women International.*

Kneipp, S. (in press). The health of women in transition from welfare to employment. *Western Journal of Nursing Research.*

Krach, P., & Brooks, J. A. (1995). Identifying the responsibilities & needs of working adults who are primary caregivers. *Journal of Gerontological Nursing, 21,* 41–50.

Lee, K. A. (1992). Self-reported sleep disturbances in employed women. *Sleep, 15,* 493–498.

Lee, K. A., & DeJoseph, J. F. (1992). Sleep disturbances, vitality, and fatigue among a select group of employed childbearing women. *Birth, 19,* 208–213.

Lee, K. A., Lentz, M. J., Taylor, D. L., Mitchell, E. S., & Woods, N. F. (1994). Fatigue as a response to environmental demands in women's lives. *Image: Journal of Nursing Scholarship, 26,* 149–154.

Lee, K. A., Portillo, C. J., & Miramontes, H. (1999). The fatigue experience for women with human immunodeficiency virus. *Journal of Obstetrics, Gynecology and Neonatal Nursing, 28,* 193–200.

Lee, K. A., & Rittenhouse, C. (1991). Prevalence of perimenstrual symptoms in employed women. *Women and Health, 17,* 17–32.

Lee, K. A., & Rittenhouse, C. A. (1992). Health and perimenstrual symptoms: health outcomes for employed women who experience perimenstrual symptoms. *Women and Health, 19,* 65–78.

Lee, K. A., & Taylor, D. L. (1996). Is there a generic midlife women? The health and symptom experience of employed midlife women. *Menopause, 3,* 154–164.

Lee, K. A., & Zaffke, M. E. (1999). Longitudinal changes in fatigue and energy during pregnancy and the postpartum period. *Journal of Obstetrics, Gynecology and Neonatal Nursing, 28,* 183–191.

Lee, K. A., Zaffke, M. E., McEnany, G., & Hoehler, K. (1994). Sleep and fatigue: Before, during and after pregnancy. *Sleep Research, 23,* 416.

Levin, P. F., Hewitt, J. B., & Misner, S. T. (1996). Workplace violence: Female occupational homicides in metropolitan Chicago. *American Association of Occupational Health Nursing Journal, 44,* 326–331.

Levin, P. F., Hewitt, J. B., & Misner, S. T. (1998). Insights of nurses about assault in hospital-based emergency departments. *Image: Journal of Nursing Scholarship, 30,* 249–254.

Logsdon, M. C., McBride, A. B., & Birkimer, J. C. (1994). Social support and postpartum depression. *Research in Nursing & Health, 17,* 449–457.

Lombardi, E. L., & Ulbirch, P. M. (1997). Work conditions, mastery and psychological distress: Are housework and paid work contexts conceptually similar? *Women and Health, 26,* 17–39.

Luke, B., Memelle, N., Keith, L., Monuz, F., Minogue, J., Papiernik, E., & et al. (1995). The association between occupational factors and preterm birth: A United States Nurses' Study. *American Journal of Obstetrics and Gynecology, 173,* 849–862.

Lusk, S. L. (1992). Violence in the workplace. *American Association of Occupational Health Nursing Journal, 40,* 212–213.

Lusk, S. L. (1997). Workers and worker populations. In M. K. Salazar (Ed.), *Core curriculum for occupational health nursing.* Philadelphia: W. B. Saunders.

McAbee, R. R., Gallucci, B. J., & Checkoway, H. (1993). Adverse reproductive outcomes and occupational exposures among nurses: an investigation of multiple hazardous exposures. *American Association of Occupational Health Nursing Journal, 41,* 110–119.

McCloskey, J. C. (1990). Two requirements for job contentment: Autonomy and social integration. *Image: Journal of Nursing Scholarship, 22,* 140–143.

Melcis, A. I., Norbeck, J. S., & Laffrey, S. C. (1989). Role integration and health among female clerical workers. *Research in Nursing and Health, 12,* 355–364.

Meleis, A. I., & Stevens, P. E. (1992). Women in clerical jobs: Spousal role satisfaction, stress, and coping. *Women and Health, 18,* 23–40.

Messias, D. K., Regev, H. I., Im, E. O., Spiers, J. A., Van, P., & Meleis, A. (1997). Expanding the visibility of women's work: Policy implications. *Nursing Outlook, 45,* 258–264.

Mike, D., McGovern, P., Kochevar, L., & Roberts, C. (1994). Role function and mental health in postpartum working women: a pilot study. *American Association of Occupational Health Nursing Journal, 42,* 214–229.

Miller, A. M., Wilbur, J., Montgomery, A., & Chandler, P. (1998). Social role quality and psychological well-being in employed Black and White midlife women. *American Association of Occupational Health Nursing Journal, 46,* 371–378.

Miller, S. (1996). Questioning, resisting, acquiescing, balancing: New mothers' career reentry strategies. *Health Care for Women International, 17,* 109–131.

Morris, J. A. (1999). Injury experiences of temporary workers in a manufacturing setting. Factors that increase vulnerability. *American Association of Occupational Health Nursing Journal, 47,* 470–478.

Murphy, S. A., Beaton, R. D., Cain, K. C., & Pike, K. C. (1994). Gender differences in fire fighter job stressors and symptoms of stress. *Women and Health, 22,* 55–69.

Napholz, L. (1994). Indices of psychological well-being and sex role orientation among working women. *Health Care for Women International, 15,* 307–316.

Nelson, M. A. (1997). Health practices and role involvement among low-income working women. *Health Care for Women International, 18,* 195–205.

Nies, M. A., Vollman, M., & Cook, T. (1999). African-American women's experiences with physical activity in their daily lives. *Public Health Nursing, 16,* 23–31.

O'Campo, P., Faden, R. R., Gielen, A. C., & Wang, M. C. (1992). Prenatal factors associated with breastfeeding duration: recommendations for prenatal interventions. *BIRTH, 19,* 195–201.

Parks, P. L., Lenz, E. R., Milligan, R. A., & Han, H. R. (1999). What happens when fatigue lingers for 18 months after delivery? *Journal of Obstetric, Gynecologic and Neonatal Nursing, 28,* 87–83.

Paul, M. E. (1994). Disorders of reproduction. *Occupational Health, 21,* 367–385.

Pender, N. J., Walker, S. N., Sechrist, K. R., & Frank-Stromborg, M. (1990). Predicting health-promoting lifestyles in the workplace. *Nursing Research, 39,* 326–332.

Phillips, L., Morrison, E., Steffl, B., Chae, Y., Cromwell, S., & Russell, C. (1995). Effects of the situational context and interactional process on the quality of family caregiving. *Research in Nursing and Health, 18,* 205–216.

Rankin, E. D. (1993). Stresses and rewards experienced by employed mothers. *Health Care for Women International, 14,* 527–537.

Reviere, R., & Eberstein, I. W. (1992). Work, marital status, and heart disease. *Health Care for Women International, 13,* 393–399.

Riegel, B., & Gocka, I. (1995). Gender differences in adjustment to acute myocardial infarction. *Heart Lung, 24,* 457–466.

Rogers, J. L., & Maurizio, S. L. (1993). Prevalence of sexual harassment among rural community care workers. *Home Healthcare Nurse, 11,* 37–40.

Ross, M. M., Rideout, E., & Carson, M. (1994). Nurses' work: Balancing personal and professional caregiving careers. *Canadian Journal of Nursing Research, 26,* 43–59.

Sampselle, C. M., Seng, J., Yeo, S., Killion, C., & Oakley, D. (1999). Physical activity and postpartum well-being. *Journal of Obstetric, Gynecologic and Neonatal Nursing, 28,* 41–49.

Sarna, L. (1994). Functional status in women with lung cancer. *Cancer Nursing, 17,* 87–93.

Schaefer, J. A., & Moos, R. H. (1996). Effects of work stressors and work climate on long-term care staff's job morale and functioning. *Research in Nursing & Health, 19,* 63–73.

Schroeder, C. & Ward, D. (1998). Women, welfare, and work: One view of the debate. *Nursing Outlook, 46,* 226–232.

Smith, M., Droppleman, P., & Thomas, S. P. (1996). Under assault: The experience of work-related anger in female registered nurses. *Nursing Forum, 31,* 22–33.

Sorensen, G., & Verbrugge, L. M. (1987). Women, work, and health. *Annual Review of Public Health, 8,* 235–251.

Sorenson, D. L., & Tschetter, L. (1994). Reasons for employment or non-employment during pregnancy. *Health Care for Women International, 15*, 453–463.

Sowell, R. L., Seals, B. F., Moneyham, L., Demi, A. S., Cohen, L., & Brake, S. (1997). Quality of life in HIV-infected women in the south-eastern United States. *AIDS Care, 9*, 501–512.

Spratlen, L. P. (1994). Perceived workplace mistreatment in higher education . . . characteristics and consequences. *American Association of Occupational Health Nursing Journal, 42*, 548–554.

Stevens, P. E., Hall, J. M., & Meleis, A. I. (1992). Examining vulnerability of women clerical workers from five ethnic/racial groups. *Western Journal of Nursing Research, 14*, 754–774.

Stevens, P. E., & Meleis, A. (1991). Maternal role of clerical workers: A feminist analysis. *Social Science and Medicine, 32*, 1425–1433.

Stone, R., & Stone, P. (1990). The completing demands of employment and informal caregiving to disabled elders, *Medical Care, 28*, 513–529.

Strasser, P. B., Lusk, S. L., Franzblau, A., & Armstrong, T. J. (1999) Perceived psychological stress and upper extremity cumulative trauma disorders. *American Association of Occupational Health Nursing Journal, 47*, 22–30.

Thomas, L., Riegel, B., Gross, D., & Andrea, J. (1992). Job stress among emergency department nurses. *Heart and Lung, 21*, 294.

Thomas, S. P. (1995). Psychosocial correlates of women's health in middle adulthood. *Issues in Mental Health Nursing, 16*, 285–314.

Tiedje, L. B., & Darling-Fisher, C. S. (1993). Factors that influence fathers' participation in child care. *Health Care for Women International, 14*, 99–107.

Trinkoff, A. M., Zhou, Q., Storr, C. L., & Soeken, K. L. (2000). Workplace access, negative proscriptions, job strain, and substance use in registered nurses. *Nursing Research, 49*, 83–90.

Tulman, L., & Fawcett, J. (1990). Maternal employment following childbirth. *Research in Nursing & Health, 13*, 181–188.

Tulman, L., Fawcett, J., Groblewski, L., & Silverman, L. (1990). Changes in functional status after childbirth. *Nursing Research, 39*, 70–75.

U.S. Department of Labor Bureau of Labor Statistics. (1995). *BLS releases new 1994–2005 employment projections* (Rep. No. Bulletin 95-485). Washington: U.S. Government Printing Office.

Verbrugge, L. M. (1986). Role burdens and physical health of women and men. *Women and Health, 11*, 47–77.

Visness, C. M., & Kennedy, K. I. (1997). Maternal employment and breast-feeding: findings from the 1988 National Maternal and Infant Health Survey. *American Journal of Public Health, 87*, 945–950.

Walker, L. O., & Best, M. A. (1991). Well-being of mothers with infant children: a preliminary comparison of employed women and homemakers. *Women and Health, 17*, 71–89.

Wang, X., Crosby, L. G., Harris, M. G., & Liu, T. (1999). Major concerns and need of breast cancer patients. *Cancer Nursing, 22*, 157–163.

Ward, D. (1990). Gender, time, and money in caregiving. *Scholarly Inquiry for Nursing Practice, 4,* 223–236.

Ward, D., & Brown, M. A. (1994). Labor and cost in AIDS family caregiving. *Western Journal of Nursing Research, 16,* 10–22.

Wilbur, J., Miller, A. M., Montgomery, A., & Chandler, P. (1998). Women's physical activity patterns: Nursing implications. *Journal of Obstetrics, Gynecology and Neonatal Nursing, 27,* 383–392.

Williams, M. F. (1996). Violence and sexual harassment: impact on registered nurses in the workplace. *American Association of Occupational Health Nursing Journal, 44,* 73–77.

Women's Bureau U.S. Department of Labor. (1994). *1993 Handbook on Women Workers: Trends & Issues.* U.S. Department of Labor.

Woods, N. F., Lentz, M., & Mitchell, E. (1993). The new woman: Health-promoting and health-damaging behaviors. *Health Care for Women International, 14,* 389–405.

Woods, N. F., Lentz, M., Mitchell, E. S., & Oakley, L. D. (1994). Depressed mood and self-esteem in young Asian, Black, and White women in America. *Health Care for Women International, 15,* 243–262.

Woods, N. F., & Mitchell, E. S. (1996). Patterns of depressed mood in midlife women: Observations from the Seattle midlife women's health study. *Research in Nursing and Health, 19,* 111–123.

Woods, N. F., & Mitchell, E. S. (1997a). Women's images of midlife: Observations from the Seattle Midlife Women's Health Study. *Health Care for Women International, 18,* 439–453.

Woods, N. F., & Mitchell, E. S. (1997b). Pathways to depressed mood for midlife women: Observations from the Seattle Midlife Women's Health Study. *Research in Nursing and Health, 20,* 119–129.

Youngblut, J., Singer, L. T., Madigan, E., & Swegart, L. A. (1997). Mother, child, and family factors related to employment of single mothers with LBW preschoolers. *Psychology of Women Quarterly, 21,* 247–263.

Youngblut, J. M. (1995). Consistency between maternal employment attitudes and employment status. *Research in Nursing and Health, 18,* 501–513.

Youngblut, J. M., & Ahn, S. (1997). How does maternal employment affect preterm infants? *MCN: American Journal of Maternal Child Nursing, 22,* 204–208.

Youngblut, J. M., Brady, N. R., & Brooten, D. (2000). Factors influencing single mother's employment status. *Health Care for Women International, 21,* 125–136.

Youngblut, J. M., Loveland-Cherry, C. J., & Horan, M. (1993). Maternal employment, family functioning, and preterm infant development at 9 and 12 months. *Research in Nursing and Health, 16,* 33–43.

Youngblut, J. M., Loveland Cherry, C. J., & Horan, M. (1990). Factors related to maternal employment status following the premature birth of an infant. *Nursing Research, 39,* 237–240.

Youngblut, J. M., Loveland Cherry, C. J., & Horan, M. (1991). Maternal employment effects on family and preterm infants at three months. *Nursing Research, 40,* 272–275.

Youngblut, J. M., Loveland Cherry, C. J., & Horan, M. (1994). Maternal employment effects on families and preterm infants at 18 months. *Nursing Research, 43,* 331–337.

Youngblut, J. M., Singer, L. T., Madigan, E. A., Swegart, L. A., & Rodgers, W. L. (1998). Maternal employment and parent-child relationships in single-parent families of low-birth-weight preschoolers. *Nursing Research, 47,* 114–121.

Chapter 5

Interventions for Women As Family Caregivers

MARGARET J. BULL

ABSTRACT

Family caregivers are the mainstay of long-term care, as they enable chronically ill elders and children to remain at home. The majority of family caregivers are women and historically their caregiving role has been viewed as an extension of their roles as wife and mother. Although numerous studies report the stresses associated with family caregiving and are predictors of burden, less attention has been given to interventions for family caregivers. The objective of this review is to examine reports of interventions to reduce family caregiver burden, to consider their implications for nursing practice, and to identify directions for future nursing research.

Key words: family caregiving, intervention studies, women's roles

In our changing health care systems, family caregivers assume an increasingly important role in providing assistance to elders and children who have chronic illnesses. With the emphasis in health care on cost containment, family caregivers are the mainstay for long-term care as they enable chronically ill elders and children to remain at home. The majority of family caregivers are women (Robinson, 1997; Stone, Cafferata, & Sangl, 1987; Warner & Wexler, 1998). Since elders and children with disabilities comprise the groups most often in need of assistance, the role of women as family caregivers has historically been viewed as an extension of their roles as wife and mother (Hoffmann &

Mitchell, 1998; Schroeder & Ward, 1998). The objective of this review is to examine reports of interventions to reduce family caregiver burden and their implications for nursing practice and to identify directions for future research.

CAREGIVING ROLES

Caregiving is a multidimensional concept. The role includes the provision of direct care, such as the time and tasks involved, and indirect care activities, such as care management and coordination (Swanson, Jensen, Specht, Johnson, Maas, & Saylor, 1997). For some, the role of caregiver might be unexpected, unwanted, and assumed out of a sense of obligation rather than personal desire to assist with care; others might slip into the role because they are not employed outside the home. Some family caregivers viewed the role as an opportunity to reciprocate for assistance the care recipient provided at an earlier time (Whitbeck, Hoyt, & Huck, 1994; Wright & Aquilino, 1998). Irrespective of how they come to the caregiving role, women often experience multiple role demands.

Research on the effects of family caregiver's multiple roles suggests two different perspectives. On the one hand, the competing demands perspective posits that women have a finite amount of time, energy, and commitment to dedicate to role responsibilities and that role strain and burden result from trying to balance multiple roles of wife, mother, employee, and caregiver (Goode, 1960). An alternate perspective contends that multiple roles are associated with better physical health and well-being, higher self-esteem, and less psychological stress (Waldron & Jacobs, 1989). Evidence from studies of caregivers for elders support each perspective. For instance, numerous studies document the strain and burden of caring for an impaired elder (Clyburn, Stones, Hadjistavropoulos, & Tuikko, 2000; Mui, 1995; Wilkins, Castle, Heck, Tanzy, & Fahey, 1999; Zarit, Reever, & Bach-Peterson, 1980). A few studies reported that women caregivers' multiple roles have rewards as well as stresses (Nolan & Lundh, 1999; Picot, 1995; Scharlach, 1994; Stephens, Franks, & Townsend, 1994). Although the multiple role perspective has been examined in relation to caregivers for elders, it has not been addressed in relation to mothers who provide care for a child who has a chronic illness.

CAREGIVER BURDEN

Although the research on caregiving has not consistently attended to issues related to multiple roles, findings of studies indicate that demands of caregiving can result in burden. Caregiver burden has been recognized as a multidimensional construct that includes objective and subjective dimensions. Objective burden has been defined as time spent providing care, tasks performed for the care recipient, and financial burden. Subjective burden has been defined as caregiver's feelings, attitudes and emotions expressed about providing care (Montgomery, Gonyea, & Hooyman, 1985). Most studies of caregiving include measures of both dimensions.

Much attention has been focused on predictors of caregiver strain and burden and subsequent health risks. Poor health of the caregiver, poor health of the care recipient, and more time providing care have been identified most often as predictors of stress or burden across caregiving situations, including elders with dementia and elders and children with chronic illness (Bull, Maruyama, & Luo, 1995; Cossette & Levesque, 1993; King, King, Rosenbaum, 1999; Pohl, Given, Collins, & Given, 1994; Zarit, Reever, & Bach-Peterson, 1980). In fact, the physical and mental health of the caregiver was identified as a primary factor in determining whether they were able to continue in their caregiving role (Ostwald, Leonard, Choi, Keenan, Hepburn, & Aroskar, 1993). Caregivers for elders who live in the same household and daughters have been identified as being at greater risk for burden than those who live apart from the elder (Pohl et al., 1994). Findings from a few studies suggested that female caregivers report more burden than male caregivers (Mittelman et al., 1995; Sparks, Farran, Donner, & Keane-Hagerty, 1998). Lack of preparedness for the caregiving role and conflict in the relationship with the care recipient also have been recognized as predictors of strain or burden (Archbold, Stewart, Greenlilck, & Harvath, 1990; Martire, Stephens, & Franks, 1997). Although less attention has been given to the predictors of burden for parents caring for chronically ill children, the child's functional dependency, time demands, health insurance, and income have been identified as factors influencing burden (Leonard, Dwyer & Sapienza, 1992). In addition, relationships among family members can be affected by the time demands on the mother providing care for the ill child (Sherman, 1995).

Coping and social support have been identified as potential mediators of burden. Coping refers to things that persons do, their concrete efforts to deal with life strains, stressful situations, or events. Coping is conceptually distinct from social resources, which refer not to what people do but to what is available to them in developing their coping repertoire (Pearlin, Mullan, Semple, & Skaff, 1990). Coping may be directed at managing or altering a problem causing distress or regulating the emotional response to the problem. The use of problem-solving strategies has been found to correlate with a more positive emotional state (Folkman & Lazarus, 1988); however, other investigators found that an individual's ability to use a variety of coping strategies was critical to survival (Pearlin et al., 1990). Although there are a variety of definitions and a number of ways of measuring social support, the concept is often viewed in terms of emotional and tangible support. Research on social support has produced inconclusive findings on the impact of network size on burden; however, caregivers that reported either dissatisfaction with social support or a discrepancy between their ideal and actual support scored higher on burden (Bull et al., 1995; Fiore, Coppel, Becker, & Cox, 1986).

The findings of previous studies indicated that the burdens of caregiving were positively correlated with caregiver depression and suggested that physical health risks might also be associated with providing care for family members over an extended period of time. Immunosuppression was linked with chronic stress among family caregivers of dementia patients and wound healing took nine days longer in caregivers than in matched controls (Kiecolt-Glaser, Marucha, Malarkey, Mercado, & Glaser, 1995). While the literature abounds with information on the predictors of caregiver burden and the health risks associated with caregiving, less attention has been given to interventions for family caregivers.

METHOD OF RETRIEVAL

The following databases were used in reviewing the literature: Cumulative Index to Nursing and Allied Health Literature (1990–1999), Medline (1990–1999), Healthstar (1990–1999), and the Cochrane Library database (1990–1999). The search was limited to English language articles. The years 1990–1999 were selected to focus on current studies as earlier review articles indicated that study designs often did not include random assignment or control groups (Knight, Lutzky, & Macofsky-Urban, 1993; Toseland & Rositer, 1990).

Use of the search term "family caregivers" resulted in 3,700 retrievals. The addition of the term, "research or study," narrowed the retrieval to 503 articles. The search was limited further by adding the terms "intervention" and then "elders." Similarly, the terms "intervention and child" were combined to identify caregiving interventions at opposite ends of the life cycle. A total of 27 articles were identified in which the abstract included a description of an intervention. Articles that described an intervention but did not provide evaluation data, studies that lacked a control group, and case studies that evaluated the intervention using only qualitative data were eliminated from the sample. In addition, two studies related to children with disabilities were deleted because they did not include a measure related to outcomes for the family caregiver. The final sample consisted of 14 intervention studies. These studies were summarized in Table 5.1.

TABLE 5.1   Intervention Studies with Control Group of Family Caregivers

Study	Design	Sample	Measures	Findings
Mittelman, M. S. et al. (1995) Evaluate the effect of individual and family counseling on spouse caregiver depression	Longitudinal (12 mo.); Random assignment to intervention or control group	$N = 206$ caregivers, 103 intervention; 103 controls 58% female	Geriatric Depression Scale Social Network Scale OARS-Physical Health FACES III-family cohesion Memory and Behavior Problem Checklist	Intervention group less depressed over time than control with significant differences at 4, 8 and 12 months. Intervention group significantly more satisfied with social network and less troubled by patient behaviors.
Newcomer, R. et al. (1999) Evaluate two case management models to improve access to community-based care	Longitudinal (3 yr.); Random assignment to group	$N = 5,307$ caregivers 36% of sample remained at 3 yr. 60% female	Burden (Zarit) Depression Scale (Yesavage)	No differences in burden at 12, 18, 24, or 36 months. At 6 months less than 1 point difference between intervention and control group scores on burden and depression.
Chang (1999) Test 8-week cognitive educational intervention	Before–After; Random assignment to intervention or control group	$N = 65$ dyads, all female caregivers for persons with dementia	Ways of Coping Burden Brief Symptom Inventory Memory Behavior Checklist	No differences between groups in use of problem-focused coping over time. No significant difference between groups on satisfaction or anxiety.

(continued)

TABLE 5.1 *(continued)*

Study	Design	Sample	Measures	Findings
Buckwalter, K. et al. (1999) Test the PLST Model for caregivers of persons with dementia	Longitudinal (12 mo); Random assignment to intervention or control group	*N* = 245, primarily female caregivers	POMS Geriatric Depression Scales	PLST group reported significantly lower scores on depression at 6 months but no difference between groups at 12 months.
Chen, M. (1999) Test the effectiveness of health promotion counseling for family caregivers	Before–After; Random assignment to group	*N* = 78, 75% female caregivers, average age was 45.8 yr. Sample from China	Chinese version of Health Promoting Behavior	Significant improvements were found in intervention group scores on exercise, responsibility, self-actualization, stress, and total score. No significant difference in nutrition or support.
Bartholomew, L. K. et. al. (1997) Test a Cystic fibrosis family education program for parents & child	Longitudinal (2 yr.); Nonequivalent control group	*N* = 199 parent/child dyads, 104 intervention; 95 controls 92% female parent, Child ages < 1–18 yr	Parent knowledge Management of illness Impact on Family Parenting Stress Index	Intervention group scored better on parent knowledge, self-efficacy and problem-solving area of management of illness scale. No differences between groups on parenting stress or impact on family.

TABLE 5.1   *(continued)*

Study	Design	Sample	Measures	Findings
Ostwald, S. et al. (1999) Test the effectiveness of an interdisciplinary psycho-educational family group intervention for caregivers of persons with dementia	Longitudinal (5 mo.); Random assignment to intervention or control group	$N = 117$ families; 72 intervention; 45 controls. Sample mortality—lost 23 families, leaving 60 in intervention and 34 in control group 65% were female	CES-D Depression Scale Burden (Zarit) Memory Behavior Checklist	Burden decreased for intervention group at 5 months but not at 3 months, suggesting delayed effect of intervention ($F = 5.53$, $p = .005$). Depression—no significant difference. Behavior-intervention effect alone not significant but time effect and intervention × time was significant.
Jepson, C. et al. (1999) Determine whether caregivers for cancer patients who received standardized home care intervention experienced any change in psychosocial status	Longitudinal (6 mo.); Randomized clinical trial At discharge, 3 mo., and 6 mo.	$N = 161$ caregivers living with person with cancer 67.7% female	CES-D Depression Scale Caregiver Reaction (Given)	No significant differences between groups on depression or caregiver reaction.

(continued)

TABLE 5.1   *(continued)*

Study	Design	Sample	Measures	Findings
Roberts, J., Browne, G., et al. (1999) Determine effectiveness of individualized problem-solving counseling by community health nurses for caregivers of persons with dementia	Longitudinal (12 mo.); All 140 persons with dementia referred to visiting nurse in 16-month period eligible; Random assignment to group	*N* = 77 caregivers, 38 experimental; 39 controls Canada 70% female	Burden (Zarit) Duke Social Support Psychological Adjustment to Illness Scale (Morrow) Indices of Coping (Moos) Health and Social Utilization Questionnaire	No significant differences in psychosocial adjustment to relative's illness or psychological distress between groups and 1 year later. No main effect of treatment. No differences between groups on burden or social support At 6 months no differences in expenditures between groups.
Goodman, D., & Pynoos, J. (1990) Evaluate 12-week information and support program for caregivers	Before–After 2 group	*N* = 66 caregivers for persons with Alzheimer's disease; 31 in network group; 35 in lecture group 77% female	Burden (Zarit) Social support network Memory Behavior Problem Checklist Caregiver-elder relationship scale	Lecture group reported receipt of more information and emotional support. Network group scored higher on satisfaction with social support.

TABLE 5.1 *(continued)*

Study	Design	Sample	Measures	Findings
Mant, J., Carter, J., & Wade, D. (1998) Assess the impact of information packets on patients with stroke and their family carers	Longitudinal (6 months); Randomized controlled trial	$N = 49$ family carers; 29 intervention; 20 controls United Kingdom	SF-36 Carer Strain Index Satisfaction Knowledge about stroke	Carers in intervention group significantly younger. Analysis adjusted for age on knowledge variable but not on other variables. No significant differences between groups on carer knowledge, satisfaction, or strain.
Archbold, P. et al. (1995). Test the PREP nursing intervention compared to usual home care provided by HMO	Longitudinal (12 mo.); Random assignment to group when possible	$N = 25$ families, 13 intervention; 12 controls Mean age 68 yr., 77% female, caregivers in experimental group significantly older	Role Strain Caregiving Rewards Scale Depression Care Effectiveness Scale	Intervention group scored significantly higher on Care Effectiveness Scale than control group, indicating greater preparedness, enrichment, and predictability. No differences between groups on depression, caregiving rewards, or role strain.

(continued)

TABLE 5.1   *(continued)*

Study	Design	Sample	Measures	Findings
Coleman, G. J., & Reddihough, D. S. (1995) Evaluate education program for children with cerebral palsy and their parents	Longitudinal (6 month) with control group	N = 20 children, 11 intervention 9 controls, 20 parents Mean age of child 45 months, no demographics for parents Australia	QRS-F parental coping	No significant main effects; control-group parents perceived their child's physical incapacitation as less troublesome than did the intervention group.
Robinson, K., & Yates, K. (1994) Determine whether a behavior-management or social-skills program was most beneficial to family caregivers	Pretest–posttest, 12 wk. Convenience sample; random assignment to one of 3 groups	N = 33 caregivers of adults with dementia n = 10 social skills; n = 11 behavior group; n = 12 controls 76% female	Burden (Montgomery) Attitude toward using day care (semantic differential) Satisfaction with social support	No significant differences among the 3 groups postintervention.

RESULTS

Design

Ten of the 14 studies employed longitudinal designs and random assignment of caregivers to either the intervention or control group. Although sample mortality might be anticipated in longitudinal studies, only two studies mentioned sample attrition. In one study, 36% of the 5,307 caregivers remained at the 3-year follow-up (Newcomer, Yordi, DuNah, Fox, & Wilkinson, 1999). The extent to which sample mortality was similar in the intervention and control group was not discussed. In another study, 94 of the 117 family caregivers remained at the 5-month follow-up with similar attrition in the intervention and control groups (Ostwald, Hepburn, Caron, Burns, & Mantell, 1999).

Study samples were obtained from the United States, China, Australia, Canada, and the United Kingdom, thereby giving credence to the global nature of family caregiving issues. It was not surprising to find that the majority of caregivers in all the studies were women. Sample size varied from 20 to 5,307. The proportion of female caregivers in the samples ranged from 58% to 100%. Only one study provided information on power to detect differences between groups in relation to the sample size (Roberts et al., 1999). The majority (85.7%) of the studies focused on family caregivers for elders. Of these, approximately half were specific to caregivers for elders who had dementia.

Interventions

The majority (78%) of the interventions were psycho-educational with an emphasis on providing caregivers with information about the care recipient's diagnosis, illness management, coping skills, and social support. Most of the interventions (92.8%) aimed to reduce caregiver burden and improve mental health. None of the studies reported gender differences in caregiver outcomes or response to the intervention.

Three studies employed systems level interventions. Newcomer and colleagues (1999) tested the effectiveness of two case management models. The main differences between the models were the case manager/client ratios (1:30 in the intervention; 1:100 in the control) and the capitation limit, with $200 more allowed in the intervention group than the control group. The two other studies that employed systems level interventions tested a home health care protocol against usual home care practices. While Jepson and colleagues' (1999) home care intervention focused primarily on patient care, Archbold and colleagues (1995) specifically targeted family caregivers with the goal of preparing family members for the caregiving role.

Only one study (Chen, 1999) used an intervention to promote healthy self-care practices among family caregivers. Caregivers in this study received three hours of counseling on an initial visit and also three months later from trained professional home health nurses. The counseling focused on nutrition, stress management, exercise, and responsibility for health with the goal of improving healthy behaviors.

It is important to note that, in the two studies of children with disabilities, the intervention focused on education related to the illness and disease management (Bartholomew et al., 1997; Coleman & Reddihough, 1995). Content targeted specifically to reduce parent stress was not mentioned even though a measure of parental stress was used to evaluate the effectiveness of the intervention.

Measures

The majority of the instruments used to measure outcomes for family caregivers had extensive information on reliability and validity. For instance, the Zarit Burden Scale and Behavior Problem Checklist were commonly used in studies of caregivers for elders with dementia. The geriatric depression scale and profile of mood scales were used often to measure mental health. Only two studies employed measures of family health such as family cohesion—FACES III (Mittelman et al., 1995) and impact of caregiving on the family (Bartholomew et al., 1997). Questions related to caregiver knowledge about the care recipient's illness were developed specifically for the intervention study, and psychometric properties were not reported. None of the studies summarized in Table 5.1 used physiologic measures to ascertain the impact of providing care on family caregivers.

Findings

The majority of studies found no significant differences between the intervention and control groups on depression, burden, and parental stress. The two studies that employed measures of impact on family did not find significant differences between the intervention and control groups on these measures.

Only two studies found that caregivers in the intervention group were less depressed over time than the controls (Mittelman et al., 1995; Buckwalter et al., 1999). Mittelman and colleagues reported that the intervention group was significantly less depressed at 4, 8, and 12 months following the intervention. In addition, intervention group caregivers were more satisfied with their social network and less troubled by behaviors of elders with dementia. Buckwalter and colleagues (1999) found caregivers in the intervention group were less depressed than the controls at 6 months but found no differences between groups at 1 year. Both of these studies targeted caregivers for persons with dementia, a group recognized as particularly vulnerable or at risk for depression, and therefore more likely to show a difference in response to an intervention.

In contrast, Chen's study (1999) of effectiveness of health promotion by community health nurses found that family caregivers in the intervention group reported significant improvements in scores on exercise, responsibility for health, stress, and self-actualization subscales as well as the total score on the Health Promoting Behavior Scale. Although Chen noted that, at entry to the study, 40% of the caregivers were either too slim or too heavy according to a body mass index measure, there was no report of body mass in the intervention and control groups at the end of the intervention.

Only one of the three studies that employed a systems level intervention found significant differences between the intervention and control groups. Caregivers participating in the PREP system of nursing intervention in home health care (Archbold et al., 1995) reported significantly higher scores on care effectiveness. The intervention group indicated better preparedness, enrichment of the caregiving experience, and more predictability than the controls, however, the investigators did not find significant differences between groups on caregiving rewards. The sensitivity of the measures to the intervention might account for the difference in significance. Jepson and colleagues (1999) employed a home care protocol that targeted patient care and did not find significant differences between caregivers in the intervention and control groups. Similarly, there were no significant differences between caregivers in the two case management models (Newcomer et al., 1999).

DISCUSSION AND RECOMMENDATIONS FOR FUTURE RESEARCH

A strength of the studies reviewed included the use of longitudinal designs and random assignment to intervention and control groups. Since most of the samples were convenience or purposive type, investigators usually compared the two groups of caregivers on baseline data and employed appropriate statistical controls when the groups differed on baseline data. It is disappointing that the majority of studies did not find a significant difference in outcomes between caregivers who received an intervention and those in the control groups. According to Lipsey (1990), several factors might influence design sensitivity and impede detection of group differences. Sample size, selection of control groups, specificity of outcome measures, and the dose of the intervention might account for the lack of statistically significant findings in the studies reviewed. The majority of studies did not provide a power analysis or discuss the effect size (how big a difference might be detected), given the sample employed. A sample with more than 5,000 caregivers detected small differences between groups but lacked practical significance (Newcomer et al., 1999). With such a large sample it would be possible to have a significance level of .01, power of .99, and an effect size of less than .10 (Cohen, 1969). On the other hand, an intervention that employed a small sample size such as Goodman and Pynos (1990) would need to have an effect size greater than .50 to show statistically significant differences at an alpha level of .05 with a power of .90.

Although a small sample size might contribute to the lack of significant findings, the sensitivity of measures is equally important. For instance, the study by Archbold and colleagues (1995) employed a sample of 25 families, 13 in the intervention and 12 in the control group. Yet, statistically significant differences between groups were found on measures specific to the intervention, such as preparedness and enrichment. In future research, investigators might give more attention to the sample size necessary to detect differences between groups in discussing their findings and to the sensitivity of measures to the proposed intervention. Global measures of caregiver health might not be appropriate when the goal of the intervention is to prepare family members for the caregiver role. Presentation of this information might help other researchers decide whether to employ a similar intervention with a larger sample or whether the intervention requires modification for future studies.

Selection of control groups is another important consideration. A key question to address is how different the intervention and control groups are. For the three systems level interventions it is unclear how much the usual practice in case management or home health care varied from the intervention. It might be that any intervention that provided services was beneficial to caregivers. On the other hand, the services in two studies (Jepson et al., 1999; Newcomer et al., 1999) did not specifically target the caregivers. Instead, the interventions focused on services to the care recipient which might not have a direct effect on the family caregiver's health and well-being.

The specificity of outcome measures in relation to the intervention is another factor that might explain the lack of significant differences between groups. Stewart and Archbold (1992) contend that outcome measures need to be selected that are sensitive to the effects of the intervention. For instance, an intervention that specifically targeted health promoting behaviors (Chen, 1999) showed improvement on a health behavior inventory. Similarly, the two studies that found caregivers in the intervention group were less depressed focused a component of the intervention on managing the troublesome behaviors of the persons with dementia. These behaviors were known to impact on caregivers mental health. In contrast, interventions that focused on providing education about the illness might improve knowledge but not necessarily result in fewer burdens, decrease parental stress, change behavior, or improve caregiver health. It is surprising that physiologic measures were not used in any of the studies, given the abundant literature on the stressful nature of caregiving and evidence that stress effects the immune system (Kiecolt-Glaser, Marucha, Malaskey, Mercado, & Glaser, 1995; Wilkins et al., 1999). Deterioration in immune function was associated with increases in perceived burden and depressed mood in caregivers for persons with dementia (Wilkins et al., 1999). In future studies, measures of physiologic changes might provide a more comprehensive understanding of the impact of caregiving on women's health. Physiologic measures might be particularly useful in studies in which interventions include stress management or health promotion components. Also, none of the studies examined gender differences in response to the intervention or discussed the extent to which interventions might require modification for male and female caregivers. Future research might examine gender differences in caregiving and response to interventions.

The dose or strength of the intervention is another factor to consider in relation to design sensitivity. The dose includes the extent to which all study participants received the complete intervention as well as consideration of the period of time needed to produce an effect. The psycho-educational interventions in the studies reviewed were conducted over an 8 to 12 weeks. In some studies measures were taken before and after; in others measures were collected over an extended time following the intervention. In the studies that found significant differences, data were collected for an extended time following the intervention. It is possible that a longer time is needed for an intervention to show an effect, particularly if the intervention requires that the family caregiver practice or acquire mastery of specific strategies.

The findings of this review suggest that intervention strategies focused on the caregiver, such as health promotion counseling, merit further research. Strategies that aim to improve the health of the caregiver and increase their resilience might be particularly fruitful since poor health of the caregiver has been identified as a factor contributing to institutionalization of the care recipient. Different health promotion strategies might be tested with different age groups and different cultural groups of family caregivers. In promoting healthy behaviors one might also ask whether caregivers that are in better health are also able to manage multiple role demands more effectively. Strengthening the caregivers' health and personal resources might also be effective in protecting caregivers from the stress of caregiving.

REFERENCES

Archbold, P. A., Stewart, B. J., Greenlick, M. R., & Harvath, T. A. (1990). Mutuality and preparedness as predictors of caregiving role strain. *Research in Nursing and Health, 13*, 375–384.

Archbold, P. G., Stewart, B. J., Miller, L. L., Harvath, T. A., Greenlick, M. R., VanBuren, L., Kirschling, J. M., Valanis, B. G., Brody, K. K., Schook, J. E., &

Hagan, J. M. (1995). The PREP system of nursing interventions: A pilot test with families caring for older members. *Research in Nursing and Health, 18*, 3–16.

Bartholomew, L. K., Czyzewski, D. I., Parcel, G. S., Swank, P. R., Sockrider, M. M., Mariotto, M. J., Schidlow, D. V., Rink, R. J., & Seilheimer, D. K. (1997). Self-management of Cystic Fibrosis: Short-term outcomes of the Cystic Fibrosis family education program. *Health Education and Behavior, 224*, 652–666.

Buckwalter, K. C., Gerdner, L., Kohout, F., Hall, G. R., Kelly, A., Richards, B., & Sime, M. (1999). A nursing intervention to decrease depression in family caregivers of persons with dementia. *Archives of Psychiatric Nursing, 13*(2), 80–88.

Bull, M. J., Maruyama, G., & Luo, D. (1995). Testing a model for posthospital transition of family caregivers for elderly persons. *Nursing Research, 44*, 132–138.

Chang, B. (1999). Cognitive-behavioral intervention for homebound caregivers of persons with dementia. *Nursing Research, 48*, 173–182.

Chen, M. (1999). The effectiveness of health promotion counseling to family caregivers. *Journal of Public Health Nursing, 16*, 125–132.

Clyburn, L. D., Stones, M. J., Hadjistavropoulos, T., & Tuokko, H. (2000). Predicting caregiver burden and depression in Alzheimer's Disease. *Journal of Gerontology, 55B*(1), S2–S13.

Cohen, J. (1969). *Statistical Power Analysis for the Behavioral Sciences.* New York: Academic Press.

Coleman, G., King, J., & Reddihough, D. (1995). A pilot evaluation of conductive education-based intervention for children with cerebral palsy: The Tongala project. *Journal of Paediatrics and Child Health, 31*, 412–417.

Cossette, S., & Levesquie, L. (1993). Caregiving tasks as predictors of mental health of wife caregivers of men with chronic obstructive pulmonary disease. *Research in Nursing and Health, 16*, 251–263.

Fiore, J., Coppel, D., Becker, J., & Cox, G. (1986). Social support as a multifaceted concept: Examination of important dimensions for adjustment. *American Journal of Community Psychology, 14*, 93–111.

Folkman, S., & Lazarus, R. (1988). Coping as a mediator of emotion. *Journal of Personality and Social Psychology, 54*, 466–475.

Goode, W. J. (1960). A theory of role strain. *American Sociological Review, 25*, 483–496.

Goodman, C. C., & Pynoos, J. (1990). A model telephone information and support program for caregivers of Alzheimer's patients. *Gerontologist, 30*, 399–404.

Hoffmann, R. L., & Mitchell, A. M. (1998). Caregiver burden: Historical development. *Nursing Forum, 33*(4), 5–11.

Jepson, C., McCorkle, R., Adler, D., Nuamak, I., & Lusk, E. (1999). Effects of home care on caregiver psychosocial status. *Image: Journal of Nursing Scholarship, 31*, 115–120.

Kiecolt-Glaser, J. K., Marucha, P. T., Malarkey, W. B., Mercado, A. M., & Glaser, R. (1995). Slowing of wound healing by psychological stress. *Lancet, 346*, 1194–1196.

King, G., King, S., Rosenbaum, P., & Goffin, R. (1999). Family-centered caregiving and well-being of children with disabilities: Linking process with outcome. *Journal of Pediatric Psychology, 24*(1), 41–53.

Knight, B. G., Lutzky, S. M., & Macofsky-Urban, F. (1993). A meta-analytic review of interventions for caregiver distress: Recommendations for future research. *Gerontologist, 33*, 240–248.

Leonard, B., Dwyer, B. J., & Sapienza, J. (1992). Financial and time costs to parents of severely disabled children. *Public Health Reports, 107*, 302–312.

Lipsey, M. W. (1990). *Design sensitivity.* Newbury Park, CA: Sage.

Mant, J., Carter, J., & Wade, D. T. (1998). The impact of an information pack on patients with stroke and their carers: A randomized controlled trial. *Clinical Rehabilitation, 12*, 465–476.

Martire, L. M., Stephens, M., & Franks, M. M. (1997). Multiple roles of women caregivers: Feelings of mastery and self-esteem as predictors of psychosocial well-being. *Journal of Women and Aging, 9*(1/2), 117–131.

Mittleman, M. S., Ferris, S. H., Shulman, E., Steinberg, G., Ambinder, A., Mackell, J. A., & Cohen, J. (1995). A comprehensive support program: Effect on depression in spouse caregivers of AD patients. *Gerontologist, 35*, 792–802.

Montgomery, R. J., Gonyea, J. G., & Hooyman, N. R. (1985). Caregiving and the experience of objective and subjective burden. *Family Relations, 34*, 19–26.

Mui, A. C. (1995). Caring for frail elderly parents: A comparison of adult sons and daughters. *Gerontologist, 35*, 86–93.

Newcomer, R., Yordi, C., DuNah, R., Fox, R., & Wilkinson, A. (1999). Effects of the Medicare Alzheimer's Disease Demonstration on caregiver burden and depression. *Health Services Research, 34*, 669–689.

Nolan, M., & Lundh, U. (1999). Satisfactions and coping strategies of family carers. *British Journal of Community Nursing, 4*, 470–475.

Ostwald, S., Hepburn, K., Caron, W., Burns, T., & Mantell, R. (1999). Reducing caregiver burden: A randomized psychoeducational intervention for caregivers of persons with dementia. *Gerontologist, 39*, 299–309.

Ostwald, S., Leonard, B., Choi, T., Keenan, J., Hepburn, K., & Aroskar, M. (1993). Caregivers of frail elderly and medically fragile children: Perceptions of ability to continue to provide home health care. *Home Health Care Services Quarterly, 14*(1), 55–80.

Pearlin, L. I., Mullan, J. T., Semple, S. J., & Skaff, M. M. (1990). Caregiving and the stress process: An overview of concepts and their measures. *Gerontologist, 30*(5), 583–594.

Picot, S. J. (1995). Rewards, costs, and coping of African-American caregivers. *Nursing Research, 44*, 147–152.

Pohl, J., Given, C., Collins, C., & Given, B. (1994). Social vulnerability and reactions to caregiving in daughters and daughters-in-law caring for disabled aging parents. *Health Care for Women International, 15*, 385–395.

Roberts, J., Browne, G., Milne, C., Spooner, L., Gafni, A., Drummond-Young, M., LeGris, J., Watt, S., LeClair, K., Beaumont, L., & Roberts, J. (1999). Problem-solving counseling for caregivers of the cognitively impaired: Effective for whom? *Nursing Research, 48*, 162–172.

Robinson, K., & Yates, K. (1994). Effects of two caregiver-training programs on burden and attitude toward help. *Archives of Psychiatric Nursing, 8*, 312–319.

Robinson, K. M. (1997). Family caregiving: Who provides the care, and at what cost? *Nursing Economics, 15,* 243–247.

Scharlach, A. E. (1994). Caregiving and employment: Competing or complementary roles? *Gerontologist, 34,* 378–385.

Schroeder, C., & Ward, D. (1998). Women, welfare, and work: One view of the debate. *Nursing Outlook, 46,* 226–232.

Sherman, B. (1995). Impact of home-based respite care on families of children with chronic illnesses. *Child Health Care, 24*(1), 33–45.

Sparks, M. B., Farran, C. J., Donner, E., & Keane-Hagerty, E. (1998). Wives, husbands, and daughters of dementia patients: Predictors of caregivers' mental and physical health. *Scholarly Inquiry for Nursing Practice, 12,* 221–234.

Stephens, M. A., Franks, M. M., & Townsend, A. L. (1994). Stress and rewards in women's multiple roles: The case of women in the middle. *Psychology and Aging, 9,* 454–52.

Stewart, B. J., & Archbold, P. G. (1992). Nursing intervention studies require outcome measures that are sensitive to change: Part one. *Research in Nursing and Health, 15,* 477–481.

Stone, R. I., Cafferata, G. L., & Sangl, J. (1987). Caregivers of the frail elderly: A national profile. *Gerontologist, 27*(5), 616–626.

Swanson, E. A., Jensen, D. P., Specht, J., Johnson, M. L., Maas, M., & Saylor, D. (1997). Caregiving: Concept analysis and outcomes. *Scholarly Inquiry for Nursing Practice, 11*(1), 65–79.

Toseland, R. W., Rossiter, C. M., Peak, T., & Smith, G. C. (1990). Comparative effectiveness of individual and group interventions to support family caregivers. *Social Work, 35,* 209–217.

Waldron, I., & Jacobs, J. A. (1989). Effects of multiple roles on women's health: Evidence from a national longitudinal study. *Women and Health, 15,* 3–19.

Warner, L., & Wexler, S. (1998). *Eight Hours a Day and Taken for Granted?* London: The Princess Royal Trust for Carers.

Whitbeck, L., Hoyt, D. R., & Huck, S. M. (1994). Early family relationships, intergenerational solidarity, and support provided to parents by their adult children. *Journal of Gerontology, 49*(2), S85–S94.

Wilkins, S. S., Castle, S., Heck, E., Tanzy, K., & Fahey, J. (1999). Practical geriatrics: Immune function, mood, and perceived burden among caregivers participating in a psychoeducational intervention. *Psychiatric Services, 50,* 747–749.

Wright, D. L., & Aquilino, W. S. (1998). Influence of emotional support exchange in marriage on caregiving wives' burden and marital satisfaction. *Family Relations, 47,* 195–204.

Zarit, S., Reever, K., & Bach-Peterson, J. (1980). Relatives of the impaired elderly: Correlates of feelings of burden. *Gerontologist, 20,* 649–655.

PART III

Research on Diversity and Women's Health

Chapter 6

Lesbian Health and Health Care

LINDA A. BERNHARD

ABSTRACT

Research on lesbian health and health care is very limited, but is beginning to increase. Evidence of limited access to care, homophobic attitudes of health care professionals, and expected or actual negative experiences in interactions with health care professionals help to explain why lesbians are less likely than other women to seek health care. Lesbians have many of the same physical health needs that other women do, but the most prevalent topics on which research could be found were screening for breast and cervical cancer, sexually transmitted infections (STIs), and HIV. More research has been conducted in areas related to mental health, such as stress, use of therapy, alcohol abuse and recovery, and violence. The chief conclusion from this review is that there is a need for all types of research in all areas of lesbian health.

Key words: AIDS, artificial insemination, bisexual women, childhood sexual abuse, disclosure, eating disorders, intimate partner violence, lesbian motherhood, pregnancy, women who have sex with women

Lesbians are a diverse group of women who differ from one another by demographic variables, such as age, race, and class. Lesbians also differ from one another by less obvious variables, such as the label they use for self-identification (e.g., lesbian, gay, dyke), degree of outness (i.e., number of people who know they are lesbian), and sexual partners (i.e., women, men, or both). Lesbians have in common a love for women.

Women's health research has finally come of age, but lesbians are still largely invisible in most women's health research. Now that women's health is an accepted area of study, however, it is important to study the diversity within women's health. Lesbian health is an important part of that diversity. Lesbian health for this review includes the physical, mental, social, and spiritual health of women who consider themselves lesbian, or who might be considered lesbian by others, because of their sexual or affectional preferences or practices.

In a major review of research about lesbians, Tully (1995) noted that research on lesbians since 1950 has gone through five major periods: etiology of lesbianism, personality and psychological functioning of lesbians, social functioning of lesbians, life span development of lesbians, and professional interventions with lesbians and their families. Very few of the studies in her review dealt with health. This review will add to her review and expand its use by nurses and other health care professionals.

METHODS OF RETRIEVAL

The selected time period for this review is 1980 to 1999. To search for articles on lesbian health, I searched the MEDLINE, CINAHL, and PsychINFO databases using terms and variables associated with lesbian health generally and with specific areas of lesbian health. I handsearched newer journals, such as the *Journal of Lesbian Studies*, that are not indexed well. Finally, to find any additional articles, I also reviewed the bibliography in the first Institute of Medicine report on lesbian health (Solarz, 1999) and other published reviews of topics related to aspects of lesbian health care included in this review (e.g., Stevens, 1992). I searched widely to find as many articles as possible, because it has often been difficult to have lesbian research published.

Although a few nurses have been at the forefront of women's health and lesbian health research, scholars in other fields have conducted many of the germinal studies. For example, social scientists Bradford and Ryan (1987) conducted the National Lesbian Health Care Survey (NLHCS), the most important and widely quoted study of lesbian health to date. It was important to include non-nursing literature because many of the earlier studies have formed the basis for the studies that nurses are now conducting.

Inclusion criteria for studies were published research, on any topic related to health, with lesbian participants only or with lesbians and any comparison group, so long as data were analyzed by gender and sexual orientation in comparison studies (e.g., lesbians and gay men or lesbian and heterosexual women). One exception is that studies were retained if the principal focus of the study was some aspect of lesbian health, even though bisexual women were included and the analysis was not separate for lesbian and bisexual women because so many of the studies did not separate lesbian and bisexual women. Case studies were also excluded.

HEALTH CARE SERVICES FOR LESBIANS

Access to Care

An important issue in lesbian health care is access. Access includes many components; one is financial. Lesbians consistently report money as a problem (Roberston, 1992; Sorensen & Roberts, 1997). In the NLHCS (Bradford & Ryan, 1987), the most frequently reported barrier to receiving health care (by 16% of the sample) was financial. In another study (Trippet & Bain, 1990), 37% said cost was the most important reason for not obtaining care. More recently, 28% of a sample of older lesbians reported that the greatest obstacles to access of health care were poverty and lack of health insurance (Butler & Hope, 1999).

Stevens (1993b) noted that the presence and type of health care coverage was the strongest indicator of access to care for her racially diverse sample of lesbians in San Francisco. Thirty-six percent of her sample had no insurance and had to rely on public sources of care; without any choice in providers, these lesbians felt humiliated, powerless, hopeless, and resigned to not having a relationship with a health care provider.

Per White and Dull (1997), 65% to 80% of lesbians (Cochran & Mays, 1988) report having a primary provider. Geographic location is also important to access. Even if they have a provider, rural lesbians report that distance is a barrier to access and limits choice (Butler & Hope, 1999; Tiemann, Kennedy, & Haga, 1997).

Regardless of access issues, lesbians are less likely to seek, or more likely to delay seeking, health care than other women. They are afraid of being discriminated against because of their lesbianism. Their fear may be due to their own bad experiences or to bad experiences they have heard described to them by their friends.

Lesbians in a variety of studies report that they are reluctant to seek health care (Stevens & Hall, 1988), have delayed seeking health care (Reagan, 1981; Zeidenstein, 1990), have only sought care for the worst problems (White & Dull, 1997), do not seek routine health care (Robertson, 1992), or avoid care (Trippet & Bain, 1992). Hall (1994) reported that lesbians in alcoholic treatment programs were skeptical about entering treatment because they believed the programs to be unsafe for lesbians. Older lesbians worry about having to go to a nursing home, fearing the discrimination they might experience there with no one to protect them (Butler & Hope, 1999).

Ellingson and Yarber (1997) found that lesbians were significantly less likely to report having regular check-ups than heterosexual women. Rankow, Cambre, and Cooper (1998) also found that, in a sample of lesbian, bisexual, and transgendered women, women who had experienced child sexual abuse (CSA) were the least likely to seek health care. White and Dull (1997) used linear regression and found that difficulty obtaining care, difficulty communicating with the primary care provider, discomfort discussing depression, and increased comfort in discussing menopause were associated with delay in seeking health care in Oregon lesbians with an average age of 41.

HEALTH CARE PROFESSIONALS' ATTITUDES

Attitudes of health care professionals affect the quality of care they provide to lesbians. Lesbians' beliefs that health care professionals are homophobic or have negative attitudes about lesbians are an important reason why they do not readily seek health care. Studies have examined homophobic attitudes of physicians (Douglas, Kalman, & Kalman, 1985; Mathews, Booth, Turner, & Kessler, 1986), registered nurses (Douglas et al., 1985; Harris, Nightengale, & Owen, 1995), nurse educators (Randall, 1989), and nursing students (Eliason, 1998; Eliason & Randall, 1991; Eliason, Donelan, & Randall, 1992), as well as psychologists and social workers (Harris et al., 1995).

All of these studies demonstrate negative attitudes and inaccurate beliefs about lesbians, such as that lesbianism is unnatural, wrong, immoral, perverted, or disgusting; lesbians try to seduce heterosexual women; and lesbians are a common source for transmission of HIV. Nurses' attitudes are similar to physicians' (Douglas et al., 1985) but more negative than psychologists' or social workers' (Harris et al., 1995). Knowing someone gay (Douglas et al., 1985; Eliason & Randall, 1991), and being a younger, female physician (Mathews et al., 1986) were associated with less negative attitudes.

HEALTH CARE INTERACTIONS

The most frequent problem that lesbians report in their actual experiences with health care providers is the assumption by the provider that the client is heterosexual (Hall, 1994; Paroski, 1987; Reagan, 1981; Robertson, 1992;

Ryan & Bradford, 1993; Stevens, 1995; Stevens & Hall, 1990; White & Dull, 1998). This assumption makes lesbians feel forced to disclose their identity, to actively lie and deny their identity, or to passively lie by accepting procedures or treatments that are unnecessary.

Some lesbians report positive experiences of health care (Butler & Hope, 1999; Ryan & Bradford, 1993; Stevens, 1993a, 1994b; Stevens & Hall, 1988). In these instances, lesbians reported feeling like they were treated with respect, like human beings, like they were heard. They felt like they could collaborate with the health care providers and be believed (Stevens, 1994b). Providers who were positive, sensitive, and compassionate also made lesbians feel accepted (Reagan, 1981). The most positive situation was if health care providers treated lesbians as if their care was routine, "like anybody else" (Stevens & Hall, 1988).

Unfortunately, negative stories predominate in lesbians' reports about their experiences of health care (Stevens, 1994b; Stevens & Hall, 1990; Zeidenstein, 1990). Most often negative experiences are with male physicians (Geddes, 1994; Reagan, 1981; Stevens, 1996). Lesbians experience prejudice in their care because of their gender (Robertson, 1992), race, and class (Stevens, 1998) in addition to their sexual identity.

Negative experiences with care include poor communication and feeling disrespected (Trippet & Bain, 1992). Negative stories that lesbians told Stevens (1994b) included being abandoned, dismissed, silenced, dominated, and disregarded. They reported feeling like snap judgments were made about them, like they were intruding, and that health care providers were not present to them. They felt humiliated and in danger.

Disclosure

Fear of provider responses to one's disclosure ("coming out") is one of the main reasons why lesbians avoid seeking health care. Lesbians report that health care professionals have responded to disclosure of their lesbianism with reactions of pity, shock, or unfriendliness as well as by breaching confidentiality, mistreating partners, and making the lesbian wait (Stevens & Hall, 1988).

Several studies note the prevalence of disclosure by lesbians to health care providers. Anywhere from 31% of lesbian college students in West Virginia (mean age = 23 years) (Lehmann, Lehmann, & Kelly, 1998) and 33% of African American lesbians (mean age = 33 years) (Cochran & Mays, 1988) to 90% of mostly White lesbians (mean age = 41 years) in Oregon (White & Dull, 1998) have disclosed their sexual identity to providers.

In only one study (Martinson, Fisher, & DeLapp, 1996) were lesbians asked to respond to an ordinal scale about the effects of disclosure on care received: 65% reported no difference, 28% said care was better, and 7% said it was worse. Others believe that care would be enhanced if they could be out (Reagan, 1981) or that there are situations where being out to a provider is necessary (Stevens & Hall, 1988).

Other lesbians indicate that they would like to disclose but do not (Allen, Glicken, Beach, & Naylor, 1998). Between 33% (Smith, Johnson, & Guenther, 1985) and 68% (Lehmann et al., 1998) of lesbians would like to disclose but do not because they think it is dangerous. Still, not being able to disclose leaves lesbians feeling invisible. The more persons to whom a lesbian is out in general, the more likely it is that she will also come out to health care providers (Martinson et al., 1996), and being out to the provider results in greater likelihood of seeking regular health care (White & Dull, 1998).

There are three types of disclosure: planned, passive, and unplanned. Planned, or active, disclosure occurs when a lesbian decides that she will reveal her sexual orientation to the health provider even though it may be risky.

Hitchcock and Wilson (1992) developed a grounded theory of "personal risking" that lesbians use to deal with the problem of deciding whether to disclose. The two-phase process consists of the anticipatory phase and the interactional phase. In the anticipation phase the lesbian imagines what will happen during the interaction with a provider. In addition, she may collect information about the provider to decide whether the provider is safe. The interactional phase begins while the lesbian is waiting to be seen. She scans the environment to identify any further clues about whether disclosure will be safe. Even as she begins to disclose, she continues to monitor the reaction of the provider to determine her own safety.

Passive disclosure can occur when a lesbian assumes that the provider knows she is a lesbian, often because of her personal appearance (Geddes, 1994; Stevens & Hall, 1988). Passive disclosure also occurs commonly when a lesbian does not specifically identify herself, or when she neither denies nor confirms a provider's veiled suggestion that she is, or might be, lesbian (Hitchcock & Wilson, 1992).

Unplanned disclosure is the most risky (Tiemann, Kennedy, & Haga, 1998). It occurs in a situation where the lesbian had planned for non-disclosure, or perhaps had not even thought about it. As a result of some occurrence during the health care interaction, however, the lesbian may feel forced to come out to avoid negative consequences of some unnecessary procedure or treatment.

Lesbians have described strategies they use to protect or defend themselves from health care providers (Hitchcock & Wilson, 1992; Stevens, 1994c; Stevens & Hall, 1988). In addition to screening providers by obtaining information about possible providers from friends or other lesbian-friendly providers, they often bring witnesses with them. They also maintain vigilance during interactions and control the information they reveal. Some lesbians have simply walked out to escape the danger they perceived in a given situation (Stevens, 1994c).

In an attempt to respond to the negative experiences they have had, some lesbians have challenged the mistreatment they received (Stevens, 1994c). Some negotiate immediately with a provider when an incident happens; others register their complaints to administrators, either verbally or in writing.

PREFERENCES FOR HEALTH CARE PROVIDERS

Lesbians consistently report a preference for female providers (Johnson, Guenther, Laube, & Keettel, 1981; Lucas, 1992; Paroski, 1987; Robertson, 1992; Trippet & Bain, 1993). Although many would like lesbian providers (Johnson et al., 1981; Lucas, 1992; Trippet & Bain, 1993), they want someone who is comfortable with and sensitive to lesbian health concerns (Robertson, 1992). They want providers who are knowledgeable, understanding, and who listen. Lesbian adolescents want providers to use "gentleness" when touching them (Paroski, 1987).

Lesbians also want holistic care (Trippet & Bain, 1992). They report frequent use of alternative/complemental providers, from 13% (Trippet & Bain, 1993) to 32% (White & Dull, 1998). Oregon lesbians said it was easier to be open with alternative providers than with allopathic providers.

INTERVENTIONS WITH HEALTH CARE PROVIDERS

If health care providers are educated about lesbians and lesbian health care issues, we could expect them to provide better care. Only one intervention study is published. Rankow (1997) provided an educational intervention to 103 North Carolina providers of health services to lesbians. Most were physicians, nurses and nurse practitioners, and either nursing or medical assistants. Most (93%) were women, with almost half Caucasian and half African American. The median age was 37 years. The intervention consisted of a 90-minute class consisting of three components: diversity among lesbians, barriers to care for lesbians, and strategies for providing sensitive, culturally competent care. Using a tool developed for the study, knowledge and sensitivity scores improved from pre- to post-intervention. No attempt was made, however, to determine the relationship between improved knowledge and sensitivity and actual practice. Still, the results suggest that improvement is possible.

HEALTH RISK AND HEALTH SCREENING

If lesbians delay seeking health care, it follows that risks for some diseases may be increased. White and Dull (1997) compiled a health risk score and found that younger age, belief in the importance of lung cancer (which they interpreted as a proxy for smoking, since smoking history was not measured), difficulty obtaining care when needed, reliance on partners for health support, and having fewer male sex partners predicted greater health risk in Oregon lesbians.

CANCER SCREENING

Lucas (1992) surveyed lesbians about their health care needs and preferences for a planned gay community health center in a large city. The most desired service was cancer screening. This is consistent with the findings of White and Dull (1998) in which lesbians indicated that the most important health issue they wanted to discuss with health care providers was breast cancer. Cervical and ovarian cancers were also in the top 10 issues they wanted to discuss.

Nonetheless, there has been a general perception among health care providers and lesbians alike that lesbians do not need Pap smears because they are not at risk for cervical cancer. This belief is perpetuated by the assumption that lesbians do not have sex with men, however, four of five lesbians have had sex with men (Diamant, Schuster, McGuigan, & Lever, 1999; Johnson et al., 1981).

In recent studies 92% (Rankow & Tessaro, 1998a) to 98% (Kunkel & Skokan, 1998; White & Dull, 1997) of lesbians reported ever having had a Pap smear, however, only 43% (Rankow & Tessaro, 1998a) to 68% (White & Dull, 1997) had had one in the past year. An average 32 months had passed since the last Pap smear (Kunkel & Skokan, 1998). Buenting (1992) did not report the prevalence of Pap screening, but found that heterosexual women were significantly more likely to have regular Pap smears than lesbians.

Two studies used the Health Belief Model (HBM) to explain cervical screening behavior among lesbians. Price, Easton, Telljohann, and Wallace (1996) used a random sample from the National Women's Mailing List and found that lesbians perceived themselves less susceptible to cervical cancer than either bisexual or heterosexual women. Kunkel and Skokan (1998) found self-efficacy and barriers to be the strongest predictors of compliance with current guidelines for cervical cancer screening in a sample of lesbians.

Price et al. (1996) also studied knowledge of risks for cervical cancer. Knowledge was poor in the entire sample. Although half of the women in the study could identify one of the risk factors for cervical cancer, about 20% were unable to identify any of the risk factors. The only difference across groups was that lesbians were more likely than either heterosexual or bisexual women to recognize that sexual intercourse with men is a risk factor for cervical cancer.

In 1992, Suzanne Haynes, an epidemiologist at the National Cancer Institute, reviewed results of studies about lesbian health practices and concluded that the risk of breast cancer in lesbians was about three times that of the general population. Her report was not based on any empirical data, but it resulted in a virtual panic among lesbians. Even though Haynes' report was never peer reviewed or published, the perception remains that the risk for breast cancer in lesbians is high.

There still are no longitudinal, prospective epidemiologic studies that investigate the question of whether lesbians are at higher risk for breast cancer. One large retrospective record review of risks for breast cancer, however, showed no differences between lesbian and heterosexual women on the risk factors of alcohol and family history of breast cancer (Roberts, Dibble, Scanlon, Paul, & Davids, 1998). Charts of 586 heterosexual and 433 lesbian women 35 years of age and over who visited a women's clinic between 1995 and 1997 were examined. Most were White and all were poor. Heterosexual women were more likely to smoke, have been pregnant, and use birth control pills. Lesbians were more likely to have had breast biopsies and higher body mass index (BMI).

The practice of breast self-examination (BSE) among lesbians is reportedly low. Measurement of BSE is probably unreliable, both among women and among researchers. Results of the two large national surveys in the 1980s showed that 21% of lesbians perform BSE every month (Bradford & Ryan, 1987) and 44% of lesbians always or sometimes practice monthly BSE (Roberts & Sorensen, 1999). More recently, 21% (Ellingson & Yarber, 1997) to 29% (Rankow & Tessaro, 1998b) of lesbians report regular practice.

There is only one study of BSE in lesbians (Ellingson & Yarber, 1997). Lesbians with an average age of 48 were significantly less likely than heterosexual women to practice BSE regularly, however, about one-third of both groups never or rarely practiced BSE. In addition, the frequency of BSE was associated with having regular gynecological exams, which is consistent with lesbians' lack of cervical screening.

All adult women should practice BSE, but the recommendations for mammography screening vary with age. Nonetheless, Trippet and Bain (1990) reported that 65% of the lesbians in their study had had a mammogram, however, most participants in the study were under 40 years of age. Roberts and Sorensen (1999) reported that 58% of women in their 40s and 79% of women in their 50s had had a mammogram. White and Dull (1997) noted that 91% of lesbians 40 and over, and 93% of those 50 and over had had a mammogram, with 53% of those 40 and over, and 76% of those 50 and over, having one in the past year.

Studies of lesbians and mammography screening have also examined factors that are associated with screening and barriers to screening. Variables associated with seeking mammography by lesbians include older age and Caucasian race (Rankow & Tessaro, 1998b), having insurance and higher income (Burnett, Steakley, Slack, Roth, & Lerman, 1999; Rankow & Tessaro, 1998b), and greater worry about breast cancer or perceiving self at risk (Burnett et al., 1999; Lauver et al., 1999).

Barriers to mammography screening include cost or lack of insurance (Lauver et al., 1999; Rankow & Tessaro, 1998), lack of motivation, and feeling not at risk (Lauver et al., 1999; Robertson, 1992). Lauver concludes that barriers to mammography for lesbians are similar to women in general.

One study examined the attitudes about genetic testing for breast cancer in lesbians who had at least one first-degree relative with breast cancer (Durfy, Bowen, McTiernan, Sporleder, & Burke, 1999). Women were only eligible to participate in the study if they were willing to participate in counseling about breast cancer risk. Lesbians, as well as the other women in the study, had significantly higher perceived than actual risk for breast cancer and high levels of worry about breast cancer. Women in the study strongly favored ready access to genetic testing, and indicated that, with a positive result, they would increase frequency of BSE, mammograms, and clinical breast exams but probably not undergo prophylactic mastectomy.

OSTEOPOROSIS

One recent study on health screening behaviors other than cancer was found. The purpose was to compare risks for osteoporosis between lesbian and heterosexual women. Premenopausal lesbian and heterosexual women between 30 and 50 years in good health were studied. The principal variable was ultrasound measures of bone density in the heel. There were no differences between groups in age, BMI, exercise, calcium intake, alcohol use, or calcaneal ultrasound measures. However, antidepressant use in both groups was associated with a significant reduction in calcaneal bone mass, suggesting a possible relationship between the treatment of depression and bone density (Patton et al., 1998).

LESBIAN HEALTH CONCERNS

Physical Concerns

Lesbians generally report themselves to be in good or excellent health (Buenting, 1992; Stevens & Hall, 1988). The most commonly reported physical health problems among lesbians are vaginitis (Moran, 1996; Trippet & Bain, 1990), menstrual problems (Trippet & Bain, 1993), and weight (Ryan & Bradford, 1993; Trippet & Bain, 1990). Older lesbians report arthritis (Kehoe, 1986; 1988), physical handicaps (Kehoe, 1986), and hypertension (Kehoe, 1988), as their most common problems. Studies of specific physical health problems, however, are extremely limited.

PREGNANCY AND MOTHERHOOD/PARENTING

Lesbians have always been mothers. In the NLHCS (Ryan & Bradford, 1993), 30% had been pregnant and 16% had borne children. Results of a large 1987 survey of Minnesota adolescents suggest that lesbian teens are no more likely to have had heterosexual intercourse but are more likely to become pregnant than heterosexual teens (Saewyc, Bearinger, Blum, & Resnick, 1999). Lesbian teens use less effective contraception.

Prior to the 1980s most lesbians who had children had them during a heterosexual marriage. When those women recognized their lesbian identity, they often brought their children with them into the families they created as lesbians. Around 1980, increasing numbers of lesbians began to acknowledge their right to have children even if they did not want heterosexual marriage, and they began to seek alternative approaches to having children. Some obtained fresh sperm from their gay male friends and inseminated themselves. Others engaged in intercourse with men for the sole purpose of becoming pregnant. After the onset of the AIDS epidemic, lesbians claimed and gained greater access to artificial insemination (AI) and, as a result, increasing numbers of young lesbians are becoming pregnant and creating families, using AI. Only one study (Eskenazi, Pies, Newstetter, Shepard, & Pearson, 1989) investigated the risks of HIV transmission via sperm to lesbians. In that study of 98 lesbians who had been inseminated between 1979 and 1987, no lesbians were seropositive, even though 11 may have received semen from HIV-infected donors.

Three studies (Brewaeys, Ponjaert-Kristoffersen, Van Steirteghem, & Devroey, 1993; Leiblum, Palmer, & Spector, 1995; Wendland, Byrn, & Hill, 1996) compared lesbian and heterosexual women users of artificial insemination at infertility programs. Although different variables were measured in each study, lesbian and heterosexual women were more similar than different on the variables in each study. The one difference was that more lesbians than heterosexual women planned to disclose the fact of AI to their children.

Lesbians have the same health needs related to pregnancy that other women do; they attend childbirth education classes and have many of the same questions and concerns as heterosexual parents. Because they are lesbians, however, they have additional needs, many of which are related to health care interactions (Stewart, 1999).

The month when prenatal care begins is a way to evaluate obstetrical care for its availability, accessibility, and acceptability (Harvey, Carr, & Bernheine, 1989; Olesker & Walsh, 1984). All women in these two studies sought care in the first trimester, so care was apparently available and accessible. In both studies, however, lesbians indicated that their care could have been better with more knowledgeable providers.

Lesbian mothers are particularly concerned about inclusion of their partners throughout the pregnancy and birth process. All seven lesbian mothers that Stewart (1999) interviewed had problems with acknowledgement of their partners by health care providers. When these mothers felt unaccepted by health providers, they judged their maternity care to be poor, and vice versa.

Lesbian mothers appear to adapt successfully to the roles and responsibilities of motherhood. The social support that lesbian mothers receive from extended family networks, friends, and others (Ainslie & Feltey, 1991; Coleman, Strapko, Zubrzycki, & Broach, 1993; Levy, 1989) appears to be adequate in meeting their own and their children's needs.

There are two studies of lesbian couples who used AI and, at the time of the study, had children between one and two years of age (Brewaeys, Devroey, Helmerhorst, Van Hall, & Ponjaert, 1995), and between four and eight years of age (Brewaeys, Ponjaert, Van Hall, & Golombok, 1997). Most lesbian parents in these studies shared child care responsibilities equally, and they made it clear to the children that there were two parents in the family. The quality of parent-child interaction did not differ significantly between the two mothers. By ages 4 to 8, the child had been told that a sperm donor was used in all but 1 of the 30 families.

WEIGHT, BODY IMAGE, AND EATING DISORDERS

The most common hypotheses in studies of lesbians and body image or eating is that lesbians have less body dissatisfaction, dieting, and disordered eating behaviors than do gay men or heterosexual women. The theory is that lesbians reject the socially constructed image of the ideal woman as extremely thin, so they are more open to a range of body types and less likely to diet. Studies consistently show that lesbians have higher weights (Brand, Rothblum, & Solomon, 1992) or higher BMI (Beren, Hayden, Wilfley, & Grilo, 1996; Roberts et al., 1998; Siever, 1994) than heterosexual women.

Results of studies that tested these hypotheses, however, are mixed. Lesbian and heterosexual women do not differ (Beren et al., 1996; Heffernan, 1996; Striegel-Moore, Tucker, & Hsu, 1990) or differ on some variables but not all (French, Story, Remafedi, Resnick, & Blum, 1996; Siever, 1994). For example, lesbians and bisexual women with the most feminine identity have lower body satisfaction (Ludwig & Brownell, 1999); more than half of older lesbians view themselves as too fat (Kehoe, 1986; 1988), and 25% of lesbian and bisexual teens had been on a diet at least once a month in the past year (Saewyc, Bearinger, Heinz, Blum, & Resnick, 1998). These inconsistent findings suggest that gender may be more important than sexual orientation for body esteem and that lesbians are not immune to the unrealistic ideal body images advocated in society.

SEXUALLY TRANSMITTED INFECTIONS

Very few studies have been conducted on sexually transmitted infections (STIs) in lesbians because of the common belief that lesbians are unlikely to have these problems or to transmit them to other women, largely on the basis of one old study in which no cases of syphilis, gonorrhea, chlamydia, or herpes simplex virus were identified (Robertson & Schachter, 1981). Johnson, Smith, and Guenther (1987) supported that view when they reported that bisexual women were more likely than lesbians to report herpes, gonorrhea, trichomoniasis, and vaginitis. When sexual orientation was controlled in their study, however, most of the STIs were associated with a difference in reported heterosexual intercourse. Skinner, Stokes, Kirlew, Kavanagh, and Forster (1996) noted no significant differences between lesbian and heterosexual women in the frequency and types of STIs diagnosed in their clinic, and they conclude that lesbians are at risk of STIs.

Other researchers have tried to determine whether lesbians can transmit STIs. Cochran and Mays (1996) concluded that STIs are transmitted between lesbian partners when they found that the number of female partners was associated with the number of self-reported vaginal infections in a sample of young women who have sex with women (WSW). Several researchers who studied specific STIs concluded that bacterial vaginosis (BV) can be sexually transmitted by lesbians (Berger et al., 1995; Carroll, Goldstein, Lo, & Mayer, 1997; Edwards & Thin, 1990). Although McCaffrey, Varney, Evans, and Taylor-Robinson (1999) diagnosed BV in 52% of the lesbians in their study, however, they could not find evidence to support female-to-female transmission.

Edwards and Thin (1990) also noted a high incidence of viral STIs in their sample of lesbians, and they concluded that these diseases can be transmitted between lesbians. The most methodologically sophisticated study (Marrazzo et al., 1998) used type-specific DNA probes for nine human papillomavirus (HPV) types and a universal probe to detect other types of HPV. They identified HPV in 30% of a sample of WSW. Although presence of HPV was associated with recent sexual intercourse with men and a higher lifetime number of male sexual partners, HPV was also detected in women who had never had sex with men. Consequently, these researchers concluded that HPV is sexually transmitted between women.

HUMAN IMMUNOVIRUS INFECTION AND ACQUIRED IMMUNODEFICIENCY SYNDROME

Just as lesbians have been considered at low risk for STIs, they have been considered at low risk for HIV infection. Lampon's (1995) qualitative study of lesbians' perceptions about risks for HIV and the availability of information on HIV for lesbians affirms that many lesbians do not consider themselves at risk for HIV. None of the lesbians in Raiteri's et al. (1994) study reported using safer sex.

Since there is no Centers for Disease Control and Prevention (CDC) category for women who have sex with women, and since transmission is based on a hierarchy of categories, little is known about woman-to-woman transmission of HIV. Chu, Hammet, and Buehler (1992) identified a very small number of women in the United States who had developed AIDS and reported sex with women only since 1978 (i.e., the CDC definition of lesbian). Most cases of AIDS in lesbians are attributed to injection drug use.

With HIV (and STIs) it is important to examine sexual behaviors rather then sexual identity (i.e., lesbian) because women who have sex with women do not always call themselves lesbian, and women who identify as lesbian may also have sex with men. In Moore et al.'s (1996) study of HIV infected women, 11% of women who identified as heterosexual and 98% of women who identified as bisexual reported having had sex with women. Moreover, 19% of women who identified as lesbian and 75% of women who identified as bisexual reported having had sex with a man in the past 6 months.

Simple seroprevalence rates of HIV among lesbians and WSW were reported in four studies in the early 1990s. The seroprevalence rates for WSW and women who had sex with men only (WSM) attending a New York City sexually transmitted disease clinic between 1988 and 1992 were 17% and

11%, respectively (Bevier, Chiasson, Heffernan, & Castro, 1995). The overall seroprevalence rate for a sample of lesbian and bisexual women in the San Francisco Bay Area in 1993 was 1.2% (Lemp et al., 1995). Among women who were tested at HIV clinics in New York State between 1993 and 1994, the seroprevalence rate was 3.7% for WSW, 4.8% for women who reported sex with both women and men (WSWM), and 2.9% for WSM (Shotsky, 1996). Between 1992 and 1994, Kral, Lorvick, Bluthenthal, and Watters (1997) studied women injection drug users and crack cocaine users in 19 cities across the United States. In the women who reported sex with women in the previous 30 days, the overall seroprevalence rate was 13%.

The large variations in these rates may be due to the definitions used for the participants, for example, WSW can include women who have sex only with women or any women who have sex with women (but who may also have sex with men). Bevier et al (1995) used the latter definition and, in fact, referred to them as bisexual women. Shotsky (1996) classified the women on the basis of their reported partners only, for example, WSW were women who reported only female sexual partners. Hence, making comparisons or conclusions about these data are difficult, if not inappropriate. In addition, it is not surprising to find high seroprevalence rates at STD clinics or in injection drug users, and the low rates in the Lemp et al. (1995) study may be because data were collected from participants at community events rather than from a clinic population.

Studies have also examined risk behaviors of WSW for transmission of HIV. In each of the seroprevalence studies just cited, injection drug use was associated with HIV infection in WSW (Bevier et al., 1995; Kral et al., 1997; Lemp et al., 1995; Shotsky, 1996). Raiteri et al. (1994) could find no evidence of female-to-female transmission of HIV in their study; injection drug use was most associated with HIV. Risky behaviors, in addition to injection drug use, include unprotected vaginal and anal sex with male partners (Cochran & Mays, 1996; Lemp et al., 1995; Norman, Perry, Stevenson, Kelly, & Roffman, 1996), exchange of sex for money or drugs (Bevier et al., 1995; Moore et al., 1996), giving or receiving oral sex with female partners (Kral et al., 1997), and unprotected sex with someone known to be HIV positive (Einhorn & Polgar, 1994).

Perry (1995) demonstrated an association between the frequency of alcohol and marijuana use and a number of risky sexual behaviors and injection drug use. In her study of lesbian and bisexual women in Houston, even though these women practiced many risky behaviors, 95% thought they would not contract HIV in their lifetime.

Women who have sex with women seem to have a high prevalence of risk behaviors that could put them at increased risk for HIV. Cochran, Bybee,

Gage, and Mays (1996) compiled the results of three large studies (with more than 8,500 women) to identify behaviors that put lesbians at risk for HIV. Those identified were injection drug use, including heroin, and sex with men. Lower education and income were most associated with drug use. Self-identification as bisexual, being younger, and not being in a lesbian relationship were most associated with having sex with men.

It appears, however, that women who have sex exclusively with women have lower risks than bisexual women or WSWM. Women who have sex with both women and men may be having the most sex and thus are also at the highest risk. Ziemba-Davis, Sanders, and Reinisch (1996) asked women who identified as lesbians at the time of the study if they had ever identified themselves as bisexual or heterosexual. Lesbians who previously considered themselves bisexual or heterosexual were more than twice as likely to report having had STI than lesbians who always considered themselves lesbian.

Einhorn and Polgar (1994) surveyed a large national sample of lesbian and bisexual women. They found a significantly higher prevalence of high-risk sexual behaviors among bisexual women (49%) than among lesbians (21%). In Cochran and Mays' study (1996), the highest frequency of risky sexual behaviors was among teen women who identified as bisexual.

Gomez, Garcia, Kegebein, Shade, and Hernandez (1996) studied self-identified lesbian and bisexual women, and classified them into three groups based on the gender of their sexual partners in the past three years: lesbians who had sex only with women (LSW), lesbians who had sex with women and men (LSWM), and bisexual women who had sex with women and men (BSWM). Bisexual women who reported sex only with women (17%) were excluded from the analysis. LSWM were significantly younger than LSW and more likely to have a history of injecting drugs; otherwise, they did not differ in sexual behaviors. All women reported a wider range of unprotected sexual behaviors with primary partners than with non-primary partners. LSWM had significantly more female partners and were more likely to have female partners who injected drugs. BSWM had significantly more male partners as well as male partners who injected drugs or had sex with other men.

Finally, Deren et al. (1996) matched pairs of women who identified as lesbian and who identified as bisexual with heterosexual women to compare risk behaviors for HIV. Bisexual women had significantly more risk behaviors than their heterosexual matches, but lesbians did not differ from their matches in the frequency of risk behaviors, suggesting that bisexual women have the most risky behaviors.

INTERVENTIONS

Interventions for lesbians and WSW to prevent HIV infection have been limited, however, one major study was conducted in San Francisco and reported by Stevens (1994a) and Stevens and Hall (1997; 1998). The project was conducted for 2 years between 1992 and 1994 at gay bars and clubs. A large team of peer educators provided one-to-one, individualized, culturally specific HIV education to 1189 individual women and group presentations to about 3500 women. The purpose of the study was to abolish the notion that lesbians and bisexual women are not at risk for HIV, and in doing so, to save lives.

The lesbians and bisexual women in the study (Stevens & Hall, 1998) engaged in many risk behaviors, such as unprotected oral, vaginal, and anal sex with women and men, and injection drug use. These women often rationalized the use of such behaviors because they considered themselves not at risk. Although they defined "monogamy" in quite diverse ways, they often trusted in monogamy to protect them. They also let the "passion of the moment" prohibit them from use of safer sex practices. Women who participated in the study greatly valued the intervention and often encouraged their friends to participate. Researchers considered the continuity of peer educators and the length of time to be extremely valuable in making the program a success.

Mental Health Concerns

Lesbians are thought to have more mental health problems because of the stress of living as marginalized individuals in society. Lesbians in the NLHCS reported major problems suggestive of high stress and mental health problems (Bradford, Ryan, & Rothblum, 1994). More than one-third reported having had a "long depression or sadness" at some point in their lives. Another national survey, the Boston Lesbian Health Project (Sorensen & Roberts, 1997), reveals similar results.

Gillow and Davis (1987) studied sources of stress and coping methods in another small, national sample of lesbians. The most frequently reported primary stressor for lesbians was job-related (27%), followed closely by primary relationship issues (25%). The most frequently reported coping methods included seeing the humor in the situation, crying, and temporarily withdrawing. Use of alcohol and recreational drugs as coping methods had decreased. In Trippet and Bain's (1994) study, the most frequent mental health concerns were relationship problems (77%), conflict between being in the closet at work and out socially, and depression (66% each).

Cochran and Mays (1994) examined depressive distress in African American women and men who had at least one same sex sexual experience. Probable clinical depression was identified in 38% of the women; only symptomatic HIV positive gay men had worse scores. Hughes, Haas, and Avery (1997) found no differences in depression between lesbian and heterosexual women

Bernhard and Applegate (1999) compared lesbian and heterosexual women on mental health issues. They found no differences between the groups on a single item measure of stress, although more than 80% of both groups reported having moderate or severe stress. When presented with a list of 18 possible stressors, however, lesbians reported significantly more stress than heterosexual women, but there were no differences between the groups in use of stress management measures.

Most of the lesbians in the previous studies were in their 30's. Studies of mental health in older lesbians, however, show them well adjusted (Kehoe, 1986) and in excellent or good mental health (Deevey, 1990; Kehoe, 1988).

USE OF THERAPY BY LESBIANS

Lesbians are heavy users of mental health counseling services. Anywhere from 56% (Trippet & Bain, 1990) to 86% (Bernhard & Applegate, 1999) of lesbians in various studies report having used therapy. Lesbians are significantly more likely to have used therapy than are heterosexual women (Hughes et al., 1997).

Morgan (1992; 1997; Morgan & Eliason, 1992) conducted a number of studies to explain the high use of therapy by lesbians. In the first study (Morgan, 1992) she found that lesbians have more positive responses to therapy than heterosexual women do. Morgan and Eliason (1992) interviewed lesbians who had used and who had not used therapy as a tool that was then used in the third study.

Lesbians indicated whether they had experienced each of a list of 27 issues that might be discussed with a therapist (Morgan, 1997). If they had experienced it, they indicated whether they had discussed it with a therapist; if they had not experienced it, they indicated the likelihood that they would discuss it with a therapist. Results showed that lesbians were very likely to have experienced the issues and to either have taken them or be willing to take them to therapy.

ALCOHOL AND SUBSTANCE USE

Older research suggests that lesbians drink alcohol at higher rates than heterosexual women (Lewis, Saghir, & Robins, 1982), however, such studies are now criticized because of methodological problems, such as collecting data in bars (Bloomfield, 1993). Still, results are conflicting. Some studies show that lesbians are more likely than heterosexual women to drink daily and are less likely to abstain from alcohol (Bradford & Ryan, 1987; McKirnan & Peterson, 1989). Data from a random household sample of women in San Francisco, however, showed no statistically significant differences in alcohol consumption and drinking patterns between lesbian and heterosexual women (Bloomfield, 1993). Buenting (1992) also found no significant difference between lesbian and heterosexual women in alcohol consumption.

Smoking cigarettes may be a problem among lesbians, but data are conflicting. Ryan and Bradford (1993) reported that 41% of the lesbians in NLHCS smoked cigarettes, and half of them worried about their smoking. More recently, White and Dull (1997) found that only 11%, and Burnett et al. (1999) found that only 12% of their samples were current smokers. Although Skinner (1994) found that lesbians smoke cigarettes more than gay men, Buenting (1992) did not find a significant difference between lesbian and heterosexual women.

Welch, Howden-Chapman, and Collings (1998) noted that young lesbians were most likely to smoke. That is consistent with findings of a study of lesbian and bisexual teens in which 83% reported their onset of smoking at an average age of 13 years (Rosario, Hunter, & Gwadz, 1997).

Lesbians also seem to have high use of illicit drugs. Skinner and Otis (1996) reported the lifetime use of a number of illicit drugs among lesbians (mean age = 34) to be 86%. Buenting (1992) found that lesbians were significantly more likely to use recreational drugs than heterosexual women. Marijuana, however, is the most frequently used illicit drug (Ryan & Bradford, 1993; Rosario et al., 1997; Skinner & Otis, 1996; Welch et al., 1994), and use of drugs appears to decrease with age (Skinner & Otis, 1996).

Alcohol Recovery.   Lesbians also appear to have high rates of being in recovery from alcohol and/or other drugs (Bloomfield, 1993; Hughes et al., 1997; Sorensen & Roberts, 1997). Although lesbians participate in Alcoholics Anonymous (AA) to achieve recovery, their participation causes them considerable tension (Hall, 1994a), as it does for many women. Hall (1992) notes that the principal image of recovery in AA is conversion, and although lesbians discuss conversion in their recovery, they also consider many more aspects. For lesbians, recovery also includes a physical transition, personal growth, struggle with compulsivity, reclaiming the self, connection with women and lesbians, vocational change, and empowerment. McNally and Finnegan (1992) developed a model of how lesbians integrate their experiences of alcoholism with their experiences of being an out lesbian to achieve a positive identity as a "lesbian recovering alcoholic."

In the only study of social support for lesbians in recovery, Mays, Beckman, Oranchak, and Harper (1994) compared the sources of support among Black heterosexual, bisexual, and lesbian women in alcohol treatment programs. Heterosexual women had many more sources of support than lesbian and bisexual women, but the quality of support did not differ between the groups.

Childhood Sexual Abuse.   Almost half of the lesbians in Hall's (1996b) dissertation study spontaneously reported that they were survivors of CSA. These women, unlike the others, described their alcoholism as pervasive in every aspect of their lives. All of them reported frequent suicidal and self-harm behaviors.

For her postdoctoral work, Hall (1996a, 1998, 1999) studied lesbian recovering alcoholics who were also CSA survivors. These women lived in unstable, chaotic homes where they not only experienced but also witnessed sexual, physical, and emotional violence. In reflection they described their experiences with a great deal of loss, specifically the loss of being a child. These experiences caused them to struggle as adults and in recovery, however, they can be described as resilient because they did survive. Rankow et al. (1998) described emotional barriers of CSA survivors that affect their use of health care.

VIOLENCE

While about one-fourth of lesbians who have been surveyed report CSA (Hughes et al., 1997; Ryan & Bradford, 1993), lesbians also experience many other forms of violence against them. In the NLHCS, 37% of the lesbians reported experiencing physical abuse, and women of color were more likely than White women to have been abused (Ryan & Bradford, 1993).

Brand and Kidd (1986) compared the experiences of lesbian and hetero-sexual women to determine whether physical aggression was more frequent in opposite or same sex dyads (i.e., committed and dating relationships). Opposite sex dyads had significantly more violence than same sex dyads, however, 25% of the lesbians had experienced physical abuse in same sex committed relationships.

Intimate Partner Violence.   Lesbians experience intimate partner violence and abuse in the same ways and probably with the same frequencies as heterosexual women (Hughes et al., 1997; Moran, 1996; Renzetti, 1992). Renzetti (1992) was one of the first to study systematically violence in lesbian couples. She surveyed 100 lesbians who reported having been the victim of lesbian battering. Most lesbians indicated that the abuse increased over time. Partners' mutual dependency was most strongly associated with abuse.

Scherzer (1998) studied lesbians in San Francisco, most of whom were in their 30's. One in three women reported emotional abuse in her current or most recent lesbian relationship, and one in six reported physical abuse. There were no differences between women of color and White women in the prevalence of abuse.

A few studies have used the Conflict Tactics Scale (CTS), which facilitates comparisons among studies and also allows measurement as both victim and perpetrator of aggressive acts. Lockhart, White, Causby, and Isaac (1994) surveyed lesbians for their experiences of violence only. About one-third (31%) reported having been the victim of physical violence (e.g., being pushed or shoved, having something thrown at them) in the past year; 12% reported "severe" physical violence (e.g., kicking, biting, and being hit with a fist) against them; 90% reported at least one act of verbal aggression (e.g., verbal insults, refusing to talk) from a partner in the past year. Having been emotionally or physically abused by parents was associated with both verbal and physical aggression now.

Lie and Gentlewarrior (1991) studied lesbians as both victim and perpetrator. Half of those surveyed reported having been abused by a female partner, and one-third had abused a female partner. One-fourth had been both abused and abuser. The most frequent form of abuse was a combination of physical and psychological abuse.

Waldner-Haugrud, Gratch, and Magruder (1997) compared lesbians and gay men as victims and perpetrators. Almost half (48%) of the lesbians and 30% of the gay men had been the victim of same sex partner violence; 38% of the lesbians and 22% of the gay men had acted against a same sex partner.

Lie, Schilit, Bush, Montagne, and Reyes (1991) examined the abuse histories of lesbians who were aggressive in their current relationships and concluded that a history of aggression is a risk factor for subsequent aggression. Eighty-six percent of the sample had observed or been the target of at least one act of physical, sexual, or verbal aggression in their family of origin. Two thirds had experienced some form of aggression in past relationships with men, and three-fourths had experienced some form of aggression in past relationships with women. In their current relationships with women, 9% experienced sexual, 12% physical, and 24% verbal abuse. Alcohol (Perry, 1995; Schilit, Lie, Montagne, 1990) and marijuana (Perry, 1995) use are also associated with lesbian partner abuse.

Two studies specifically examined sexual coercion, comparing lesbians with gay men. Waterman, Dawson, and Bologna (1989) found no significant differences, although 31% of lesbians and 12% of gay men reported being forced into sex by their current or most recent same sex partner. Eight percent of lesbians and 6% of gay men had forced a partner to have sex. More recently, Waldner-Haugrud and Gratch (1997) reported that 45% of lesbians and 57% of gay men had experienced at least one act of sexual coercion. The most common was persistent undesired touching. Gay men had significantly more coercive incidents than lesbians, but there were no differences between the tactics used. Differences between these studies may be due to operational definitions of sexual coercion.

Tuel and Russell (1998) compared mental health consequences of women battered by women and women battered by men. Heterosexual women reported significantly more of both physical and nonphysical abuse, but did not differ from lesbians on depression or self-esteem. Physical abuse predicted depression, and nonphysical abuse predicted self-esteem; gender was not a predictor. Heterosexual battering relationships lasted significantly longer than did lesbian battering relationships.

Hate Crimes.   Lesbians are also the victims of hate crimes, that is, crimes against them because of their sexual orientation. More than one-third of lesbian and bisexual college students reported experiencing physical or verbal abuse at school because of their sexuality (Lehmann et al., 1998).

Two studies compared the experiences of hate crimes by lesbians and gay men (Herek, Gillis, Cogan, & Glunt, 1997; Otis & Skinner, 1996). In each study, half of the sample had experienced at least one crime or attempted crime. They concluded that these crimes were committed because of their sexual orientation due to statements made by the perpetrators or because of their own visibility as a lesbian or gay individual at the time of the incident. The most prevalent crimes were threats/verbal abuse and theft/vandalism (Otis & Skinner, 1996).

The experience of hate crimes may be related to mental health of lesbians. Otis and Skinner (1996) found that sexual assault by men (but not by women), physical attacks, threats/verbal abuse, and multiple victimization predicted depression (measured with the CES-D) in lesbians. Self-esteem (measured with the Rosenberg self-esteem scale), however, was the best predictor of depression in their study.

SUICIDE

Lesbians and gay men, particularly youth, are thought to be at increased risk for suicide. Relatively large numbers of lesbians, up to 67%, report having suicidal thoughts (Hammelman, 1993; Sorensen & Roberts, 1997), however, the number of actual attempts is much smaller, from 11% (Trippet & Bain, 1994) to 27% (Lehmann et al., 1998). In a study of adolescent lesbian and bisexual girls, 12% of those ages 14 and under, and 31% of those 15 and over, reported suicidal attempts (Saewyc et al., 1998).

Hughes et al. (1997) reported that lesbians had a significantly higher rate of attempted suicide than heterosexual women. Bradford et al. (1994) noted that women of color were more likely to have attempted suicide than White women. D'Augelli and Hershberger (1993) reported that predictors for suicidal attempts in the lesbian teens in their study were loss of friends due to being lesbian and frequenting gay bars. Garofalo, Wolf, Wissow, Woods, and Goodman (1999) used data from the 1995 Massachusetts Youth Risk Behavior Survey to identify suicide risk in lesbian, gay, bisexual, and "not sure" (GLBN) high school students. Less than 4% of the sample were GLBN, but GLBN youth were significantly more likely to report a suicide attempt than heterosexual students were. GLBN females were twice as likely and GLBN males were 6.5 times more likely to report a suicide attempt than their heterosexual peers.

SUMMARY AND RECOMMENDATIONS

The principal conclusion of this review is that very little is known about lesbian health. It is difficult to generalize on any particular topic because there are so few studies on any topic. Consequently, the knowledge base is limited in many ways. First, nearly all the studies were descriptive or survey designs that merely begin to name and describe variables. Second, few comparisons can be made across studies due to the use of different definitions and measurement of variables, including the definition of lesbian. Third, only a small number of studies have comparison groups. The most frequent comparison group is heterosexual women, but bisexual women, and both gay and heterosexual men, are included in some studies. Unfortunately, however, bisexual women are included in several studies in the lesbian group, making interpretations difficult.

Fourth, convenience samples are used in almost every study. Hence, no generalizations can be made. Moreover, the samples include only the most "visible" lesbians and not the diversity among lesbians. In these studies, the majority of participants are White, well-educated lesbians who are in their 30s and have social or political connections to other lesbians. A few studies included lesbian youth or college students, and even fewer had older lesbians. Only Cochran and Mays have regularly studied Black lesbians. Deeply closeted lesbians, who are extremely difficult to identify, are not included in these studies. Fifth, very few studies used established, reliable, and valid instruments. Most survey questionnaires were developed for the studies and were rarely described in the articles. Sixth, only the most basic forms of data analysis were used. In many cases no statistical tests were used.

Finally, there are only two intervention studies in this review. One educated health care providers about lesbianism and lesbian concerns with health care in an attempt to improve the provider side of the client-provider relationship. Although an increase in knowledge occurred, no outcomes related to an improvement in practice were measured. The other intervention educated lesbian and bisexual women about their risks for HIV. In this case there were no measures to show either an increase in knowledge or behavior.

Some conclusions can be drawn from this review. First, many lesbians feel unsafe in health care interactions. Care does matter. Second, lesbians want access to health care but have low usage rates, except for psychotherapy. Third, much more is known about mental health issues, including alcohol use and violence, than about physical health concerns of lesbians. Fourth, younger lesbians (and bisexual women) appear to be at the greatest risk for many mental and physical health problems. Fifth, most researchers in this review have one publication. This can be viewed positively, that increasing numbers of researchers are involved in lesbian health research. It can also be viewed less positively, in that researchers are not continuing to do studies to build a body of knowledge in a substantive area. Finally, there are many discrepancies and conflicts among these studies, suggesting the need for more research, particularly using the same measures.

Thus, the need for lesbian health research is great. We need large probability samples of women with prospective and longitudinal designs to obtain epidemiological data about lesbians in areas of health risks and behaviors. We need to identify the health needs of subpopulations among lesbians. We need to better understand the lesbian client/health care provider interaction. How do lesbians actually access care, and what are the outcomes of the care they receive? Do lesbians really use more alternative/complemental sources of care? For what conditions? And what are the outcomes? What interventions work best to encourage lesbians to participate in health screening in particular, and in health care in general? We also need to know whether different interventions work better for different subpopulations of lesbians? We also need to emphasize research on focused problems so that bodies of knowledge in specific areas of lesbian health can be developed.

The 1980s was a decade in which women's health activism enabled the acceptance of women's health research in the 1990s. The 1990s also saw activism in lesbian health that has laid the groundwork for this decade to become the one in which lesbian health research will become a valued part of the national health agenda. Recommendations in the Institute of Medicine report on lesbian health include greater funding for research on lesbian health and for the training of researchers in lesbian health, research to identify the risks and protective factors of lesbians for both physical and mental health problems, and methodological research to improve measurement of sexual orientation (Solarz, 1999). With this impetus, research on lesbian health is likely to expand greatly.

REFERENCES

Ainslie, J., & Feltey, K. M. (1991). Definitions and dynamics of motherhood and family in lesbian communities. *Marriage and Family Review, 17*(1/2), 63–85.

Allen, L. B., Glicken, A. D., Beach, R. K., & Naylor, K. E. (1998). Adolescent health care experience of gay, lesbian, and bisexual young adults. *Journal of Adolescent Health, 23*, 212–220.

Beren, S. E., Hayden, H. A., Wilfley, D. E., & Grilo, C. M. (1996). The influence of sexual orientation on body dissatisfaction in adult men and women. *International Journal of Eating Disorders, 20*, 135–141.

Berger, B. J., Kolton, S., Zenilman, J. M., Cummings, M. C., Feldman, J., & McCormack, W. M. (1995). Bacterial vaginosis in lesbians: A sexually transmitted disease. *Clinical Infectious Diseases, 21*, 1402–1405.

Bernhard, L. A., & Applegate, J. M. (1999). Comparison of stress and stress management strategies between lesbian and heterosexual women. *Health Care for Women International, 20*, 335–347.

Bevier, P. J., Chiasson, M. A., Heffernan, R. T., & Castro, K. G. (1995). Women at a sexually transmitted disease clinic who reported same-sex contact: Their HIV seroprevalence and risk behaviors. *American Journal of Public Health, 85*, 1366–1371.

Bloomfield, K. (1993). A comparison of alcohol consumption between lesbians and heterosexual women in an urban population. *Drug and Alcohol Dependence, 33*, 257–269.

Bradford, J., & Ryan. C. (1987). *The National Lesbian Health Care Survey.* Washington, DC: National Lesbian and Gay Health Foundation.

Bradford, J., Ryan, C., & Rothblum, E. D. (1994). National Lesbian Health Care Survey: Implications for mental health care. *Journal of Consulting and Clinical Psychology, 62*, 228–242.

Brand, P. A., & Kidd, A. H. (1986). Frequency of physical aggression in heterosexual and female homosexual dyads. *Psychological Reports, 59*, 1307–1313.

Brand, P. A., Rothblum, E. D., & Solomon, L. J. (1992). A comparison of lesbians, gay men, and heterosexuals on weight and restrained eating. *International Journal of Eating Disorders, 11*, 253–359.

Brewaeys, A., Devroey, P., Helmerhorst, F. M., Van Hall, E. V., & Ponjaert, I. (1995). Lesbian mothers who conceived after donor insemination: A follow-up study. *Human Reproduction, 10*, 2731–2735.

Brewaeys, A., Ponjaert-Kristoffersen, I., Van Steirteghem, A. C., & Devroey, P. (1993). Children from anonymous donors: An inquiry into homosexual and heterosexual parents' attitudes [Special issue]. *Journal of Psychosomatic Obstetrics and Gynaecology, 14*, 23–35.

Brewaeys, A., Ponjaert, I., Van Hall, E. V., & Golombok, S. (1997). Donor insemination: Child development and family functioning in lesbian mother families. *Human Reproduction, 12*, 1349–1359.

Buenting, J. A. (1992). Health life-styles of lesbian and heterosexual women. *Health Care for Women International, 13*, 165–171.

Burnett, C. B., Steakley, C. S., Slack, R., Roth, J., & Lerman, C. (1999). Patterns of breast cancer screening among lesbians at increased risk for breast cancer. *Women and Health, 29*(4), 35–55.

Butler, S. S., & Hope, B. (1999). Health and well-being for late middle-aged and old lesbians in a rural area. *Journal of Gay & Lesbian Social Services, 9*(4), 27–46.

Carroll, N., Goldstein, R. S., Lo, W., & Mayer, K. H. (1997). Gynecological infections and sexual practices of Massachusetts lesbian and bisexual women. *Journal of the Gay and Lesbian Medical Association, 1*, 15–23.

Chu, S. Y., Hammett, T. A., & Buehler, J. W. (1992). Update: Epidemiology of reported cases of AIDS in women who report sex only with other women, United States, 1980–1991. *AIDS, 6*, 518–519.

Cochran, S. D., Bybee, D., Gage, S., & Mays, V. M. (1996). Prevalence of HIV-related self-reported sexual behaviors, sexually transmitted diseases, and problems with drugs and alcohol in three large surveys of lesbian and bisexual women: A look into a segment of the community. *Women's Health: Research on Gender, Behavior, and Policy, 2*(1&2), 11–33.

Cochran, S. D., & Mays, V. M. (1988). Disclosure of sexual preference to physicians by Black lesbian and bisexual women. *Western Journal of Medicine, 149*, 616–619.

Cochran, S. D., & Mays, V. M. (1994). Depressive distress among homosexually active African American men and women. *American Journal of Psychiatry, 151*, 524–529.

Cochran, S. D., & Mays, V. M. (1996). Prevalence of HIV-related sexual risk behaviors among young 18- to 24-year old lesbian and bisexual women. *Women's Health: Research on Gender, Behavior, and Policy, 2*(1&2), 75–89.

Coleman, E., Strapko, N., Zubrzycki, M. R., & Broach, C. L. (1993). Social and psychological needs of lesbian mothers. *Canadian Journal of Human Sexuality, 2*(1), 13–17.

D'Augelli, A. R., & Hershberger, S. L. (1993). Lesbian, gay, and bisexual youth in community settings: Personal challenges and mental health problems. *American Journal of Community Psychology, 21*, 421–448.

Deevey, S. (1990). Older lesbian women an invisible minority. *Journal of Gerontological Nursing, 16*(5), 35–39.

Deren, S., Goldstein, M., Williams, M., Stark, M., Estrada, A., Friedman, S. R., Young, R. M., Needle, R., Tortu, S., Saunders, L., Beardsley, M., Jose, B., & McCoy, V. (1996). Sexual orientation, HIV risk behavior, and serostatus in a multisite sample of drug-injecting and crack-using women. *Women's Health: Research on Gender, Behavior, and Policy, 2*(1&2), 35–47.

Diamant, A. L., Schuster, M. A., McGuigan, K., & Lever, J. (1999). Lesbians' sexual history with men. *Archives of Internal Medicine, 159*, 2730–2736.

Douglas, C. J., Kalman, C. M., & Kalman, T. P. (1984). Homophobia among physicians and nurses: An empirical study. *Hospital and Community Psychiatry, 36*, 1309–1311.

Durfy, S. J., Bowen, D. J., McTiernan, A., Sporleder, J., & Burke, W. (1999). Attitudes and interest in genetic testing for breast and ovarian cancer susceptibility in diverse groups of women in western Washington. *Cancer Epidemiology, Biomarkers & Prevention, 8,* 369–375.

Einhorn, L., & Polgar, M. (1994). HIV-risk behavior among lesbians and bisexual women. *AIDS Education and Prevention, 6,* 514–523.

Eliason, M. J. (1998). Correlates of prejudice in nursing students. *Journal of Nursing Education, 37,* 27–29.

Eliason, M., Donelan, C., & Randall, C. (1992). Lesbian stereotypes. *Health Care for Women International, 13,* 131–144.

Eliason, M. J., & Randall, C. E. (1991). Lesbian phobia in nursing students. *Western Journal of Nursing Research, 13,* 363–374.

Ellingson, L. A., & Yarber, W. L. (1997). Breast self-examination, the Health Belief Model, and sexual orientation in women. *Journal of Sex Education and Therapy, 22*(3), 19–24.

Eskenazi, B., Pies, C., Newstetter, A., Shepard, C., & Pearson, K. (1989). HIV serology in artificially inseminated lesbians. *Journal of Acquired Immune Deficiency Syndromes, 2,* 187–193.

French, S. A., Story, M., Remafedi, G., Resnick, M. D., & Blum, R. W. (1996). Sexual orientation and prevalence of body dissatisfaction and eating disordered behaviors: A population-based study of adolescents. *International Journal of Eating Disorders, 19,* 119–126.

Garofalo, R., Wolf, R. C., Wissow, L. S., Woods, E. R., & Goodman, E. (1999). Sexual orientation and risk of suicide attempts among a representative sample of youth. *Archives of Pediatrics and Adolescent Medicine, 153,* 487–493.

Geddes, V. A. (1994). Lesbian expectations and experiences with family doctors. *Canadian Family Physician, 40,* 908–920.

Gillow, K. E., & Davis, L. L. (1987). Lesbian stress and coping methods. *Journal of Psychosocial Nursing and Mental Health Services, 25*(9), 28–32.

Gomez, C. A., Garcia, D. R., Kegebein, V. J., Shade, S. B., & Hernandez, S. R. (1996). Sexual identity versus sexual behavior: Implications for HIV prevention strategies for women who have sex with women. *Women's Health: Research on Gender, Behavior, and Policy, 2*(1&2), 91–109.

Hall, J. M. (1992). An exploration of lesbians' images of recovery from alcohol problems. *Health Care for Women International, 13,* 181–198.

Hall, J. M. (1994a). The experiences of lesbians in Alcoholics Anonymous. *Western Journal of Nursing Research, 16,* 556–576.

Hall, J. M. (1994b). Lesbians recovering from alcohol problems: An ethnographic study of health care experiences. *Nursing Research, 43,* 238–244.

Hall, J. M. (1996a). Geography of childhood sexual abuse: Women's narratives of their childhood environments. *Advances in Nursing Science, 18*(4), 29–47.

Hall, J. M. (1996b). Pervasive effects of childhood sexual abuse in lesbians' recovery from alcohol problems. *Substance Use & Misuse, 31,* 225–239.

Hall, J. M. (1998). Lesbians surviving childhood sexual abuse: Pivotal experiences related to sexual orientation, gender, and race. *Journal of Lesbian Studies, 2*(1), 7–28.

Hall, J. M. (1999). Lesbians in alcohol recovery surviving childhood sexual abuse and parental substance abuse. *International Journal of Psychiatric Nursing Research, 5*, 507–515.

Hammelman, T. L. (1993). Gay and lesbian youth: Contributing factors to serious attempts or considerations of suicide. *Journal of Gay & Lesbian Psychotherapy, 2*(1), 77–89.

Harris, M. B., Nightengale, J., & Owen, N. (1995). Health care professionals' experience, knowledge, and attitudes concerning homosexuality. *Journal of Gay & Lesbian Social Services, 2*(2), 91–107.

Harvey, S. M., Carr, C., & Bernheine, S. (1989). Lesbian mothers: Health care experiences. *Journal of Nurse-Midwifery, 34*, 115–119.

Heffernan, K. (1996). Eating disorders and weight concern among lesbians. *International Journal of Eating Disorders, 19*, 127–138.

Herek, G. M., Gillis, J. R., Cogan, J. C., & Glunt, E. K. (1997). Hate crime victimization among lesbian, gay, and bisexual adults. *Journal of Interpersonal Violence, 12*(2), 195–215.

Hitchcock, J. M., & Wilson, H. S. (1992). Personal risking: Lesbian self-disclosure of sexual orientation to professional health care providers. *Nursing Research, 41*, 178–183.

Hughes, T. L., Haas, A. P., & Avery, L. (1997). Lesbians and mental health: Preliminary results from the Chicago Women's Health Survey. *Journal of the Gay and Lesbian Medical Association, 1*, 137–148.

Johnson, S. R., Guenther, S. M., Laube, D. W., & Keettel, W. C. (1981). Factors influencing lesbian gynecologic care: A preliminary study. *American Journal of Obstetrics and Gynecology, 140*, 20–28.

Johnson, S. R., Smith, E. M., & Guenther, S. M. (1987). Comparison of gynecologic health care problems between lesbian and bisexual women: A survey of 2,345 women. *Journal of Reproductive Medicine, 32*, 805–811.

Kehoe, M. (1986). Lesbians over 65: A triply invisible minority. *Journal of Homosexuality, 12*, 139–152.

Kehoe, M. (1988). *Lesbians over 60 speak for themselves.* New York: Harrington Park Press.

Kral, A. H., Lorvick, J., Bluthenthal, R. N., & Watters, J. K. (1997). HIV risk profile of drug-using women who have sex with women in 19 United States cities. *Journal of Acquired Immune Deficiency Syndromes and Human Retrovirology, 16*, 211–217.

Kunkel, L. E., & Skokan, L. A. (1998). Factors which influence cervical cancer screening among lesbians. *Journal of the Gay and Lesbian Medical Association, 2*(1), 7–15.

Lampon, D. (1995). Lesbians and safer sex practices. *Feminism and Psychology, 5*, 170–176.

Lauver, D. R., Karon, S. L., Egan, J., Jacobson, M., Nugent, J., Settersten, L., & Shaw, V. (1999). Understanding lesbians' mammography utilization. *Women's Health Issues, 9*, 264–274.

Lehmann, J. B., Lehmann, C. U., & Kelly, P. J. (1998). Development and health care needs of lesbians. *Journal of Women's Health, 7*, 379–387.

Leiblum, S. R., Palmer, M. G., & Spector, I. P. (1995). Non-traditional mothers: Single heterosexual/lesbian women and lesbian couples electing motherhood via donor insemination. *Journal of Psychosomatic Obstetrics and Gynasoecology, 16*(1), 11–20.

Lemp, G. F., Jones, J., Kellogg, T. A., Nieri, G. N., Anderson, L., Withum, D., & Katz, M. (1995). HIV seroprevalence and risk behaviors among lesbians and bisexual women in San Francisco and Berkeley, California. *American Journal of Public Health, 85,* 1549–1552.

Levy, E. F. (1989). Lesbian motherhood: Identity and social support. *Affilia, 4*(4), 40–53.

Lewis, C. E., Saghir, M. T., & Robins, E. (1982). Drinking patterns in homosexual and heterosexual women. *Journal of Clinical Psychiatry, 43,* 277–279.

Lie, G., & Gentlewarrior, S. (1991). Intimate violence in lesbian relationships: Discussion of survey findings and practice implications. *Journal of Social Service Research, 15*(1/2), 41–59.

Lie, G., Schillt, R., Bush, J., Montagne, M., & Reyes, L. (1991). Lesbians in currently aggressive relationships: How frequently do they report aggressive past relationships? *Violence and Victims, 6,* 121–135.

Lockhart, L. L., White, B. W., Causby, V., & Isaac, A. (1994). Letting out the secret: Violence in lesbian relationships. *Journal of Interpersonal Violence, 9,* 469–492.

Lucas, V. A. (1992). An investigation of the health care preferences of the lesbian population. *Health Care for Women International, 13,* 221–228.

Ludwig, M. R., & Brownell, K. D. (1999). Lesbians, bisexual women, and body image: An investigation of gender roles and social group affiliation. *International Journal of Eating Disorders, 25,* 89–97.

Marrazzo, J. M., Koutsky, L. A., Stine, K. L., Kuypers, J. M., Grubert, T. A., Galloway, D. A., Kiviat, N. B., & Handsfield, H. H. (1998). Genital human papillomavirus infection in women who have sex with women. *Journal of Infectious Diseases, 178,* 1604–1609.

Martinson, J. C., Fisher, D. G., & DeLapp, T. D. (1996). Client disclosure of lesbianism: A challenge for health care providers. *Journal of Gay & Lesbian Social Services, 4*(3), 81–94.

Mathews, W. C., Booth, M. W., Turner, J. D., & Kessler, L. (1986). Physicians' attitudes toward homosexuality—Survey of a California county medical society. *Western Journal of Medicine, 144,* 106–110.

Mays, V. M., Beckman, L. J., Oranchak, E., & Harper, B. (1994). Perceived social support for help-seeking behaviors of Black heterosexual and homosexually active women alcoholics. *Psychology of Addictive Behaviors, 8,* 235–242.

McCaffrey, M., Varney, P., Evans, B., & Taylor-Robinson, D. (1999). Bacterial vaginosis in lesbians: Evidence for lack of sexual transmission. *International Journal of STD & AIDS, 10,* 305–308.

McKirnan, D. J., & Peterson, P. L. (1989). Alcohol and drug use among homosexual men and women: Epidemiology and population characteristics. *Addictive Behaviors, 14,* 545–553.

McNally, E. B., & Finnegan, D. G. (1992). Lesbian recovering alcoholics: A qualitative study of identity transformation—A report on research and applications to treatment. *Journal of Chemical Dependency Treatment, 5*(1), 93–103.

Moore, J., Warren, D., Zierler, S., Schuman, P., Solomon, L., Schoenbaum, E. E., & Kennedy, M. (1996). Characteristics of HIV-infected lesbians and bisexual women in four urban centers. *Women's Health: Research on Gender, Behavior, and Policy, 2*(1&2), 49–60.

Moran, N. (1996). Lesbian health care needs. *Canadian Family Physician, 42,* 879–884.

Morgan, K. S. (1992). Caucasian lesbians' use of psychotherapy. *Psychology of Women Quarterly, 16,* 127–130.

Morgan, K. S. (1997). Why lesbians choose therapy: Presenting problems, attitudes, and political concerns. *Journal of Gay & Lesbian Social Services, 6*(3), 57–75.

Morgan, K. S., & Eliason, M. J. (1992). The role of psychotherapy in Caucasian lesbians' lives. *Women and Therapy, 13*(4), 27–52.

Norman, A. D., Perry, M. J., Stevenson, L. Y., Kelly, J. A., & Roffman, R. A. (1996). Lesbian and bisexual women in small cities—At risk for HIV? *Public Health Reports, 111,* 347–352.

Olesker, E., & Walsh, L. V. (1984). Childbearing among lesbians: Are we meeting their needs? *Journal of Nurse-Midwifery, 29,* 322–329.

Otis, M. D., & Skinner, W. F. (1996). The prevalence of victimization and its effect on mental well-being among lesbian and gay people. *Journal of Homosexuality, 30*(3), 93–121.

Paroski, P. A. (1987). Health care delivery and the concerns of gay and lesbian adolescents. *Journal of Adolescent Health Care, 8,* 188–192.

Patton, C. L., Millard, P. S., Kessenich, C. R., Storm, D., Kinnicutt, E., & Rosen, C. J. (1998). Screening calcaneal ultrasound and risk factors for osteoporosis among lesbians and heterosexual women. *Journal of Women's Health, 7,* 909–915.

Perry, S. M. (1995). Lesbian alcohol and marijuana use: Correlates of HIV risk behaviors and abusive relationships. *Journal of Psychoactive Drugs, 27,* 413–419.

Price, J. H., Easton, A. N., Telljohann, S. K., & Wallace, P. B. (1996). Perceptions of cervical cancer and Pap smear screening behavior by women's sexual orientation. *Journal of Community Health, 21,* 89–105.

Raiteri, R., Fora, R., Gioannini, P., Russo, R., Lucchini, A., Terzi, M. G., Giacobbi, D., & Sinicco, A. (1994). Seroprevalence, risk factors and attitude to HIV-1 in a representative sample of lesbians in Turin. *Genitourinary Medicine, 70,* 200–205.

Randall, C. E. (1989). Lesbian phobia among BSN educators: A survey. *Journal of Nursing Education, 28,* 302–306.

Rankow, E. J. (1997). Lesbian health issues and cultural sensitivity training for providers in the primary care setting: Results of a pilot intervention. *Journal of the Gay and Lesbian Medical Association, 1,* 227–234.

Rankow, E. J., Cambre, K. M., & Cooper, K. (1998). Health care-seeking behavior of adult lesbian and bisexual survivors of childhood sexual abuse. *Journal of the Gay and Lesbian Medical Association, 2,* 69–76.

Rankow, E. J., & Tessaro, I. (1998). Cervical cancer risk and Papanicolaou screening in a sample of lesbian and bisexual women. *Journal of Family Practice, 47,* 139–143.

Rankow, E. J., & Tessaro, I. (1998). Mammography and risk factors for breast cancer in lesbian and bisexual women. *American Journal of Health Behavior, 22,* 403–410.

Reagan, P. (1981). The interaction of health professionals and their lesbian clients. *Patient Counselling and Health Education, 3*(1), 21–25.

Renzetti, C. M. (1992). *Violent betrayal: Partner abuse in lesbian relationships.* Newbury Park, CA: Sage.

Roberts, S. A., Dibble, S. L., Scanlon, J. L., Paul, S. M., & Davids, H. (1998). Differences in risk factors for breast cancer: Lesbian and heterosexual women. *Journal of the Gay and Lesbian Medical Association, 2*, 93–101.

Roberts, S. J., & Sorensen, L. (1999). Health related behaviors and cancer screening of lesbians: Results from the Boston Lesbian Health Project. *Women and Health, 28*(4), 1–12.

Robertson, M. M. (1992). Lesbians as an invisible minority in the health services arena. *Health Care for Women International, 13*, 155–163.

Robertson, P., & Schachter, J. (1981). Failure to identify venereal disease in a lesbian population. *Sexually Transmitted Diseases, 8*, 75–76.

Rosario, M., Hunter, J., & Gwadz, M. (1997). Exploration of substance use among lesbian, gay, and bisexual youth: Prevalence and correlates. *Journal of Adolescent Research, 12*, 454–476.

Rush, M. M. (1997). A study of the relations among perceived social support, spirituality, and power as knowing participation in change among sober female alcoholics within the science of unitary human beings. *Journal of Addictions Nursing, 9*, 146–155.

Ryan, C., & Bradford, J. (1993). The National Lesbian Health Care Survey: An overview. In L. D. Garnets & D. C. Kimmel (Eds.), *Psychological perspectives on lesbian and gay male experiences* (pp. 541–556). New York: Columbia University Press.

Saewyc, E. M., Bearinger, L. H., Blum, R. W., & Resnick, M. D. (1999). Sexual intercourse, abuse and pregnancy among adolescent women: Does sexual orientation make a difference? *Family Planning Perspectives, 31*, 127–131.

Saewyc, E. M., Bearinger, L. H., Heinz, P. A., Blum, R. W., & Resnick, M. D. (1998). Gender differences in health and risk behaviors among bisexual and homosexual adolescents. *Journal of Adolescent Health, 23*, 181–188.

Scherzer, T. (1998). Domestic violence in lesbian relationships: Findings of the Lesbian Relationships research project. *Journal of Lesbian Studies, 2*(1), 29–47.

Schilit, R., Lie, G., & Montagne, M. (1990). Substance use as a correlate of violence in intimate lesbian relationships. *Journal of Homosexuality, 19*, 51–65.

Shotsky, W. J. (1996). Women who have sex with other women: HIV seroprevalence in New York state counseling and testing programs. *Women and Health, 24*(2), 1–15.

Siever, M. D. (1994). Sexual orientation and gender as factors in socioculturally acquired vulnerability to body dissatisfaction and eating disorders. *Journal of Consulting and Clinical Psychology, 62*, 252–260.

Skinner, C. J., Stokes, J., Kirlew, Y., Kavanagh, J., & Forster, G. E. (1996). A case-controlled study of the sexual health needs of lesbians. *Genitourinary Medicine, 72*, 277–280.

Skinner, W. F. (1994). The prevalence and demographic predictors of illicit and licit drug use among lesbians and gay men. *American Journal of Public Health, 84*, 1307–1310.

Skinner, W. F., & Otis, M. D. (1996). Drug and alcohol use among lesbian and gay people in a southern U.S. sample: Epidemiological, comparative, and methodological findings from the Trilogy Project. *Journal of Homosexuality, 30*(3), 59–92.

Smith, E. M., Johnson, S. R., & Guenther, S. M. (1985). Health care attitudes and experiences during gynecologic care among lesbians and bisexuals. *American Journal of Public Health, 75,* 1085–1087.

Solarz, A. L. (Ed.). (1999). *Lesbian health: Current assessment and directions for the future.* Washington, DC: National Academy Press.

Sorensen, L., & Roberts, S. J. (1997). Lesbian uses of and satisfaction with mental health services: Results from Boston Lesbian Health Project. *Journal of Homosexuality, 33,* 35–49.

Stevens, P. E. (1992). Lesbian health care research: A review of the literature form 1970 to 1990. *Health Care for Women International, 13,* 91–120.

Stevens, P. E. (1993a). Health care interactions as experienced by clients: Lesbians' narratives. *Communicating Nursing Research, 26,* 93–100.

Stevens, P. E. (1993b). Marginalized women's access to health care: A feminist narrative analysis. *Advances in Nursing Science, 16*(2), 39–56.

Stevens, P. E. (1994a). HIV prevention education for lesbians and bisexual women: A cultural analysis of a community intervention. *Social Science and Medicine, 39,* 1565–1578.

Stevens, P. E. (1994b). Lesbians' health-related experiences of care and noncare. *Western Journal of Nursing Research, 16,* 639–659.

Stevens, P. E. (1994c). Protective strategies of lesbian clients in health care environments. *Research in Nursing and Health, 17,* 217–229.

Stevens, P. E. (1995). Structural and interpersonal impact of heterosexual assumptions on lesbian health care clients. *Nursing Research, 44,* 25–30.

Stevens, P. E. (1996). Lesbians and doctors: Experiences of solidarity and domination in health care settings. *Gender & Society, 10*(1), 24–41.

Stevens, P. E., & Hall, J. M. (1988). Stigma, health beliefs and experiences with health care in lesbian women. *Image: Journal of Nursing Scholarship, 20,* 69–73.

Stevens, P. E., & Hall, J. M. (1990). Abusive health care interactions experienced by lesbians: A case of institutional violence in the treatment of women. *Response to the Victimization of Women, 13*(3), 23–27.

Stevens, P. E., & Hall, J. M. (1997). Emotional and social contingencies affecting HIV risk reduction among lesbians and bisexual women. *Journal of the Gay and Lesbian Medical Association, 1*(1), 5–14.

Stevens, P. E., & Hall, J. M. (1998). Participatory action research for sustaining individual and community change: A model of HIV prevention education. *AIDS Education and Prevention, 10,* 387–402.

Stewart, M. (1999). Lesbian parents talk about their birth experiences. *British Journal of Midwifery, 7*(2), 96–101.

Striegel-Moore, R. H., Tucker, N., & Hsu, J. (1990). Body image dissatisfaction and disordered eating in lesbian college students. *International Journal of Eating Disorders, 9,* 493–500.

Tiemann, K. A., Kennedy, S. A., & Haga, M. P. (1997). Lesbians' experiences with helping professionals. *Affilia, 12*(1), 84–95.

Tiemann, K. A., Kennedy, S. A., & Haga, M. P. (1998). Rural lesbians' strategies for coming out to health care professionals. *Journal of Lesbian Studies, 2,* 61–75.

Trippet, S. E., & Bain, J. (1994). Lesbians' mental health concerns. *Health Care for Women International, 15,* 317–323.

Trippet, S. E., & Bain, J. (1993). Physical health problems and concerns of lesbians. *Health Care for Women International, 20,* 59–70.

Trippet, S. E., & Bain, J. (1990). Preliminary study of lesbian health concerns. *Health Values, 14*(6), 30–36.

Trippet, S. E., & Bain, J. (1992). Reasons American lesbians fail to seek traditional health care. *Health Care for Women International, 13,* 145–153.

Tuel, B. D., & Russell, R. K. (1998). Self-esteem and depression in battered women. *Violence Against Women, 4,* 344–362.

Tully, C. T. (1995). In sickness and in health: Forty years of research on lesbians. *Journal of Gay and Lesbian Social Services, 3,* 1–18.

Waldner-Haugrud, L. K., & Gratch, L. V. (1997). Sexual coercion in gay/lesbian relationships: Descriptives and gender differences. *Violence and Victims, 12,* 87–98.

Waldner-Haugrud, L. K., Gratch, L. V., & Magruder, B. (1997). Victimization and perpetration rates of violence in gay and lesbian relationships: Gender issues explored. *Violence and Victims, 12,* 173–184.

Waterman, C. K., Dawson, L. J., & Bologna, M. J. (1989). Sexual coercion in gay male and lesbian relationships: Predictors and implications for support services. *Journal of Sex Research, 26,* 118–124.

Welch, S., Howden-Chapman, P., & Collings, S. C. D. (1998). Survey of drug and alcohol use by lesbian women in New Zealand. *Addictive Behaviors, 23,* 543–548.

Wendland, C. L., Byrn, F., & Hill, C. (1996). Donor insemination: A comparison of lesbian couples, heterosexual couples and single women. *Fertility and Sterility, 65,* 764–770.

White, J. C., & Dull, V. T. (1997). Health risk factors and health-seeking behavior in lesbians. *Journal of Women's Health, 6,* 103–112.

White, J. C., & Dull, V. T. (1998). Room for improvement: Communication between lesbians and primary care providers. *Journal of Lesbian Studies, 2*(1), 95–110.

Zeidenstein, L. (1990). Gynecological and childbearing needs of lesbians. *Journal of Nurse-Midwifery, 35*(1), 10–18.

Ziemba-Davis, M., Sanders, S. A., & Reinisch, J. M. (1996). Lesbians' sexual interactions with men: Behavioral bisexuality and risk for sexually transmitted disease (STD) and human immunodeficiency virus (HIV). *Women's Health: Research on Gender, Behavior, and Policy, 2*(1&2), 61–74.

Chapter 7

Immigrant Women and Their Health

KAREN J. AROIAN

ABSTRACT

Immigrant women's health is a relatively new research area. At the beginning of the 1990s, nurse scholars concluded that there was insufficient research on this topic. They recommended broadening the overly narrow research foci on immigrant women's childbearing and on select populations, developing national data bases, identifying high-risk groups, and developing population-specific interventions. This chapter reviews 292 research articles published in journals during the 1990s about adult immigrant women's health. It: (1) summarizes research findings on topics that were the major foci of research conducted in the 1990s, (2) evaluates progress over the last decade in the research agenda proposed above, and (3) makes recommendations for research in the new millennium.

Key words: breastfeeding, female genital mutilation, health service use and screening behavior, menopause, mental health, parity and family planning, pregnancy outcomes, sexually transmitted diseases

The late 20th century has been characterized as the "age of migration" and a time of increased migration for women (Castles & Miller, 1996). In 1990, about 47.7% of the 120 million of the world's immigrants[1] were women

---

[1]The term "immigrant" is used to indicate people who move from one country to another with the intention of permanent residence. This usage is more inclusive than the legal definition and includes refugees and other types of international migrants (e.g., undocumented persons).

(Zlotnik, 1999). The prevalence of immigration and the percentage of women immigrants continues to grow into the 21st century (Zlotnik, 1999).

Over the last two decades, research on immigrant health has been burgeoning in nursing as well as other disciplines. Research that specifically addresses immigrant women and their health, however, is a more recent development. Regarding the state of the science in the 1980s, feminist scholars in nursing concluded that immigrant women were neglected, both in studies about women at large as well as in studies of immigration (Anderson, 1985; Boyd, 1984; Kulig, 1990; Lynam, 1985; Meleis & Rogers, 1987). During the 1990 keynote address for the Fourth International Congress on Women's Health Issues, Meleis (1991) proposed an agenda for future study of immigrant women, including identifying high-risk groups and developing population-specific interventions. An overly narrow research focus on childbearing was also noted, and a major recommendation was to broaden this focus to the multiple roles women fulfill in their daily lives (Meleis, Lipson, Muecke, & Smith, 1998). In the mid 1990s, nurse scholars stated that we still have inadequate information to promote immigrant women's health, in part because national data bases are lacking and studies are limited to select populations (Lipson, McElmurry, & LaRosa, 1997).

SCOPE OF THE REVIEW

In this chapter I will review research articles published in journals during the 1990s about adult immigrant women's health. I evaluate progress in the research agenda proposed above, summarize generalizations from the research, and recommend direction for future research. The literature was located through on-line computer searches of select abstracting services and citation indexes. Key search terms were "women" or "female" or "gender" or "sex difference" AND "immigrant(s)/immigration" or "refugee(s)" AND "health" or "depression" or "anxiety" or "stress." The indexes were the Cumulative Index to Nursing and Allied Health Literature (CINAHL), MEDLINE, SOCIAL SCIENCES, and Public Affairs Information Service (PAIS). PAIS was included because it is international in scope, however, for practical reasons, non-English articles were excluded. This strategy yielded articles that were exclusively as well as not exclusively about immigrant women. In the latter case, the articles were included in the review if gender and immigrant status were study variables. Although an exclusive focus on immigrant women is a valuable feminist research strategy to offset how women have been neglected, comparative studies were included to explore gender differences in immigrants as well as similarities and differences among immigrant and non-immigrant minority women.

This search yielded a total of 292 articles for review, which may be an underestimate from a manual search or tracking citations from one study to another. Therefore, this chapter is a summary of the state of the science on immigrant women's health for studies reported in English and indexed by the above sources.

SUBSTANTIVE FOCI ON IMMIGRANT WOMEN'S HEALTH

The reviewed articles are listed in Table 7.1 by primary author and year (additional authors are included if needed to distinguish the citation from others). A study summary is also included in Table 7.1 according to chief substantive area(s), the primary author's academic discipline (when known), group(s) of immigrant women by country or region, and study site (usually by U.S. state or, when international, by country or region). "Varied" is used to specify immigrant group when the study sample was identified generally as foreign-born /not native language speaking or when there were more than three regionally diverse groups.

Of the 292 articles reviewed, almost half (48.5%) were of studies conducted in the U.S., followed in number by Australia, Canada, Israel, and Great Britain. Only a few studies were conducted in Puerto Rico, the Ivory Coast, Belize, Hong Kong, New Zealand, Pakistan, the Near East, and elsewhere in Europe. Study site is biased, however, by the fact that only articles published in English were included in the review. Of the studies conducted in the U.S., the highest percent (44.68%) were conducted in California, with the next largest percent (10.64%) conducted in New York. Discipline of the primary author for the largest number of articles was nursing (30.5%), followed by medicine (including psychiatry) (21.8%), and public health (17.7%).

The majority of articles pertained to the following substantive areas[2]: (1) Health Behavior (HB), including health beliefs and folk practices, illness management, health promotion, health risk, health care delivery, use of general and specialty health services, and health screening (33.3%); (2) Women's

[2]This classification was derived from the stated study focus as well as my content analysis of study findings. Alternative classifications are also valid. Percentages are based on $N = 313$, which includes dual classification of studies with more than one substantive area. Prenatal service use and postpartum depression were classified dually as Health Behavior (HB) and Women's Bodies (WB) and as Mental Health (MH) and Women's Bodies (WH), respectively.

TABLE 7.1   Summary of Studies Conducted in the 1990s

Primary author	Topical area	Discipline	Immigrant group	Study site
Ahmad, '97	HB	Social Economy	Asian	Great Britain
Alexander, '96	HB;WB	Public Health	Japanese	US
Allodi, '90	MH	Medicine	Latina	Canada
Anderson, '91	HB	Nursing	Chinese	Canada
Anderson, '93	HB	Nursing	Chinese	Canada
Anderson, '95	HB	Nursing	Chinese	Canada
Anderson, Blue, '91	HB	Nursing	Chinese	Canada
Arbesman, '93	WB	Medicine	Somali	NY
Aroian, '98	MH	Nursing	Russian	MA
Azize-Vargas, '98	HB	Women's Studies	Dominican	Puerto Rico
Baider, '96	MH	Medicine	Russian	Israel
Balarajan, '97	M/M		Bangladeshi	Great Britain
Balcazar, '97	WB	Public Health	Mexican	AZ
Beine, '95	WB	Nursing	Somali	CA
Bell, '99	HB		Varied	Great Britain
Bennett, '93	HB	Epidemiology	Varied	Australia
Berg, '99	WB	Nursing	Filipina	AZ
Berg, Lipson, '99	WB	Nursing	Filipina	CA
Bernstein, '98	MH	Sociology	Russian	Israel
Berry, '99	WB	Nursing	Mexican	CA
Bindels, '94	M/M;WB	Public Health	Varied	Netherlands
Birman, '94	MH	Psychology	Russian	Washington DC
Black, '98	MH	Medicine	Mexican	US
Blesch, '99	M/M	Epidemiology	South Asian	US
Bowes, '95	HB	Sociology	Pakistani	Great Britain
Boxall, '94	M/M	Epidemiology	Varied	Great Britain
Bridget, '93	M/M	Medicine	Chinese	Australia
Brown, '96	HB		Greek	Australia
Brown, '97	HB	Women's Health	Filipina	Australia
Brown, '99	WB	Medicine	Varied	CA
Buchwald, '93	MH	Medicine	Vietnamese	CA,HI,OR,WA
Burnette, '99	Misc.	Sociology	Latina	NY
Burton, '99	HB;WB	Public Health	Pacific Islander	Australia
Chavez, '97a	HB	Anthropology	Latina	CA
Chavez, '97b	HB	Anthropology	Latina	CA
Chavez, '95	HB	Anthropology	Mexican, Salvadoran	CA

TABLE 7.1   *(continued)*

Primary author	Topical area	Discipline	Immigrant group	Study site
Choudhry, '98	HB	Nursing	Indian	Canada
Choudhry, Srivastava, '98	HB	Nursing	Indian, Pakistani	Canada
Chow, '99	HB	Social Welfare	Russian, Varied	NY
Chung, '93	MH	Nursing	Southeast Asian	CA
Cobas, '96	WB	Sociology	Mexican	US
Condon, '93	WB	Public Health	Varied	Australia
Crane, '96	HB	Public Health	Varied	CA
Cwikel, '94	WB	Social work	Russian	Israel
D'Avanzo, '94	MH	Nursing	Cambodian	CA, MA
D'Avanzo, '98	MH	Nursing	Cambodian	France, US
Daly, '98	HB	Nursing	Lebanese	Canada
Davila, '99	MH;WB	Nursing	Mexican	Tex
De Santis, '95	Misc.	Nursing	Cuban, Haitian	FL
Dolman, '96	HB		Varied	Australia
Donato, '91	HB	Public Health	Varied	Italy
Doucet, '92	WB	Public Health	Varied	Canada
Downs, '97	HB	Nursing	Cambodian	MA
Dyck, '92	HB	Rehabilitation	Chinese	Canada
Dyck, '95	HB	Rehabilitation	Chinese, Indian	Canada
Eden, '95	HB	Medicine	Varied	Sweden
Edwards, '94	HB	Nursing	Varied	Canada
Edwards, '97	WB	Nursing	Varied	Canada
English, '97	WB	Public Health	Mexican	CA
Erickson, '99	HB	Speech	Korean	IL
Esposito, '99	WB	Nursing	Varied	NY
Ever-Hadani, '94	HB	Public Health	Varied	Israel
Eyega, '97	WB	Public Health	African	NY
Factourovich, '96	MH	Medicine	Russian	Israel
Faller, '92	WB	Nursing	Hmong	NC
Farr, '97	HB	Sociology	Mexican	OR
Farrales, '99	HB	Nutrition	Filipina	Canada
Fernandez, '98	HB	Public Health	Hispanic	Wash. D.C.
Fitch, '97	HB	Nursing	Varied	Canada
Flaskerud, '96	MH	Nursing	Latina	CA
Fornazzari, '90	MH	Medicine	Latina	Canada
Fox, '91	MH	Nursing	Vietnamese	IL
Fox, '95	MH	Nursing	Southeast Asian	Not specified

(continued)

TABLE 7.1   *(continued)*

Primary author	Topical area	Discipline	Immigrant group	Study site
Fox, '97	MH	Nursing	Southeast Asian	IL
Franks, '90	MH	Nursing	Varied	Canada
Fruchter, '90	M/M	Public Health	Caribbean	NY
Frye, '94a	MH	Nursing	Cambodian	CA,MA
Frye, '94b	MH	Nursing	Cambodian	CA,MA
Fuentes-Afflick, '98	WB	Epidemiology	Varied	CA
Fulton, '95	HB	Community Health	Hispanic	RI
Furnham, '93	MH	Psychology	Indian, Pakistani	Great Britain
Gaffney, '97	WB	Nursing	Hispanic	VA
Gagnon, '97	WB	Nursing	Varied	Canada
Gannage, '99	Misc.	Sociology	Varied	Canada
Gelfand, '94	Misc.	Gerontology	Varied	Australia
Ghaemi-Ahmadi, '92	WB	Nutrition	Varied	US
Ghaffarian, '98	MH	Psychology	Iranian	CA
Gifford, '94	WB		Australian	Australia
Glasser, '98	MH;WB		Russian	Israel
Glover, '91	MH	Public Health	Varied	Great Britain
Golding, '93	MH	Medicine	Mexican	CA
Gomez, '99	HB;WB		Latina	CA
Granot, '96	WB	Nursing	Ethiopian	Israel
Greene, '92	M/M	Public Health	Ethiopian	Israel
Grisaru, '97	WB	Medicine	Ethiopian	Israel
Harding, '95	M/M	Public Health	Varied	Great Britain
Hattar-Pollara, '95a	MH	Nursing	Jordanian	CA
Hattar-Pollara, '95b	MH	Nursing	Jordanian	CA
Hauff, '95	MH	Medicine	Vietnamese	Norway
Have, '99	HB		Varied	Netherlands
Hemingway, '97	HB	Public Health	Varied	Great Britain
Henriksen, '95	WB	Nutrition	Pakistani	Norway
Herrinton, '94	M/M	Public Health	Asian	CA,HI,WA,
Hiatt, '96	HB	Medicine	Varied	CA
Hilder, '93	WB	Epidemiology	Bangladeshi	Great Britain
Hjelm, '99	HB	Community Health	Yugoslavian	Sweden
Horswill, '99	WB	Nutrition	Chinese	CA

TABLE 7.1   *(continued)*

Primary author	Topical area	Discipline	Immigrant group	Study site
Hubbell, '95	HB	Health Policy	Mexican, Salvadoran	CA
Hubbell, '96	HB	Health Policy	Latina	CA
Hummer, '99	WB	Sociology	Varied	US
Hurh, '90	MH	Soc/Anth	Korean	IL
Hurtig, '98	WB	Medicine	Varied	Great Britain
Hyman, '96	WB	Public Health	Varied	Canada
Ibison, '96	WB	Public Health	Varied	Great Britain
Im, Meleis, '99	WB	Nursing	Korean	CA
Im, Meleis, Lee, '99	WB	Nursing	Korean	CA
Iscovich, '98	M/M	Medicine	Varied	Israel
Jackson, '95	MH	Nursing	Varied	Australia
Jackson, '96	MH	Nursing	Varied	Australia
Jacob, '98	MH	Medicine	Indian	Great Britain
Jenkins, '90	HB	Public Health	Vietnamese	CA
Jermott, '99	WB	Nursing	Asian, Pacific Islander	N.E. US city
Johansson, '97	MH	Medicine	Varied	Sweden
Jones, '97	HB	Medicine	Hispanic	Tex
Jones, '99	WB	Nursing	Mexican	Tex
Juarbe, '98	HB	Nursing	Mexican	CA
Kahler, '96	MH;WB	Nursing	Varied	NY
Kalofonos, '99	HB		Mexican	CA
Kamineni, '99	M/M	Public Health	Asian	CA,HI,WA
Kaufman, '95	HB	Medicine	Russian	Israel
Kieffer, '99	WB	Public Health	Varied	US
Kim, '94	MH	Nursing	Korean	So. US city
Kim, '99	MH	Nursing	Korean	M.W. US city
King, '99	HB		African, Caribbean	US
Kliewer, '95a	M/M	Epidemiology	Varied	Canada, Australia
Kliewer, '95b	M/M	Epidemiology	Varied	Canada, Australia
Knapp, '99	WB	Nutrition	Russian	WA
Knight, '99	WB	Medicine	African	Australia

(continued)

TABLE 7.1   *(continued)*

Primary author	Topical area	Discipline	Immigrant group	Study site
Kouris-Blazos, '96	M/M	Medicine	Greek	Australia
Kuiper, '99	Misc.		Varied	CA
Kulig, '94a	MH	Nursing	Cambodian	CA
Kulig, '94b	WB	Nursing	Cambodian	Canada
Kulig, '95	WB	Nursing	Cambodian	CA
Kulwicki, '99	MH	Nursing	Arab	M.W. US city
Kuss, '97	WB	Nursing	Vietnamese	WA
Kwan, '97	WB	Public Health	Chinese	Hong Kong
Layzell, '99	WB		Turkish	Great Britain
Leidy, '98	WB	Anthropology	Hispanic	FL,NY,S.W.
Lenart, '91	Misc.	Nursing	Cambodian	WA
Lesjak, '99	HB	Medicine	Vietnamese	Australia
Li, '90	WB	Public Health	Southeast Asian	WA
Lindenberg, '99	MH	Nursing	Hispanic	SE US city
Lipson, '94	MH	Nursing	Afghan	CA
Lipson, '95	HB;MH	Nursing	Afghan	CA
Locke, '96	MH	Medicine	Central American	SW US city
Luna, '94	HB	Nursing	Lebanese	MI
Lundberg, '99	HB	Nursing	Thai	Sweden
Ma, '96	WB	Nursing	Varied	Australia
MacIntyre, '93	M/M	Epidemiology	Varied	Australia
Mahloch, '99	HB	Nursing	Cambodian	WA
Maltby, '98	HB	Nursing	Vietnamese	Australia
Maltby, '99	HB	Nursing	Vietnamese	Australia
Mattson, '92	HB	Nursing	Southeast Asian	CA
Matuk, '96a	HB	Nursing	Varied	Canada
Matuk, '96b	HB	Nursing	Varied	Canada
McPhee, Bird, '97	HB	Medicine	Vietnamese	CA
McPhee, _, Ha, '97	HB;MH	Medicine	Vietnamese	CA
McPhee, Stewart, '97	HB	Medicine	Vietnamese	CA
McVeigh, '97	WB	Nursing	Varied	Australia
Meftuh, '91	WB	Public Health	Ethiopian	CA
Menendez, '93	M/M	Epidemiology	Puerto Rican	NY
Miller, '95	WB	Medicine	Afghan	Pakistan
Mirsky, '93	MH	Psychology	Russian	Israel
Mitchell, '95	WB	Public Health	Vietnamese	Australia
Moghaddam, '90	MH	Psychology	Indian	Canada

TABLE 7.1   *(continued)*

Primary author	Topical area	Discipline	Immigrant group	Study site
Mor, '93	WB	Public Health	Korean	HI
Morrell, '99	MH	Medicine	Varied	Australia
Morris, '96	WB	Nursing	Somali	CA
Moss, '93	WB	Sociology	Guatemalan, Salvadoran	Belize
Moss, '96	HB		Mexican, Guatemalan	CA
Mui, '96	MH	Social Work	Chinese	NY
Munet-Vilaro, '99	MH	Nursing	Latina	CA
Nahas, Nawal, '99	MH,WB			
Nahas, Hillege, '99	MH;WB	Nursing	Middle Eastern	Australia
Nedstrand, '95	WB	Medicine	South American	Sweden
Nemoto, '99	MH	Health Policy	Asian	CA
Newell, '98	WB;HB	Medicine	Yugoslavian	Great Britain
Neysmith, '97	MH	Social Work	Varied	Canada
Nilsson, '97	M/M	Epidemiology	Estonian	Sweden
Noh, '92	MH	Occup. Therapy	Korean	Canada
Nolan, '97	M/M	Medicine	Hispanic, Asian	LA
Nwadiora, '96	MH	Social Work	Amerasian	MA
O'Connor, '96	HB;WB	Medicine	Varied	Australia
O'Malley, '99	HB	Medicine	Hispanic	NY
Ogur, '90	MH	Medicine	Latina	MA
Oldenburg, '97	WB	Public Health	Varied	Sweden
Omeri, '97	HB	Nursing	Iranian	Australia
Palacios, '92	MH;HB	Medicine	Latina	Canada
Pang, '90	HB	Nursing	Korean	Wash. D.C.
Pappagallo, '96	HB		Palestinian	Near East
Peel, '96	MH	Medicine	Zairian	Great Britain
Peragallo, '98	HB	Nursing	Mexican, Puerto Rican	US city
Perez-Escamilla, '98	WB	Nutrition	Puerto Rican	CT
Peterson, '98	WB	Sociology	Mexican	AZ
Phipps, '99	HB	Medicine	Southeast Asian	PA
Pickwell, '94	HB	Medicine	Cambodian	CA
Ponizovsky, '97	MH	Medicine	Russian	Israel
Ponizovsky, '98	MH	Medicine	Russian, Ethiopian	Israel

(continued)

TABLE 7.1 *(continued)*

Primary author	Topical area	Discipline	Immigrant group	Study site
Porsch-Oezcueruemez, '99	HB	Medicine	Turkish	Germany
Raleigh, '90	MH	Public Health	Indian	Great Britain
Raleigh, '92	MH	Public Health	Indian, West Indian	Great Britain
Rapp, '97	HB	Anthropology	Varied	NY
Reichman, '98	WB		Latina	NJ
Remennick, '95	WB	Sociology	Russian	Israel
Remennick, '98	HB	Soc /Anth	Russian	Israel
Remennick, '99a	HB	Soc /Anth	Russian	Israel
Remennick, '99b	HB	Soc/Anth	Russian	Israel
Remis, '95	M/M;WB	Public Health	Varied	Canada
Reubsaet, '96	WB	Anthropology	Surinamese	Netherlands
Reynolds, '98	M/M;WB	Medicine	Varied	Canada
Rice, '98a	WB	Public Health	Thai	Australia
Rice, '98b	HB;WB	Public Health	Thai	Australia
Rice, '99	WB	Public Health	Thai	Australia
Ritsner, '98	MH	Medicine	Russian	Israel
Ritsner, '99	MH	Medicine	Russian	Israel
Rodriguez, '98	HB	Medicine	Latina, Asian	CA
Romero, '98–99	HB;WB		Latina	CA
Rossiter, '92a	WB	Nursing	Vietnamese	Australia
Rossiter, '92b	WB	Nursing	Vietnamese	Australia
Rossiter, '94	WB	Nursing	Vietnamese	Australia
Rossiter, '98	WB	Nursing	Vietnamese	Australia
Rothenburg, '99	WB	Medicine	Latina	CA
Ruskin, '96	MH	Medicine	Varied	Israel
Russell, '99	MH	Medicine	Mexican	Mexico, Tex
Santos, '98	MH	Psychology	Mexican	CA
Schreiber, '98	HB	Nursing	West Indian	Canada
Schulmeister, '99	HB	Nursing	Vietnamese	LA
Sherraden, '96a	HB	Social Work	Mexican	IL
Sherraden, '96b	WB	Social Work	Mexican	IL
Sherraden, '96c	WB	Social Work	Mexican	IL
Shin, '93;94	MH	Nursing	Korean	NY
Shin, '99	MH	Nursing	Korean	NY
Silove, '97	MH	Medicine	Varied	Australia
Singer, '96	HB;WB		Varied	Canada
Singh, '96	HB;WB		Varied	US

TABLE 7.1   *(continued)*

Primary author	Topical area	Discipline	Immigrant group	Study site
Small, '98	HB	Public Health	Varied	Australia
Small, '99	HB	Public Health	Varied	Australia
Spring, '95	HB		Hmong	MN
Stanford, '95	M/M	Public Health	Asian	CA,HI,WA
Stehr-Green, '92	M/M	Epidemiology	Varied	New Zealand
Suarez, '97	HB		Mexican	Tex
Sullivan, '97	WB		Vietnamese	Australia
Sundquist, '97	M/M	Public Health	Varied	Sweden
Sundquist, '99	HB	Medicine	Bosnian	Sweden
Swerdlow, '95	M/M	Epidemiology	Indian	Great Britain
Tabora, '97	HB	Nursing	Chinese	CA
Taylor, '99	HB	Public Health	Cambodian	WA
Thompson, '91	MH	Nursing	Cambodian	ME
Thorburn, '98	WB	Women's Health	Mexican	CA
Tran, '90	MH	Social Work	Vietnamese	US
Tran, '93	MH	Social Work	Vietnamese	MA
Tudiver, '99	HB	Medicine	Varied	Canada
Tuttle, '94	WB	Nutrition	Hmong,Vietnamese	CA
Um, '99	MH	Nursing	Korean	M.W. US city
van de Wijngaart, '97	MH	Psychology	Surinamese	Netherlands
Van der Stuyft, '93	HB	Medicine	Varied	Belgium
Van Der Zwaard, '92	HB	Women's Studies	Turkish, Moroccan	Netherlands
van Enk, '98	WB	Medicine	Varied	Netherlands
Vangen, '96	WB	Medicine	Pakistani	Norway
Vega, '91	MH	Public Health	Mexican	CA
Vega, '97	HB;WB	Public Health	Latina	CA
Vega, '99	HB	Health Policy	Mexican	CA
Wang, '96	M/M		Chinese	Denmark
Wasse, '94	HB;WB	Public Health	Ethiopian	WA
Webster, '95	MH	Psychology	Varied	Australia
Weijers, '98	M/M	Chemistry	Varied	Netherlands
Weitzman, '92	HB	Public Health	Varied	NY
Welles, '94	M/M	Public Health	Caribbean	NY
Westermeyer, '97	MH	Medicine	Hmong	MN
Wijesinghe, '91	MH	Medicine	Varied	Australia
Williams, '93	M/M	Sociology	South Asian	Great Britain

(continued)

TABLE 7.1   *(continued)*

Primary author	Topical area	Discipline	Immigrant group	Study site
Williams, '97	MH	Medical Sociology	South Asian	Great Britain
Willis, '93	WB	Public Health	Mexican	CA
Woelz-Stirling, '98	MH		Filipina	Australia
Wrightson, '97	HB	Public Health	South Asian, Caribbean	Great Britain
Yelibi, '93	HB;WB		African	Ivory Coast
Ying, '90	HB	Social Welfare	Chinese	CA
Youngshook, '99	HB	Nursing	Thai	SE US city
Yusu, '93	WB	Demography	Varied	Australia
Zambrana, '91	HB	Social Welfare	Mexican	CA
Zambrana, '97	WB	Social Work	Mexican	CA
Ziegler, '93	M/M	Epidemiology	Asian	CA,HI

Bodies (WB), including female genital mutilation, sexually transmitted diseases, and menopause as well as issues related to childbearing, including family planning, breastfeeding, and pregnancy (30.5%); (3) Mental Health (MH), specifically mental health status and psycho-social problems associated with immigration (25.1%); and (4) Morbidity or Mortality (M/M) or the epidemiology of diseases not already included in the classification of women's mental or bodily health (9.3%). For example, the epidemiology of depression, sexually transmitted diseases, and certain conditions in pregnancy are excluded from this category. A few "Miscellaneous" (Misc.) studies (1.9%) were on topics like family caregiving and occupational health. A number of topics that are commonly addressed in the general women's health literature were notably absent, including lesbian health, eating disorders, and infertility.

Research findings from the three largest substantive areas or sub areas—health service use and screening (the largest sub area of Health Behavior), Mental Health, and Women's Bodies—are reviewed next. Due to space limitations, when more than five studies support a given finding, example citations are given rather than referencing all of the studies. Exceptions to majority findings are noted.

HEALTH SERVICE USE AND SCREENING BEHAVIOR

This section includes research on health care utilization as well as self- and professional screening for disease, specifically breast and cervical cancer.

Patterns of Health Care Use

Immigrant women use general and specialty services more often than immigrant men do, most likely because of their high fertility and greater reports of psychological distress (Chow, Jaffee, & Choi, 1999; Palacios & Sheps, 1992; Van der Stuyft, Woodward, Amstrong, & De Muynck, 1993). When nonimmigrant women (including uninsured, poor women) are used as the reference group, however, it is apparent that immigrant women underuse health care. The majority or 24 of the 29 studies that addressed this topic reported that immigrant women use general or primary health care, prenatal care, mental health services, and cervical and breast cancer screening less than other women (e.g., Fulton, Rakowski, & Jones, 1995; Kalofonos & Palinkas, 1999; Lipson, Hosseini, Kabir, Omidian, & Edmonston, 1995; Matuk, 1996; McPhee, Bird, Davis, Ha, Jenkins, & Le, 1997; Peragallo, Fox, & Alba, 1998; Remennick, 1999; Vega, Kolody, Hwang, Noble, & Porter, 1997; Weitzman & Berry, 1992). For atypical cases, see Brown, Alexander, McDonald, and Mills-Evers (1997) and Faller (1992).

When findings from extant studies are not congruent with this conclusion, the explanations reinforce the more typical finding of immigrant women's underutilization of health care. For example, the finding that immigrant women use GPs more often than native-born women is confounded by their high fertility and use of GP's instead of obstetricians for prenatal care (Van der Stuyft et al., 1993). The only time immigrant women see a provider regularly is when they are pregnant (Mattson & Lew, 1992).

Immigrant women also access health care by less effective means than native-born women, including native-born minority women of their own ethnic background. They are less likely to have a regular source of health care and more likely to enter the health care system through emergency rooms, crisis centers, and clinics not requiring an appointment (Chavez, Hubbell, Mishra, & Valdez, 1997; Have & Bijl, 1999; Mattson & Lew, 1992). With regard to mental health needs, immigrant women are more apt than native-born women to seek medical rather than psychiatric care for emotional distress (e.g., Have & Bijl, 1999; Pang, 1990; Schreiber, Stern, & Wilson, 1998; Vega, Kolody, Aguilar-Gaxiola, & Catalano, 1999; Ying, 1990). This practice has been documented to lead to underdiagnosis and undertreatment of mental health problems, even when the health care provider shares the same ethnic and linguistic background as the patient (Jacob, Bhugra, Lloyd, & Mann, 1998).

Barriers to Accessing Health Care

Numerous barriers disadvantage immigrant women from accessing health care. In most instances, the barriers cut across type of health care, however, comparing barriers by type of service is not entirely possible due to lack of uniformity in how the studies are conceptualized. For example, studies on mental health service use focus on one type of cultural barrier—differing explanatory models of mental illness. In contrast, studies on breast and cervical cancer screening utilize a more extensive theoretical framework (e.g., the Health Belief Model) to identify broader cultural as well as structural barriers.

For general practitioners (GPs), obstetrical services, and cancer screening, barriers include: cost (particularly for undocumented immigrants or menial laborers without health insurance); provider relationships, such as feeling "put off" or uncared for; lack of female physicians[3]; women's lower status and men's gatekeeping; time constraints from family and immigration demands; transportation; and language (e.g., Anderson, Blue, Holbrook, & Ng, 1993; Bowes & Domokos, 1995; Chavez et al., 1997; Crane, Kaplan, Bastani, & Scrimshaw, 1996; Edwards, 1994; Juarbe, 1998; Kaufman, Shpitz, & Rozin, 1995; Lesjak, Hua, & Ward, 1999; Lipson et al., 1995; Remennick, 1999a; Spring, Ross, Etkin, & Deinard, 1995). Language barriers are more problematic for telephone triage, emergency services, and women from small ethnic communities because interpreters are not available on demand or for small language/ethnic groups (Dolman, Shackleton, Ziaian, Gay, & Yeboah, 1996). Fear of immigration authorities also deters some undocumented immigrant women from using health services (Moss, Baumeister, & Biewener, 1996).

Lack of knowledge is a major reason for immigrant women's low rate of cervical and breast cancer screening, that is, breast self-exams, clinical breast exams, mammography, and Pap smear tests (Chavez, Hubbell, McMullin, Martinez, & Mishra, 1995; Fernandez, Tortolero-Luna, & Gold, 1998; Fitch et al., 1997; Hubbell, Chavez, Mishra, Magana, & Valdez, 1995; Schulmeister & Lifsey, 1999). For example, Latina immigrants are more likely than U.S.-born Latinas or Anglo women to believe that a Pap smear is necessary only for abnormal vaginal bleeding. Latinas who hold this belief are more likely to report not receiving a Pap smear within the past three years (Hubbell, Chavez, Mishra, & Valdez, 1996).

Certain attitudes, beliefs, and fears are also associated with lower screening rates. For instance, fate and karma (which have been documented in Hispanics and Southeast Asians) are inversely related to breast and cervical screening (Hubbell et al., 1996; Taylor et al., 1999). Fear of losing virginity from a Pap smear test is also inversely associated with cervical and breast screening (Schulmeister & Lifsey, 1999).

Cues to action (i.e., recommendations from peers or health care providers) are another class of strong predictors of cervical and breast screening

---

[3]Females are preferred when there is a cultural emphasis on modesty and the separation of men and women.

(Choudhry, Srivastava, & Fitch, 1998; Crane et al., 1996; Fulton et al., 1995). For instance, screening is higher among immigrant women who have regular health care providers and among immigrant women who have been married (e.g., Hubbell et al., 1996; Remennick, 1999a; Tudiver & Fuller-Thompson, 1999). Marital status may serve as a proxy for pregnancy, which provides a reason for immigrant women to access the health care system and receive cues to action. In some studies, however, having a primary health care provider is not associated with cervical and breast screening when the resettlement country (e.g., Israel) and/or the provider have a weak preventative focus (Lesjak et al., 1999; McPhee et al., 1997; Remennick, 1999a). Immigrant providers usually have a weak preventative focus because they are often trained in countries that lack preventive health care or practice in settings (e.g., walk-in clinics) that are more conducive to acute rather than preventative care.

Reasons for under-utilization of mental health services include stigma, preference for relying on self, God, and family, and attributing emotional symptoms to physical causes (Schreiber et al., 1998; Tabora & Flaskerud, 1997; Vega et al., 1999; Ying, 1990).

For all types of health services, immigrant women with the greatest barriers are those who are unemployed, less acculturated, more recent arrivals, less educated, poorer, of lower social status, and not comfortable with their language skills (e.g., Hemingway, Saunders, & Parsons, 1997; Hiatt & Pasick, 1996; Matuk, 1996b; Peragallo et al., 1998; Tabora & Flaskerud, 1997; Van der Stuyft et al., 1993). Language and other cultural barriers are more problematic for older women, whereas younger women attribute not using health services to shortage of time and energy (Remennick, 1999a).

When immigrant women are compared with immigrant men, there is some evidence that women face even greater barriers to using health services. For example, elderly South Asian immigrant women are less informed about social services and have greater difficulty using GPs than their male counterparts (Ahmad & Walker, 1997). On the other hand, Russian immigrant women report less difficulty with using health care than Russian immigrant men (Remennick & Ottenstein-Eisen, 1998). Russian immigrant women's greater ease may be because gender inequity in education, work status, and language skills is minimal in Russians, whereas it is marked among South Asians (Ahmad & Walker, 1997; Remennick & Ottenstein-Eisen, 1998).

In summary, immigrant women are more disadvantaged and face greater barriers to using health services than nonimmigrant minority women. Although immigrant women use health care more often than immigrant men, this is likely due to their reproductive health needs rather than their having fewer barriers. Data about patterns of health care use suggest that the reproductive years offer an opportunity to educate immigrant women and provide preventative as well as other types of health care. Conversely, women who are not childbearing or not integrated in the resettlement society are at greatest risk for not having their health care needs met.

IMMIGRANT WOMEN'S HEALTH: FOCUS ON MENTAL HEALTH

This section reviews research on the prevalence and manifestation of psychological distress among immigrant women as well as the sources of their psychological distress. Research on postpartum depression is reviewed in a subsequent section on Pregnancy Outcomes.

Rates of Psychological Distress

Immigrants, regardless of their gender, have higher rates of psychological distress than their host populations (Black, Markides, & Miller, 1998; Kim & Rew, 1994; Webster, McDonald, Lewin, & Carr, 1995; Willliams & Hunt, 1997). Immigrant women are at even higher risk. The majority of studies that address gender differences in psychological distress (83% of the 30 studies that fit this category) stated that immigrant women report significantly more distress than immigrant men (e.g., Aroian, Norris, Patsdaughter, & Tran, 1998; Chung & Kagawa-Singer, 1993; Kim & Rew, 1994; Munet-Vilaro, Folkman, & Gregorich, 1999). For exceptions, see Flaskerud & Uman (1996), Hurh & Kim (1990), Mui (1996), Nwadiora & McAdoo (1996), and Ponizovsky, Safro, Ginath, & Ritsner (1997).

Although there are few comparative studies of immigrant and native-born minority women, extant studies depict immigrant women as also having higher rates of distress than subsequent generations of minority women (Black et al., 1998; Munet-Vilaro et al., 1999; Russell, Williams, Farr, Schwab & Plattsmier, 1999). Only in the area of substance abuse are first generation immigrant women at lower risk for mental health problems than later generations (Lindenberg et al., 1999; Palacios & Sheps, 1992).

Some ethnic groups of immigrant women may be particularly at risk. Higher rates of distress have been noted in Russians compared with Ethiopians (Ponizovsky et al., 1998), in Chinese and Portuguese compared with Vietnamese and Latinas (Franks & Faux, 1990), and in Middle Easterners and North Africans compared with Europeans and Americans (Ruskin et al., 1996). Ethnic background, however, was confounded with other correlates of psychological distress (e.g., time since immigration, age, or language ability) in these studies.

Manifestations of Psychological Distress

Like gender differences in general populations, immigrant women manifest their distress differently from immigrant men. Affective symptoms such as depression and anxiety are more common among women, whereas men are more likely to manifest distress through behavioral problems like substance abuse, violence, and social withdrawal (e.g., Allodi & Stiasny, 1990; D'Avanzo, Frye, & Froman, 1994; Mirsky & Barasch, 1993; Mui, 1996). Although substance abuse among immigrant women is rare (Allodi & Stiasny, 1990; Gaffney et al., 1997; Lindenberg et al., 1999; Palacios & Sheps, 1992; Vega et al., 1997), secondary depression among immigrant women who are substance abusers is over three times more likely than among immigrant men who are substance abusers (Golding, Burnam, Benjamin, & Wells, 1993). Findings from the two studies that investigated gender differences in suicidal ideation were inconsistent (Locke, Southwick, McCloskey, & Fernandez-Esquer, 1996; Ponizovsky et al., 1997). With regard to completed suicide, however, immigrant women from India are at higher risk than their male counterparts (Raleigh & Balarajan, 1992).

Gender differences in how psychological distress is manifested could be viewed as evidence that women's high rates of psychological distress are artifactual. Surveys may be biased against women because they more typically focus on affective symptoms (e.g., depression and anxiety) and omit equivalent behavioral symptoms that are more common among men. Immigrant women may also be more willing than immigrant men to report or seek help for psychological symptoms. On the other hand, research about the sources of immigrant women's distress provides ample evidence for the counter-argument that gender differences are substantive.

Sources and Correlates of Psychological Distress for Immigrant Women

Irrespective of gender, certain variables are associated with immigrants' psychological distress, including low income, unemployment or not working in one's field, less education, low acculturation or retention of traditional values, language difficulty, older age, general life stress, poor health, lack of social support and other types of coping resources (e.g., mastery, self-esteem), and pre-migration trauma (e.g., Bernstein & Shuval, 1998; Chung & Kagawa-Singer, 1993; Hurh & Kim, 1990; Peel, 1996; Tran, 1993). Many of these risk factors, however, are more prevalent in women. Compared with immigrant men, immigrant women's income, education, acculturation, language ability, and self-esteem are lower, and they are more often unemployed and widowed (e.g., Flaskerud & Uman, 1996; Ghaffarian, 1998; Kim, 1999; Tran, 1990).

There are also qualitative differences for men and women with regard to some of these variables. Although, both genders encounter pre-migration trauma (i.e., trauma in the homeland or in transit), the nature and consequences of pre-migration trauma are different for women. For instance, immigrant women from war-torn or politically repressive countries are more often raped and sexually tortured and have more extensive family loss than their male counterparts (e.g., Allodi & Stiasny, 1990; Chung & Kagawa-Singer, 1993; D'Avanzo et al., 1994; Fox, Cowell, & Johnson, 1995).

These types of pre-migration trauma are strong predictors of distress. Sexual torture is associated with greater and more long-term distress than other types of physical torture (Allodi & Stiasny, 1990; Peel, 1996). Grief over family loss has been noted to persist for up to 10 years and may worsen over time (Chung & Kagawa-Singer, 1993; Fox et al., 1995; Locke et al., 1996).

Correlates of psychological distress also vary by gender. Specifically, social support and other relational variables are of greater import for immigrant women's mental status, whereas work-related variables are stronger predictors of distress for immigrant men (Baider, Kaufman, Ever-Hadani & Kaplan De-Nour, 1996; Hurh & Kim, 1990; Ponizovsky et al., 1997). When immigrant women are distressed by work, their distress stems from relational aspects of work, specifically feeling estranged from co-workers and discrimination (Jackson, 1995, 1996). These findings are consistent with theories of women's relational orientation and further supported by studies that identify loneliness and feeling estranged due to cultural differences as major sources of distress among immigrant women (Hattar-Pollara & Meleis, 1995a; Lipson & Miller, 1994; Ogur, 1990; Shin & Shin, 1999; van de Wijngaart, 1997).

Yet another class of stressors—those that pertain to changes in female gender roles and women's differential power in relation to men—are gender-specific and in addition to the generic stressors encountered by both men and women. With regard to female gender roles, most sending countries have traditional female roles, which are more rigid than male roles. As a result, immigrant women encounter greater and more stressful role change than their male counterparts (e.g., Frye & D'Avanzo, 1994a; Hattar-Pollara & Meleis, 1995a; Omeri, 1997; Shin & Shin, 1999).

Outside employment is a common gender role change for immigrant women. Outside employment not only exposes immigrant women from traditional societies to more contemporary gender roles and changes power relationships between spouses, but also forces choices between fitting in with the new society or risking disapproval by the immigrant community (Fox, 1991). For example, immigrant women who retain a traditional gender role and do not work outside of the home are more alienated and lonely and have less well-being than immigrant women with outside employment (Birman & Tyler, 1994; Fox, 1991; Kim, 1999). On the other hand, adopting a less traditional gender role may be less important than having a choice (Kim & Rew, 1994; Russell et al., 1999; Um & Dancy, 1999; Williams & Hunt, 1997). For instance, immigrant women who are not satisfied at home and favor modern gender roles are more distressed than those who prefer traditional roles (Moghaddam, Ditto, & Taylor, 1990).

Role burden is another component of outside employment. Role burden may explain why employed immigrant women are about eight times more likely to be depressed than their male counterparts (Noh, Wu, Speechley, & Kaspar, 1992). Immigrant women are still expected to fully carry family and home responsibilities, even if they have outside employment and their spouses do not (e.g., Luna, 1994; Singer et al., 1996; Schreiber et al., 1998). Immigrant women who are widowed, have been abandoned, or have spouses with resettlement problems (e.g., unemployment) or pre-migration trauma (from being soldiers or political prisoners) have total family and economic responsibility (e.g., Farr & Wilson-Figueroa, 1997; Lipson et al., 1995; Thompson, 1991). Men with pre-migration trauma often abdicate family responsibility through abusing alcohol and withdrawing from family life.

Immigrant women are also at risk for domestic violence. Wife battering is a common response among immigrant men with resettlement problems and pre-migration trauma (Fox, 1991; Lipson & Miller, 1994; Singer et al., 1996; Thompson, 1991; Woelz-Stirling, Kelaher, & Manderson, 1998). In addition, domestic violence is sanctioned in some immigrant groups as men's right to control their wives, especially when cultural expectations about traditional female behavior are challenged (Davila & Brackley, 1999; Fox, 1991; Kulwicki & Miller, 1999; Lipson & Miller, 1994; Singer et al., 1996).

Mothering also involves new and conflicting role dimensions for immigrant women. Immigrant mothers are not only vigilant and discipline their children for cultural adherence, but also advocate for children's wish to assimilate and mediate disagreements between children and spouses (D'Avanzo & Barab, 1998; Fox et al., 1995; Hattar-Pollara & Meleis, 1995b; Lipson & Miller, 1994).

A few studies have compared ethnicity, age, or nativity group differences in stressors among immigrant women. Findings from these studies suggest that sources and correlates of psychological distress may vary across these dimensions (Black et al., 1998; Chung & Kagawa-Singer, 1993; Franks & Faux, 1990). For example, lack of insurance, functional health, and not having a confidant are significant predictors of depression among Mexican immigrant women but have less explanatory power for their U.S.-born counterparts (Black et al., 1998). Number of life events, greater age, and fewer friends are the most important predictors for immigrant women from Vietnam, whereas financial status and employment are significant predictors for immigrant women from Latin America (Frank & Faux, 1990). Elderly immigrant women are more troubled by social isolation and lack of respect, whereas immigrant women at midlife are more burdened by role conflict from being a housewife, employee, and mediator between children and spouse (Lipson & Miller, 1994).

In summary, immigrant women are at greater risk for psychological distress than immigrant men and native-born women of minority backgrounds. Research findings about sources and correlates of immigrant women's psychological distress suggest that immigrant women's mental health should be considered in the context of gender roles, differential power, and relational theories of women's development. Research findings about group differences among immigrant women and differences between immigrant and native-born minority women are less conclusive, mostly because these topics have not been studied extensively. Nonetheless, preliminary findings from extant studies suggest that there are important group differences.

FOCUS ON THE BODY

The research that has focused on immigrant women's bodies spans a number of areas, with topics related to childbearing (i.e., family planning, breastfeeding, and pregnancy) more heavily represented than topics such as female genital mutilation (FGM), sexually transmitted diseases (STDs), and menopause. However, research on less represented topics is growing, most likely due to increased migration from countries with FMG and AIDS epidemics and because immigrant populations are aging.

Female Genital Mutilation

FGM practices differ by country of origin and are far from homogenous (Knight, Hotchin, Bayly, & Grover, 1999). For instance, clitoridectomy and excision of the labia minora are more common in Ethiopia, whereas infibulation (i.e., excision of part or all of the external genitalia and stitching/narrowing of the vaginal opening) is more common in Somalia (Arbesman, Kahler, & Buck, 1993; Grisaru, Lezer, & Belmaker, 1997; Knight et al., 1999; Morris, 1996).

FGM may also differ for immigrants and nonimmigrants. For example, one study found fewer than anticipated complications from FGM among immigrant women when expectations were based on reports from nonimmigrants (Arbesman et al., 1993). Immigrants may have fewer complications because, by virtue of their higher social class, they are more apt than nonimmigrants to be infibulated by professionals. On one hand, immigrants may underreport complaints because FMG is stigmatized in most resettlement countries (Eyega & Conneely, 1997). On the other hand, it is possible that complications from FGM are overestimated because data on this topic typically come from women seeking care for problems.

There are a number of serious health problems associated with FGM regardless of whether problems are over- or underreported. According to a study that assessed immigrants during routine prenatal or gynecology care, most infibulated women (85%) experience dyspareunia, apareunia, and urinary tract infections; about one third (29.4%) need surgery to facilitate intercourse (Knight et al., 1999). Infibulated women are also at greater risk for AIDS. Vaginal intercourse can reopen and infect wounds and anal intercourse, often unprotected, is used as a less painful alternative to vaginal sex (Singer et al., 1996).

The problem of reinfibulation after childbirth is unique to immigrant women. FGM is a criminal offense in the United States and many women are not financially able to return home for reinfibulation. Yet, women fear that their husbands will divorce them if they are not reinfibulated (Morris, 1996). Although there is some variation in desire to continue the tradition of FGM, most immigrant women fear that their daughters will be promiscuous or not find husbands if they do not have the procedure (Arbesman et al., 1993; Eyega & Conneely, 1997; Morris, 1996). On the other hand, one study found that Ethiopian women do not wish to continue their traditional FGM practices. These women, however, may not have been candid with the interviewer because he was male (Grisaru et al., 1997).

In a study of health care providers, most providers knew about and had treated women with FGM, perhaps because the study was conducted in an area with a large African immigrant community. Nonetheless, fewer than half of the providers initiated discussion about FGM with their patients, reportedly because of language barriers, acceptance of FGM as a valid cultural practice, lack of cultural and medical knowledge of the implications of FGM, and women's reluctance to discuss the topic. Midwives, however, were more knowledgeable and more apt to initiate discussions about FMG than other health providers (Eyega & Conneely, 1997).

Sexually Transmitted Diseases

Immigrant women are less knowledgeable than immigrant men about AIDS prevention (Yelibi et al., 1993). Immigrant women are also at greater risk for contracting AIDS and other STDs than non-immigrant women (Bindels et al., 1994; O'Connor, Berry, Rohrsheim, & Donovan, 1996; Remis et al., 1995; Reynolds et al., 1998).

Women from countries where HIV is endemic or that culturally sanction men having multiple sex partners are at highest risk (Bindel et al., 1994; Remis et al., 1995; Singer et al., 1996). Many cultures value female chastity and monogamy but these standards do not apply to men (Singer et al., 1996). Specifically, unprotected, extramarital sex is normative for immigrant men, particularly when immigration results in prolonged periods of spousal separation (Romero, Wyatt, Chin, & Rodriguez, 1998–99; Singer et al., 1996).

Despite immigrant women's high risk for STDs, condom use among immigrant women is low and inconsistent. In many cultures, asking a husband to use a condom is unacceptable and a sign of mistrust. Also, immigrant women lack power in their relationships and fear abuse or abandonment if they insist on condoms (Jermott, Maula, & Bush, 1999; Romero et al., 1998–99; Singer et al., 1996). Condom use does increase, however, with interventions to promote decision making and comfort with sexual communication (Gómez, Hernández, & Faigeles, 1999).

Menopause

Studies on menopause in immigrant women address age of onset, health beliefs, and symptomatology. Berg (1999) found that age of onset is earlier in immigrant women. Leidy (1998) found that age with subsequent generations of immigrant women more closely approximates age of onset for the resettlement country. With regard to symptoms, South American immigrant women experience the same prevalence and severity of vasomotor symptoms as Swedish women in Sweden (Nedstrand, Ekseth, Lindgren, & Hammar, 1995). However, Filipina and Korean immigrant women experience fewer vasomotor and other symptoms than native-born American women (Berg, 1999; Im, Meleis, & Lee, 1999). Regardless of symptoms, immigrant women are less apt to use hormone replacement therapy and more apt to normalize rather than medicalize menopause (Brown et al., 1999; Im & Meleis, 1999; Nedstrand et al., 1995). These conclusions, however, are based on a limited number of studies and are therefore tentative.

Childbearing

Studies on childbearing include parity and family planning, infant feeding practices, and pregnancy outcomes. The latter category includes usual indicators of pregnancy outcomes as well as post-partum depression and labor and delivery outcomes.

PARITY AND FAMILY PLANNING

Research on parity and family planning addresses how parity and methods of contraception change with immigration as well as describes health beliefs, decision making, and knowledge about contraception. Findings about the relationship between immigration and parity are mixed. Short birth intervals for Bangladeshi immigrant women are twice that reported for women in Bangladesh or native-born women in the UK (Hilder, 1993). On the other hand, immigrant women in Belize have lower fertility than native born women in Belize (Moss, Stone, & Smith, 1993). Unlike women in Belize, however, most immigrant women resettle in countries with low birth rates. Since large families are the norm in most sending societies, comparison with non-immigrants portray immigrant women as highly parous. The more essential question, however, is how immigration changes family planning and preferred family size.

Speculation about changes (higher or lower) in fertility postimmigration include disruptions in birth control methods that were previously effective (e.g., replacing breast with bottle-feeding), spousal separation, and stress of immigration. Inadequate birth control among immigrant women, particularly poor knowledge and inadequate decision making, has not been substantiated. Only one study reported that immigrant women are not effective users of contraception (Reubsaet & Ineichen, 1996). Although level of knowledge differs by immigrant group and is lower for nontraditional methods, most immigrant women not only know about family planning but also actively engage in the practice (Thorburn, Harvey, & Beckman, 1998; Yusu, Siedlecky, & Byrnes, 1993). They tend to discuss options with spouses, however, rather than seek advice from health providers (Kuss, 1997; Moss et al., 1993; Remennick, Amir, Elimelech, & Novikov, 1995).

Stress of immigration, on the other hand, is a substantiated reason for decreasing parity among immigrant women. Although immigrant women typically prefer large families, they limit family size for financial and practical reasons (e.g., need for outside employment) (Kulig, 1994b; Kuss, 1997). Undocumented and poor immigrant women are among those who are most interested in constraining family growth (Moss et al., 1993). On the other hand, Somali immigrant women do not practice contraception because they view pregnancy as "a blessing from God" (Beine, Fullerton, Palinkas, & Anders, 1995).

Changes in method of family planning after immigration are due, in part, to availability and cost. For instance, Russian immigrant women attribute their increased use of the pill and condoms to greater availability, whereas they had to rely on induced abortion and more traditional methods in the former Soviet Union (Cwikel, Rozentsweig, Sofer, Ben-Tal, & Shvartzman, 1994; Remennick et al., 1995). Cultural beliefs also influence birth-control choices. Immigrant women from more traditional countries prefer less modern methods (e.g., breastfeeding, withdrawal, rhythm, douche, and abstinence) and hold negative beliefs about modern methods, including: the pill and depo provera upsets the hot and cold balance in the body and causes cancer, tubal ligations release women's passions and cause extramarital affairs, vasectomies cause impotence, condoms are for prostitutes and burn the uterus, and it is not appropriate to touch and insert a diaphragm into one's vagina (Kulig, 1994b, 1995; Kuss, 1997; Yusu et al., 1993).

BREASTFEEDING

Acculturation plays an important role in infant feeding decisions. Five of the seven studies on this topic report that immigrant women's rate and/or duration of breastfeeding decreases after immigration and is inversely related to number of years in the resettlement country (Ghaemi-Ahmadi, 1992; Meftuh, Tapsoba, & Lamounier, 1991; Perez-Escamilla et al., 1998; Rossiter, 1992a; Tuttle & Dewey, 1994). Exceptions to these findings were documented by Ever-Hadani, Seidman, Manor, and Harlap (1994) and Knapp and Houghton (1999). There are ethnic group differences, however. Iranian immigrants are more apt to breastfeed their infants than are Afghan and Southeast Asian immigrants (Ghaemi-Ahmadi, 1992).

Reasons why immigrant women do not breastfeed include receiving infant formula and bottle-feeding advice, perceptions of breastfeeding as unpopular or not supported in the resettlement country, financial reasons (needing to return to work), and lack of availability of traditional foods believed to improve breast milk (Ghaemi-Ahmadi, 1992; Perez-Escamilla et al., 1998; Rossiter, 1992a, 1992b; Tuttle & Dewey, 1994).

Findings about maternal education and breastfeeding are mixed. One study reported that less educated Ethiopian women are more apt to breastfeed, whereas two other studies reported that less educated Iranian, Afghan, and Southeast Asian women are more apt to bottle-feed (Ghaemi-Ahmadi, 1992; Rossiter, 1992a). The influence of education on infant feeding, however, is not straightforward. Among nonimmigrant women in the United States, for example, higher education is associated with longer breastfeeding. In contrast, the elite are the first to replace breast with bottle-feeding in developing countries. Immigrant women appear to bring this elite bias with them and opt to bottle-feed, in part because they perceive this as the preferred practice in the resettlement country (Meftuh et al., 1991). Breastfeeding practices, however, appear amenable to intervention. The provision of a culture- and language-specific intervention effectively increases breastfeeding as well as knowledge of and positive attitudes towards breastfeeding (Rossiter, 1994).

PREGNANCY AND BIRTHING OUTCOMES

Infant birth weight, the most commonly used indicator of pregnancy outcome, differs by immigrant group (Hummer et al., 1999; van Enk, Buitendijk, van der Paul, van Enk, & Schulpen, 1998; Singh & Yu, 1996). Nonetheless, cumulative research findings portray infant birth weight among immigrant mothers as better than or comparable to native born women in resettlement countries (e.g., Alexander, Mor, Kogan, Leland, & Kieffer, 1996; English, Kharrazi, & Guendelman, 1997; Fuentes-Afflick, Hessol, & Perez-Stable, 1998; Singh & Yu, 1996, Wasse, Holt, Daling, 1994). Only one out of nine studies on this topic found that immigrants were more likely than native-born mothers to deliver a low-birth-weight infant (Sullivan & Shepherd, 1997). Comparisons, however, were between Vietnamese immigrants and native-born Australians. The finding of low birth weight among Vietnamese could be because growth charts are based on Australians and not racially appropriate.

The incidence of infant mortality, sudden infant death, and premature birth are also low among immigrant mothers (Burton & Lancaster, 1999; Doucet Baumgarten, & Infante-Rivard, 1992; van Enk et al., 1998; Hummer et al., 1999; Oldenburg, Rasmussen, & Cotton, 1997; Singh & Yu, 1996). (See Mor, Alexander, Kieffer, & Baruffi [1993] for exception.) Some immigrant groups also have a low incidence of pre-eclampsia (Sullivan & Shepherd, 1997.)

Many of these positive pregnancy outcomes may be due to cultural practices and lifestyle. For instance, family support during pregnancy is high for immigrant women (Berry, 1999; Sherraden & Barrera, 1996b). Immigrant mothers are also less likely than mothers born in resettlement countries to smoke, use alcohol and drugs, and be teens or single parents (e.g., Alexander et al., 1996; Balcazar, Peterson, & Krull, 1997; Doucet et al., 1992; Hummer et al., 1999; Ma & Bauman, 1996; Vega et al., 1997; Wasse et al., 1994; Zambrana, Scrimshaw, Collins, & Dunkel-Schetter, 1997). Conversely, acculturation and years/generation in the resettlement country are strong predictors of risk factors and low infant birth weight (e.g., Cobas, Balcazar, Benin, Keith, & Chong, 1996; Gaffney et al., 1997; Hyman & Dussault, 1996). For example, birth outcomes are markedly worse among non-immigrant than among immigrant Latinas (English et al., 1997; Fuentes-Afflick et al., 1998; Zambrana et al., 1997).

Nonetheless, there are some pregnancy-related problems for immigrant women. These problems include gestational diabetes, hepatitis B infection, tuberculosis, intestinal parasites, high lead levels, and post-partum depression (e.g., Boxall, Skidmore, Evans, & Nightingale, 1994; Glasser et al., 1998; Kieffer, Martin, & Herman, 1999; Kwan, Ho, & Lee, 1997; Ma & Bauman, 1996; Nahas, Hillege, & Amasheh, 1999; Nolan, Espinosa, & Pastorek, 1997; Rothenberg et al., 1999; Sullivan & Shepherd, 1997). TB infection, intestinal parasites, and depression are particularly high among refugee women who are pregnant while in transit, probably due to adverse pre-migration and refugee camp conditions (Kahler, Sobota, Hines, & Griswold, 1996). Mothers from countries without vaccination programs are at high risk of having a baby with congenital rubella (Condon & Bower, 1993). Immigrant women who are heavily clothed for modesty and/or have low dietary or supplemental intake are more prone to developing vitamin D deficiency during pregnancy (Henriksen et al., 1995). Foreign-born mothers also have higher rates of Caesarean sections, postpartum hemorrhage, third-degree tears, and puerperal infection, and are less likely to receive analgesia in labor than women giving birth in the resettlement country (Ibison, Swerdlow, Head, & Marmot, 1996; Ma & Bauman, 1996; Vangen, Stoltenberg, & Schei, 1996).

Unlike infant birth weight, mortality, and prematurity, which are are superior among immigrant mothers, problems such as gestational diabetes, intestinal parasites, and birthing complications, stem from conditions in the homeland and/or care delivery issues. For instance, birthing complications such as Caesarean sections would likely decrease if language was not a barrier during childbirth. Gestational diabetes, which is likely related to the older childbearing age of immigrant mothers, could be addressed with adequate prenatal care.

In summary, immigrant women are at high risk for a number of problems related to their bodily health, including AIDS and other STDs. FGM is also a problem for select groups of immigrant women, particularly in terms of physical complications and clashes between cultural norms and attitudes in resettlement countries. In addition, there is some evidence that the experience of menopause differs for immigrant and native-born women, however, research on this topic is sparse and not conclusive.

The research on immigrant women's childbearing has been ample, particularly their parity and family planning, infant feeding practices, and pregnancy outcomes. Although birth rates are high among immigrant women, their parity decreases after immigration. Immigrant women are actively engaged in family planning. Practical consideration as well as cultural beliefs influence contraceptive choices. Even though breastfeeding is common, bottle-feeding is more the norm among immigrant women. Findings about most pregnancy outcomes

portray immigrant women as advantaged over native-born women in resettlement countries—a finding that is contrary to other areas of immigrant women's
health. Positive pregnancy outcomes are likely due to immigrant women's
lifestyle and the strong support in traditional cultures for child bearing, however, similar to the negative effect of acculturation on infant feeding decisions,
acculturation adversely affects immigrant women's life style and consequently,
their birth outcomes. When immigrant mothers have childbearing problems,
most of the problems are likely from conditions in the homeland and/or
inadequate prenatal and labor and deliver care in the resettlement country.

STATE OF THE SCIENCE AND RECOMMENDATIONS FOR FUTURE RESEARCH

Review of the 292 studies listed in Table 7.1 portrays substantial growth in
the last decade in the number of studies on immigrant women's health. The
extant body of research also addresses many of the recommendations put forth
at the beginning of the decade by nurse scholars. Not only have studies about
immigrant women proliferated, but also the scope of the studies has expanded
beyond the original focus on childbearing. Presently, studies of health behavior
exceed the number on childbearing, even when studies of prenatal service use
are considered as part of the childbearing literature. When reviewing research
on immigrant women's bodies, however, most studies focus on reproduction
and childbearing processes (i.e., pregnancy outcomes, family planning, and
breastfeeding). Nonetheless, studies of sexually transmitted diseases, female
genital mutilation, and menopause are growing.

Research on immigrant women is also no longer focused on a small
number of ethnic groups and locations but includes immigrants who are from
all over the globe and reside in various countries. This diversity reflects the
demographic characteristics during the 1990s of sending and, somewhat, of
receiving countries. Countries that are not represented in this review but
received large numbers of immigrants during the 1990s (e.g., Germany, France)
are most likely also sites for studies on immigrant women's health. Yet,
contributions from these countries may not be apparent because the findings
were not reported in English.

Despite progress, however, a number of shortcomings remain. Small,
isolated groups of immigrant women are not represented in most research
studies, perhaps because of practical problems like recruiting a critical mass
of immigrants from a particular location. Comparative studies of different
immigrant groups are still sparse and pay insufficient attention to potential
confounds. Although national data banks are available in select countries (e.g.,

Israel) or for limited topics (i.e., prenatal service use and pregnancy outcomes such as infant birth weight and mortality), they are characterized by gross measurement of a limited number of variables. Thus, these databases are superficial and lack specificity for generating clinical interventions.

The most glaring shortcoming in the state of the science on immigrant women's health pertains to the development of population-specific interventions. According to this review, only 7 of the 292 articles reporting studies conducted in the last decade were intervention studies. These included two studies to increase cancer screening (Bell, Branston, Newcombe, & Barton, 1999; Suarez et al., 1997), one study to improve mental health (Fox, Cowell, Montgomery, & Willgerodt, 1997), one study for cardiac health promotion (Brown, Lee, & Oyomopito, 1996), one study for HIV prevention (Gomez et al., 1999), and two studies to improve childbearing practices such as breastfeeding (Gagnon et al., 1994). Nurses were the primary authors of three of these seven studies.

Recommendations for future research include more comparative study of inter-group differences, including women from small immigrant groups. Research of this nature would provide greater information about conditions and groups of immigrant women who are at risk. For example, women from small immigrant groups may have different or more severe problems from their social isolation and lack of a relevant ethnic community. Similarly, comparative studies would not only disentangle how immigrant women differ from each other as well as from native-born minority women, but would also illustrate mechanisms of risk. In addition, national databases should include more complex variables and be supplemented with methods to increase depth of study findings. More emphasis should also be placed on non-childbearing aspects of women's bodies.

Lastly, the number of intervention studies should be increased. Based on this review, the descriptive base is adequate for moving research on immigrant women to the level of testing prescriptive theories. To date, nursing, has been a leading contributor to the research base on immigrant women's health. Given its focus on clinical practice, nursing is in an excellent position to forge the way for this next level of research.

A final caveat is in order. Most research on immigrant women's health has been approached from a framework that is almost exclusively problem or risk-oriented. Research on substance abuse and pregnancy outcomes among immigrant and native-born minority women suggest that a more balanced view of immigrant women is warranted. Research that investigates the beneficial health effects of gender and immigration status recognizes the strength of immigrant women and holds promise to further our overall understanding of health and disease.

ACKNOWLEDGMENTS

The author would like to acknowledge Lenny Chiang, RN, PhC, a doctoral student and research fellow at Boston College School of Nursing and Elyssa Vasas, RN, a former student and research fellow at Boston College School of Nursing and current graduate student at Tulane University School of Public Health for their assistance with the preparation of this manuscript. The author would also like to acknowledge Dr. Loretta Higgins, Associate Dean at Boston College School of Nursing and Dr. Carole A. Patsdaughter, Director of Research and Scholarship at the School of Nursing at the Northeastern University Bouvé College of Health Sciences for their reviews of an earlier version of this chapter.

REFERENCES

Ahmad, W. I. U., & Walker, R. (1997). Asian older people: Housing, health and access to services. *Aging and Society, 17*, 141–165.

Alexander, G. R., Mor, J. M., Kogan, M. D., Leland, N. L., & Kieffer, E. (1996). Pregnancy outcomes of US-born and foreign-born Japanese Americans. *American Journal of Public Health, 86*, 820–824.

Allodi, F., & Stiasny, S. (1990). Women as torture victims. *Canadian Journal of Psychiatry, 35*, 144–148.

Anderson, J. M. (1985). Perspectives on the health of immigrant women: A feminist analysis. *Advances in Nursing Science, 8*, 61–76.

Anderson, J. M. (1991). Immigrant women speak of chronic illness: The social construction of the devalued self. *Journal of Advanced Nursing, 16*, 710–717.

Anderson, J. M., Blue, C., Holbrook, A., & Ng, M. (1993). On chronic illness: Immigrant women in Canada's work force—A feminist perspective. *Canadian Journal of Nursing Research, 25*, 7–22.

Anderson, J. M., Blue, C., & Lau, A. (1991). Women's perspectives on chronic illness: Ethnicity, ideology and restructuring of life. *Social Science Medicine, 33*, 101–113.

Anderson, J. M., Wiggins, S., Rajwani, R., Holbrook, A., Blue, C., & Ng, M. (1995). Living with a chronic illness: Chinese-Canadian and Euro-Canadian women with diabetes—Exploring factors that influence management. *Social Science Medicine, 41*, 181–195.

Arbesman, M., Kahler, L., & Buck, G. M. (1993). Assessment of the impact of female circumcision on the gynecological, genitourinary and obstetrical health problems of women from Somalia: Literature review and case series. *Women and Health, 20*, 27–42.

Aroian, K. J., Norris, A. E., Patsdaughter, C. A., & Tran, T.V. (1998). Predicting psychological distress among former Soviet immigrants. *International Journal of Social Psychiatry, 44*, 284–294.

Azize Vargas, Y., & Aviles, L. A. (1998). Abortion in Puerto Rico: The limits of a colonial legality. *Puerto Rico Health Science Journal, 17,* 27–36.

Baider, L., Kaufman, B., Ever-Hadani, P., & Kaplan De-Nour, A. K. (1996). Coping with additional stresses: Comparative study of healthy and cancer patient new immigrants. *Social Science Medicine, 42,* 1077–1084.

Balarajan, R., & Raleigh, V. S. (1997). Patterns of mortality among Bangladeshis in England and Wales. *Ethnicity and Health, 2,* 5–12.

Balcazar, H., Peterson, G. W., & Krull, J. L. (1997). Acculturation and family cohesiveness in Mexican American pregnant women: Social and health implications. *Family and Community Health, 20,* 16–31.

Beine, K., Fullerton, J., Palinkas, L., & Anders, B. (1995). Conceptions of prenatal care among Somali women in San Diego. *Journal of Nurse-Midwifery, 40,* 376–381.

Bell, T. S., Branston, L. K., Newcombe, R. G., & Barton, G. R. (1999). Interventions to improve uptake of breast screening in inner city Cardiff general practices with ethnic minority lists. *Ethnicity and Health, 4,* 277–284.

Bennett, S. A. (1993). Inequalities in risk factors and cardiovascular mortality among Australia's immigrants. *Australian Journal of Public Health, 17,* 251–261.

Berg, J. A. (1999). The perimenopausal transition of Filipino American midlife women: Biopsychosociocultural dimensions. *Nursing Research, 48,* 71–77.

Berg, J. A., & Lipson, J. G. (1999). Information sources, menopause beliefs, and health complaints of midlife Filipinas. *Health Care for Women International, 20,* 81–92.

Bernstein, J. H., & Shuval, J. T. (1998). The occupational integration of former Soviet physicians in Israel. *Social Science Medicine, 47,* 809–819.

Berry, A. B. (1999). Mexican American women's expressions of the meaning of culturally congruent prenatal care. *Journal of Transcultural Nursing, 10,* 203–212.

Bindels, P. J., Mulder-Folkerts, D. K., Boer, K., Schutte, M. F., van der Velde, W. J., Wong, F. J., van den Hoek, A. J. A. R., van Doornum, G. J., & Coutinho, R. A. (1994). The HIV prevalence among pregnant women in the Amsterdam region (1988–1991). *European Journal of Epidemiology, 10,* 331–338.

Birman, D., & Tyler, F. B. (1994). Acculturation and alienation of Soviet Jewish refugees in the United States. *Genetic, Social, and General Psychology Monographs, 120,* 101–115.

Black, S. A., Markides, K. S., & Miller, T. Q. (1998). Correlates of depressive symptomatology among older community-dwelling Mexican Americans: The Hispanic EPESE. *Journal of Gerontology: Social Sciences, 53B,* S198–S208.

Blesch, K. S., Davis, F., & Kamath, S. K. (1999). A comparison of breast and colon cancer incidence rates among Native Asian Indians, U.S. immigrant Asian Indians, and Whites. *Journal of the American Dietetic Association, 99,* 1275–1277.

Bowes, A. M., & Domokos, T. M. (1995). South Asian women and their GPs: Some issues of communication. *Social Sciences in Health, 1,* 22–33.

Boxall, E., Skidmore, S., Evans, C., & Nightingale, S. (1994). The prevalence of hepatitis B and C in an antenatal population of various ethnic origins. *Epidemiology and Infection, 113,* 523–528.

Boyd, M. (1984). At a disadvantage: The occupational attainments of foreign born women in Canada. *International Migration Review XVIII,* 1091–119.

Brown, A. F., Perez-Stable, E. J., Whitaker, E. E., Posner, S. F., Alexander, M., Gathe, J., & Washington, A. E. (1999). Ethnic differences in hormone replacement prescribing patterns. *Journal of General Internal Medicine, 14*, 663–669.

Brown, W. J., Alexander, J., McDonald, B., & Mills-Evers, T. (1997). The health of Filipinas in the Hunter region. *Australian and New Zealand Journal of Public Health, 21*, 214–216.

Brown, W. J., Lee, C., & Oyomopito, R. (1996). Effectiveness of a bilingual heart health program for Greek-Australian women. *Health Promotion International, 11*(2), 117–125.

Buchwald, D., Manson, S. M., Dinges, N. G., Keane, E. M., & Kinzie, J. D. (1993). Prevalence of depressive symptoms among established Vietnamese refugees in the United States: Detection in a primary care setting. *Journal of General Internal Medicine, 8*, 76–81.

Burnette, D. (1999). Custodial grandparents in Latino families: Patterns of service use and predictors of unmet needs. *Social Work, 44*, 22–34.

Burton, A. J., & Lancaster, P. (1999). Obstetric profiles and perinatal mortality among Pacific Island immigrants in New South Wales, 1990–93. *Australian and New Zealand Journal of Public Health*, 179–184.

Castles, S., & Miller, M. J. (1996). *The age of migration: International population movements in the modern world*. London: Macmillan.

Chavez, L. R., & Hubbell, F. A. (1997). The influence of fatalism on self-reported use of Papanicolaou smears. *American Journal of Preventive Medicine, 13*, 418–424.

Chavez, L. R., Hubbell, F. A., McMullin, J. M., Martinez, R. G., & Mishra, S. I. (1995). Understanding knowledge and attitudes about breast cancer. *Archives of Family Medicine, 4*, 145–152.

Chavez, L. R., Hubbell, F. A., Mishra, S. I., & Valdez, R. B. (1997). Undocumented Latina immigrants in Orange County, California: A comparative analysis. *International Migration Review, 31*, 88–107.

Choudhry, U. K. (1998). Health promotion among immigrant women from India living in Canada. *Image: Journal of Nursing Scholarship, 30*, 269–274.

Choudhry, U. K., Srivastava, R., & Fitch, M. I. (1998). Breast cancer detection practices of South Asian women: Knowledge, attitudes, and beliefs. *Oncology Nursing Forum, 25*, 1693–1701.

Chow, J. C., Jaffee, K. D., & Choi, D. Y. (1999). Use of public mental health services by Russian refugees. *Psychiatric Services, 50*, 936–940.

Chung, R. C., & Kagawa-Singer, M. (1993). Predictors of psychological distress among southeast Asian refugees. *Social Science Medicine, 36*, 631–639.

Cobas, J. A., Balcazar, H., Benin, M. B., Keith, V. M., & Chong, Y. (1996). Acculturation and low-birthweight infants among Latino women: A reanalysis of HANES data with structural equation models. *American Journal of Public Health, 86*, 394–396.

Condon, R. J., & Bower, C. (1993). Rubella vaccination and congenital rubella syndrome in Western Australia. *Medical Journal of Australia, 158*, 379–382.

Crane, L. A., Kaplan, C. P., Bastani, R., & Scrimshaw, S. C. M. (1996). Determinants of adherence among health department patients referred for a mammogram. *Women and Health, 24*, 43–64.

Cwikel, J., Rozentsweig, A., Sofer, T., Ben-Tal, T., & Shvartzman, P. (1994). Past and present contraceptive behavior of new Soviet immigrant women in Israel. *Public Health Reviews 1994, 22*, 39–46.

Daly, J., Jackson, D., Davidson, P. M., Wade, V., Chin, C., & Brimelow, V. (1998). The experiences of female spouses of survivors of acute myocardial infarction: A pilot study of Lebanese-born women in south-western Sydney, Australia. *Journal of Advanced Nursing, 28*, 1199–1206.

D'Avanzo, C. E., & Barab, S. A. (1998). Depression and anxiety among Cambodian refugee women in France and the United States. *Issues in Mental Health Nursing, 19*, 541–556.

D'Avanzo, C. E., Frye, B., & Froman, R. (1994). Stress in Cambodian refugee families. *Image: Journal of Nursing Scholarship, 26*, 101–105.

Davila, Y. R., & Brackley, M. H. (1999). Mexican and Mexican American women in battered women's shelter: Barriers to condom negotiation for HIV/AIDS Prevention. *Issues in Mental Health Nursing, 20*, 333–335.

De Santis, L., & Ugarriza, D. N. (1995). Potential for intergenerational conflict in Cuban and Haitian immigrant families. *Archives of Psychiatric Nursing, 9*, 354–364.

Dolman, J., Shackleton, G., Ziaian, T., Gay, J., & Yeboah, D. A. (1996). A survey of health agencies' responses to non-English-speaking women's health needs in South Australia. *Australian and New Zealand Journal of Public Health, 20*, 155–160.

Donato, F., Bollani, A., Spiazzi, R., Soldo, M., Pasquale, L., Monarca, S., Lucini, L., & Nardi, G. (1991). Factors associated with non-participation of women in a breast cancer screening programme in a town in northern Italy. *Journal of Epidemiology and Community Health, 45*, 59–64.

Doucet, H., Baumgarten, M., & Infante-Rivard, C. (1992). Risk of low birthweight and prematurity among foreign-born mothers. *Canadian Journal of Public Health, 83*, 192–195.

Downs, K., Bernstein, J., & Marchese, T. (1997). Providing culturally competent primary care for immigrant and refugee women: A Cambodian case study. *Journal of Nurse-Midwifery, 42*, 499–508.

Dyck, I. (1992). Managing chronic illness: An immigrant woman's acquisition and use of health care knowledge. *American Journal of Occupational Therapy, 46*, 696–705.

Dyck, I. (1995). Putting chronic illness 'in place'. Women immigrants' accounts of their health care. *Geoforum, 26*, 247–260.

Eden, L., Ejlertsson, G., & Leden, I. (1995). Health and health care utilization among early retirement pensioners with musculoskeletal disorders. *Scandinavian Journal of Primary Health Care, 13*, 211–216.

Edwards, N. (1994). Factors influencing prenatal class attendance among immigrants in Ottawa-Carleton. *Revue Canadienne De Sante Publique, 85*, 254–258.

Edwards, N. C., & Boivin, J. F. (1997). Ethnocultural predictors of postpartum infant-care behaviours among immigrants in Canada. *Ethnicity and Health, 2*, 163–176.

English, P. B., Kharrazi, M., & Guendelman, S. (1997). Pregnancy outcomes and risk factors in Mexican Americans: The effect of language use and mother's birthplace. *Ethnicity and Disease, 7*, 229–240.

Erickson, J. G., Devlieger, P. J., & Sung, J. M. (1999). Korean-American female perspectives on disability. *American Journal of Speech-Language Pathology, 8,* 99–108.

Esposito, N. W. (1999). Marginalized women's comparisons of their hospital and freestanding birth center experiences: A contrast of inner-city birthing systems. *Health Care for Women International, 20,* 111–126.

Ever-Hadani, P., Seidman, D. S., Manor, O., & Harlap, S. (1994). Breastfeeding in Israel: Maternal factors associated with choice and duration. *Journal of Epidemiology and Community Health, 48,* 281–285.

Eyega, Z., & Conneely, E. (1997). Facts and fiction regarding female circumcision/female genital mutilation: A pilot study in New York City. *Journal of the American Medical Women's Association, 52,* 174–187.

Factourovich, A., Ritsner, M., Maoz, B., Levin, K., Mirsky, J., Ginath, Y., Segal, A., & Bar Nata, E. (1996). Psychological adjustment among Soviet immigrant physicians: Distress and self-assessments of its sources. *Israeli Journal of Psychiatry and Related Sciences, 33,* 32–39.

Faller, H. S. (1992). Hmong women: Characteristics and birth outcomes, 1990. *Birth, 19,* 144–148.

Farr, K. A., & Wilson-Figueroa, M. (1997). Talking about health and health care: Experiences and perspectives of Latina women in a farmworking community. *Women and Health, 25,* 23–40.

Farrales, L. L., & Chapman, G. E. (1999). Filipino women living in Canada: Constructing meanings of body, food, and health. *Health Care for Women International, 20,* 179–194.

Fernandez, M. E., Tortolero-Luna, G., & Gold, R. S. (1998). Mammography and Pap test screening among low-income foreign-born Hispanic women in the USA. *Cadernos de Saude Publica, 14* (Suppl. 3), 133–147.

Fitch, M. I., Greenberg, M., Levstein, L., Muir, M., Plante, S., & King, E. (1997). Health promotion and early detection of cancer in older adults: Assessing knowledge about cancer. *Oncology Nursing Forum, 24,* 1743–1748.

Flaskerud, J. H., & Uman, G. (1996). Acculturation and its effects on self-esteem among immigrant Latina women. *Journal of Behavioral Medicine, 22,* 123–133.

Fornazzari, X., & Freire, M. (1990). Women as victims of torture. *Acta Psychiatrica Scandinavica, 82,* 257–260.

Fox, P. G. (1991). Stress related to family change among Vietnamese refugees. *Journal of Community Health Nursing, 8,* 45–56.

Fox, P. G., Cowell, J. M., & Johnson, M. M. (1995). Effects of family disruption on Southeast Asian refugee women. *International Nursing Review, 42,* 27–30.

Fox, P. G., Cowell, J. M., Montgomery, A. C., & Willgerodt, M. A. (1997). Southeast Asian refugee women and depression: A nursing intervention. *International Journal of Psychiatric Nursing Research, 4,* 423–432.

Franks, F., & Faux, S. A. (1990). Depression, stress, mastery, and social resources in four ethnocultural women's groups. *Research in Nursing and Health, 13,* 283–292.

Fruchter, R. G., Nayeri, K., Remy, J. C., Wright, C., Feldman, J. G., Boyce, J. G., & Burnett, W. S. (1990). Cervix and breast cancer incidence in immigrant Caribbean women. *American Journal of Public Health, 80,* 722–724.

Frye, B. A., & D'Avanzo, C. D. (1994a). Cultural themes in family stress and violence among Cambodian refugee women in the inner city. *Advances in Nursing Science, 16*, 64–77.

Frye, B. A., & D'Avanzo, C. (1994b). Themes in managing culturally defined illness in the Cambodian refugee family. *Journal of Community Health Nursing, 11*, 89–98.

Fuentes-Afflick, E., Hessol, N. A., & Perez-Stable, E. J. (1998). Maternal birthplace, ethnicity, and low birth weight in California. *Archives of Pediatrics & Adolescents Medicine, 152*, 1105–1112.

Fulton, J. P., Rakowski, W., & Jones, A. C. (1995). Determinants of breast cancer screening among inner-city Hispanic women in comparison with other inner-city women. *Public Health Reports, 110*, 476–482.

Furnham, A., & Shiekh, S. (1993). Gender, generational and social support correlates of mental health in Asian immigrants. *The International Journal of Social Psychiatry, 39*, 22–33.

Gaffney, K. F., Choi, E., Yi, K., Jones, G. B., Bowman, C., & Tavangar, N. N. (1997). Stressful events among pregnant Salvadoran women: A cross-cultural comparison. *Journal of Obstetric, Gynecologic and Neonatal Nursing, 26*, 303–310.

Gagnon, A. J., Edgar, L., Kramer, M. S., Papageorgiou, A., Waghorn, K., & Klein, M. C. (1997). A randomized trial of a program of early postpartum discharge with nurse visitation. *American Journal of Obstetrics and Gynecology, 176*, 205–211.

Gannage, C. M. (1999). The health and safety concerns of immigrant women workers in the Toronto sportswear industry. *International Journal of Health Services, 29*, 409–429.

Gelfand, D. E., & McCallum, J. (1994). Immigration, the family, and female caregivers in Australia. *Journal of Gerontological Social Work, 22*, 41–59.

Ghaemi-Ahmadi, S. (1992). Attitudes toward breastfeeding and infant feeding among Iranian, Afghan, and Southeast Asian immigrant women in the United States: Implications for health and nutrition education. *Journal of the American Dietetic Association, 92*, 354–355.

Ghaffarian, S. (1998). The acculturation of Iranian immigrants in the United States and the implications for mental health. *The Journal of Social Psychology, 138*, 645–654.

Gifford, S. M. (1994). The change of life, the sorrow of life: Menopause, bad blood and cancer among Italian-Australian working class women. *Culture, Medicine and Psychiatry, 18*, 299–319.

Glasser, S., Barell, V., Shoham, A., Ziv, A., Boyko, V., Lusky, A., & Hart, S. (1998). Prospective study of postpartum depression in an Israeli cohort: Prevalence, incidence and demographic risk factors. *Journal of Psychosomatic Obstetrics and Gynecology, 19*, 155–164.

Glover, G. R. (1991). The use of inpatient psychiatric care by immigrants in a London borough. *International Journal of Social Psychiatry, 37*, 121–134.

Golding, J. M., Burnam, M. A., Benjamin, B., & Wells, K. B. (1993). Risk factors for secondary depression among Mexican Americans and non-Hispanic Whites: Alcohol use, alcohol dependence, and reasons for drinking. *Journal of Nervous and Mental Disease, 181*(3), 166–175.

Gomez, C. A., Hernandez, M., & Faigeles, B. (1999). Sex in the New World: An empowerment model for HIV prevention in Latina immigrant women. *Health Education & Behavior, 26,* 200–212.

Granot, M., Spitzer, A., Aroian, K. J., Ravid, C., Tamir, B., & Noam, R. (1996). Pregnancy and delivery practices and beliefs of Ethiopian immigrant women in Israel. *Western Journal of Nursing Research, 18,* 299–313.

Greene, V. W., Dolberg, O. T., Alkan, M. L., & Schlaeffer, F. C. (1992/1993). Tuberculosis cases in the Negev 1978–1987: Ethnicity, sex, and age. *Public Health Review, 20,* 53–60.

Grisaru, N., Lezer, S., & Belmaker, R. H. (1997). Ritual female genital surgery among Ethiopian Jews. *Archives of Sexual Behavior, 26,* 211–215.

Harding, M. J., Pilkington, P., & Thomas, J. (1995). Tuberculosis epidemiology in Croydon. *Public Health, 109,* 251–257.

Hattar-Pollara, M., & Meleis, A. I. (1995a). Parenting their adolescents: The experiences of Jordanian immigrant women in California. *Health Care for Women International, 16,* 195–211.

Hattar-Pollara, M., & Meleis, A. I. (1995b). The stress of immigration and the daily lived experiences of Jordanian immigrant women in the United States. *Western Journal of Nursing Research, 17,* 521–539.

Hauff, E., & Vaglum, P. (1995). Organised violence and the stress of exile: Predictors of mental health in a community cohort of Vietnamese refugees three years after resettlement. *British Journal of Psychiatry, 166,* 360–367.

Have, M. L. ten, & Bijl, R. V. (1999). Inequalities in mental health care and social services utilisation by immigrant women. *European Journal of Public Health, 9,* 45–51.

Hemingway, H., Saunders, D., & Parsons, L. (1997). Social class, spoken language and pattern of care as determinants of continuity of carer in maternity services in east London. *Journal of Public Health Medicine, 19,* 156–161.

Henriksen, C., Brunvand, L., Stoltenberg, C., Trygg, K., Haug, E., & Pedersen, J. I. (1995). Diet and vitamin D status among pregnant Pakistani women in Oslo. *European Journal of Clinical Nutrition, 49,* 211–218.

Herrinton, L. J., Stanford, J. L., Schwartz, S. M., & Weiss, N. S. (1994). Ovarian cancer incidence among Asian migrants to the United States and their descendants. *Journal of the National Cancer Institute, 86,* 1336–1339.

Hiatt, R. A., & Pasick, R. J. (1996). Unsolved problems in early breast cancer detection: Focus on the underserved. *Breast Cancer Research and Treatment, 40,* 37–51.

Hilder, A. S. (1993). Short birth intervals: The experience of Bangladeshi immigrants to the United Kingdom, 1974 through 1984. *Ethnicity and Disease, 3,* 137–144.

Hjelm, K., Nyberg, P., Isacsson, A., & Apelqvist, J. (1999). Beliefs about health and illness essential for self-care practice: A comparison of immigrant Yugoslavian and Swedish diabetic females. *Journal of Advanced Nursing, 30,* 1147–1159.

Horswill, L. J., & Yap, C. (1999). Consumption of foods from the WIC food packages of Chinese prenatal patients on the US west coast. *Journal of the American Dietetic Association, 99,* 1549–1553.

Hsu-Hage, B. H.-H., & Wahlqvist, M. L. (1993). Cardiovascular risk in adult Melbourne Chinese. *Australian Journal of Public Health, 17*, 306–313.

Hubbell, F. A., Chavez, L. R., Mishra, S. I., Magana, J. R., & Valdez, R. B. (1995). From ethnography to intervention: Developing a breast cancer control program for Latinas. *Journal of the National Cancer Institute Monographs, 18*, 109–115.

Hubbell, F. A., Chavez, L. R., Mishra, S. I., & Valdez, R. B. (1996). Beliefs about sexual behavior and other predictors of Papanicolaou smear screening among Latinas and Anglo women. *Archives of Internal Medicine, 156*, 2353–2358.

Hummer, R. A., Biegler, M., DeTurk, P. B., Forbes, D., Frisbie, W. P., Hong, Y., & Pullum, S. G. (1999). Race/ethnicity, nativity, and infant mortality in the United States. *Social Forces, 77*, 1083–1118.

Hurh, W. M., & Kim, K. C. (1990). Correlates of Korean immigrants' mental health. *Journal of Nervous and Mental Disease, 178*, 703–711.

Hurtig, A. K., Nicoll, A., Carne, C., Lissauer, T., Connor, N., Webster, J. P., & Ratcliffe, L. (1998). Syphilis in pregnant women and their children in the United Kingdom: Results from national clinician reporting surveys 1994-7. *British Medical Journal, 317*, 1617–1619.

Hyman, I., & Dussault, G. (1996). The effect of acculturation on low birthweight in immigrant women. *Revue Canadienne De Sante Publique, 87*, 158–162.

Ibison, J. M., Swerdlow, A. J., Head, J. A., & Marmot, M. (1996). Maternal mortality in England and Wales 1970–1985: An analysis by country of birth. *British Journal of Obstetrics and Gynaecology, 103*, 973–980.

Im, E. O., & Meleis, A. I. (1999). A situation-specific theory of Korean immigrant women's menopausal transition. *Image: Journal of Nursing Scholarship, 31*, 333–338.

Im, E. O., Meleis, A. I., & Lee, K. A. (1999). Symptom experience during menopausal transition: Low income Korean immigrant women. *Women and Health, 29*, 53–67.

Iscovich, J., Shushan, A., Schenker, J. G., & Paltiel, O. (1998). The incidence of borderline ovarian tumors in Israel. *Cancer, 82*, 147–151.

Jackson, D. (1995). Constructing nursing practice: Country of origin, culture and competency. *International Journal of Nursing Practice, 1*, 32–36.

Jackson, D. (1996). The multicultural workplace: Comfort, safety and migrant nurses. *Contemporary Nurse, 5*(3), 120–126.

Jacob, K. S., Bhugra, D., Lloyd, K. R., & Mann, A. H. (1998). Common mental disorders, explanatory models and consultation behaviour among Indian women living in the UK. *Journal of the Royal Society of Medicine, 91*, 66–71.

Jenkins, C. N. H., McPhee, S. J., Bird, J. A., & Bonilla, N. H. (1990). Cancer risks and prevention practices among Vietnamese refugees. *Western Journal of Medicine, 153*, 34–39.

Jermott, L. S., Maula, E. C., & Bush, E. (1999). Hearing our voices: Assessing HIV prevention needs among Asian and Pacific Islander women. *Journal of Transcultural Nursing, 10*, 102–111.

Johansson, L. M., Sundquist, J., Johansson, S.-E., Bergman, B., Qvist, J., & Traskman-Bendz, L. (1997). Suicide among foreign-born minorities and native Swedes: An epidemiological follow-up study of a defined population. *Social Science and Medicine, 44*, 181—187.

Jones, L. A., Gonzalez, R., Pillow, P. C., Gomez-Garza, S. A., Foreman, C. J., Chilton, J. A., Linares, A., Yick, J., Badrei, M., & Hajek, R. A. (1997). Dietary fiber, Hispanics, and breast cancer risk? *Annals of the New York Academy of Sciences, 837*, 524–536.

Jones, M. E., & Bond, M. L. (1999). Predictors of birth outcomes among Hispanic immigrant women. *Journal of Nursing Care Quality, 14*, 56–62.

Juarbe, T. C. (1998). Cardiovascular disease-related diet and exercise experiences of immigrant Mexican women. *Western Journal of Nursing Research, 20*, 765–782.

Kahler, L. R., Sobota, C. M., Hines, C. K., & Griswold, K. (1996). Pregnant women at risk: An evaluation of the health status of refugee women in Buffalo, New York. *Health Care for Women International, 17*, 15–23.

Kalofonos, I., & Palinkas, L. A. (1999). Barriers to prenatal care for Mexican and Mexican American women. *Journal of Gender, Culture, and Health, 4*, 135–152.

Kamineni, A., Williams, M. A., Schwartz, S. M., Cook, L. S., & Weiss, N. S. (1999). The incidence of gastric carcinoma in Asian migrants to the United States and their descendants. *Cancer Causes and Control, 10*, 77–83.

Kaufman, Z., Shpitz, B., & Rozin, M. (1995). Mastectomy as the preferred treatment for breast cancer among new immigrants from the former USSR. *Journal of Surgical Oncology, 60*, 168–173.

Kieffer, E. C., Martin, J. A., & Herman, W. H. (1999). Impact of maternal nativity on the prevalence of diabetes during pregnancy among U. S. ethnic groups. *Diabetes Care, 22*, 729–735.

Kim, O. (1999). Predictors of loneliness in elderly Korean immigrant women living in the United States of America. *Journal of Advanced Nursing, 29*, 1082–1088.

Kim, S., & Rew, L. (1994). Ethnic identity, role integration, quality of life, and depression in Korean-American women. *Archives of Psychiatric Nursing, 8*, 348–356.

King, G., Polednak, A. P., Bendel, R., & Hovey, D. (1999). Cigarette smoking among native and foreign-born African Americans. *Annals of Epidemiology, 9*, 236–244.

Kliewer, E. V., & Smith, K. R. (1995a). Breast cancer mortality among immigrants in Australia and Canada. *Journal of the National Cancer Institute, 87*, 1154-1161.

Kliewer, E. V., & Smith, K. R. (1995b). Ovarian cancer mortality among immigrants in Australia and Canada. *Cancer Epidemiology, Biomarkers & Prevention, 4*, 453–458.

Knapp, R. B., & Houghton, M. D. (1999). Breastfeeding practices of WIC participants from the former USSR. *Journal of the American Dietetic Association, 99*, 1269–1271.

Knight, R., Hotchin, A., Bayly, C., & Grover, S. (1999). Female genital mutilation— Experience of the Royal Women's Hospital, Melbourne. *Australian and New Zealand Journal of Obstetrics and Gynaecology, 39*, 50–54.

Kouris-Blazos, A., Wahlqvist, M. L., Trichopoulou, A., Polychronopoulos, E., & Trichopoulos, D. (1996). Health and nutritional status of elderly Greek migrants to Melbourne, Australia. *Age and Ageing, 25*, 177–189.

Kuiper, H., Richwald, G. A., Rotblatt, H., & Asch, S. (1999). The communicable disease impact of eliminating publicly funded prenatal care for undocumented immigrants. *Maternal and Child Health Journal, 3*, 39–52.

Kulig, J. C. (1990). A review of the health status of Southeast Asian refugee women. *Health Care for Women International, 11*, 49–63.

Kulig, J. C. (1994a). "Those with unheard voices": The plight of a Cambodian refugee woman. *Journal of Community Health Nursing, 11*, 99–107.

Kulig, J. C. (1994b). Sexuality beliefs among Cambodians: Implications for health care professionals. *Health Care for Women International, 15*, 69–76.

Kulig, J. C. (1995). Cambodian refugees' family planning knowledge and use. *Journal of Advanced Nursing, 22*, 150–157.

Kulwicki, A. D., & Miller, J. (1999). Domestic violence in the Arab American population: Transforming environmental conditions through community education. *Issues in Mental Health Nursing, 20*, 199–215.

Kuss, T. (1997). Family planning experiences of Vietnamese women. *Journal of Community Health Nursing, 14*, 155–168.

Kwan, L. F., Ho, Y. Y., & Lee, S. S. (1997). The declining HBsAg carriage rate in pregnant women in Hong Kong. *Epidemiology and Infection, 119*, 281–283.

Layzell, S., & England, R. (1999). What do Turkish women want to know about sexual health? A study to inform the production of Turkish language information leaflets. *Health Education Journal, 58*, 130–138.

Leidy, L. (1998). Menarche, menopause, and migration: Implications for breast cancer research. *American Journal of Human Biology, 10*, 451–457.

Lenart, J. C., St. Clair, P. A., & Bell, M. A. (1991). Childrearing knowledge, beliefs and practices of Cambodian refugees. *Journal of Pediatric Health Care, 5*, 299–305.

Lesjak, M., Hua, M., & Ward, J. (1999). Cervical screening among immigrant Vietnamese women seen in general practice: Current rates, predictors and potential recruitment strategies. *Australian and New Zealand Journal of Public Health, 23*, 168–173.

Li, D.-K., Ni, H., Schwartz, S. M., & Daling, J. R. (1990). Secular change in birthweight among Southeast Asian immigrants to the United States. *American Journal of Public Health, 80*, 685–688.

Lindenberg, C. S., Strickland, O., Solorzano, R., Galvis, C., Dreher, M., & Darrow, V. C. (1999). Correlates of alcohol and drug use among low-income Hispanic immigrant childbearing women living in the U.S.A. *International Journal of Nursing Studies, 36*, 3–11.

Lipson, J. G., Hosseini, T., Kabir, S., Omidian, P. A., & Edmonston, F. (1995). Health issues among Afghan women in California. *Health Care for Women International, 16*, 279–286.

Lipson, J. G., McElmurry, B., & LaRosa, J. (1997). Women across the life span: A working group on immigrant women and their health. *Proceedings of the American Academy of Nursing 1995 Annual Meeting and Conference, Health Care in Times of Global Transitions*, (#G-194), 47–65.

Lipson, J. G., & Miller, S. (1994). Changing roles of Afghan refugee women in the United States. *Health Care for Women International, 15*, 171–180.

Locke, C. J., Southwick, K., McCloskey, L. A., & Fernandez-Esquer, M. E. (1996). The psychological and medical sequelae of war in Central American refugee mothers and children. *Archives of Pediatric and Adolescent Medicine, 150,* 822–828.

Luna, L. (1994). Care and cultural context of Lebanese Muslim immigrants: Using Leininger's theory. *Journal of Transcultural Nursing, 5,* 12–20.

Lundberg, P. C. (1999). Meanings and practices of health among married Thai immigrant women in Sweden. *Journal of Transcultural Nursing, 10,* 31–36.

Lynam, M. J. (1985). Support networks developed by immigrant women. *Social Science and Medicine, 21,* 327–333.

Ma, J., & Bauman, A. (1996). Obstetric profiles and pregnancy outcomes of immigrant women in New South Wales, 1990–1992. *Australian and New Zealand Journal of Obstetrics and Gynaecology, 36,* 119–125.

MacIntyre, C. R., Dwyer, B., & Streeton, J. A. (1993). The epidemiology of tuberculosis in Victoria. *Medical Journal of Australia, 159,* 672–677.

Mahloch, J., Jackson, C., Chitnarong, K., Sam, R., Ngo, L. S., & Taylor, V. M. (1999). Bridging cultures through the development of a cervical cancer screening video for Cambodian women in the United States. *Journal of Cancer Education, 14,* 109–114.

Maltby, H. (1998). Health promotion for Vietnamese women and their families. *Nursing Standard, 12*(32), 40–43.

Maltby, H. (1999). The common thread: Health care activities of Vietnamese and Anglo-Australian women. *Health Care for Women International, 20,* 291–302.

Mattson, S., & Lew, L. (1992). Culturally sensitive prenatal care for Southeast Asians. *Journal of Obstetric, Gynecologic, and Neonatal Nursing, 21,* 48–54.

Matuk, L. C. (1996a). Pap smear screening practices in newcomer women. *Women's Health Issues, 6,* 82–88.

Matuk, L. C. (1996b). Health status of newcomers. *Canadian Journal of Public Health, 87,* 52–55.

McPhee, S. J., Bird, J. A., & Davis, T. (1997). Barriers to breast and cervical cancer screening among Vietnamese-American women. *American Journal of Preventive Medicine, 13,* 205–213.

McPhee, S. J., Bird, J. A., Davis, T., Ha, N., Jenkins, C. N. H., & Le, B. (1997). Barriers to breast and cervical cancer screening among Vietnamese-American women. *American Journal of Preventative Medicine, 13,* 205–213.

McPhee, S. J., Stewart, S., Brock, K. C., Bird, J. A., Jenkins, C. N. H., & Pham, G. Q. (1997). Factors associated with breast and cervical cancer screening practices among Vietnamese American women. *Cancer Detection and Prevention, 21,* 510–521.

McVeigh, C. (1997). Functional status after childbirth: A comparison of Australian women from English and non-English speaking backgrounds. *Australian College of Midwives Incorporated, 10,* 15–21.

Meftuh, A. B., Tapsoba, L. P., & Lamounier, J. A. (1991). Breastfeeding practices in Ethiopian women in southern California. *Indian Journal of Pediatrics, 58,* 349–356.

Meleis, A. I. (1990, November). Between two cultures: Identity, roles, and health. Keynote address for the *Fourth International Congress on Women's Health Issues*, Palmerston North, New Zealand.

Meleis, A. I. (1991). Between two cultures: Identity, roles, and health. *Health Care for Women International, 12*, 364–377.

Meleis, A. I., Lipson, J. G., Muecke, M., & Smith, G. (1998). *Immigrant women and their health: An olive paper* (pp. 1–30). Indianapolis, IN: Sigma Theta Tau International.

Meleis, A. I., & Rogers, S. (1987). Women in transition: Being versus becoming or being and becoming. *Health Care for Women International, 8*, 199–217.

Menendez, B. S., Blum, S., Singh, T. P., & Drucker, E. (1993). Trends in AIDS mortality among residents of Puerto Rico and among Puerto Rican immigrants and other Hispanic residents of New York City, 1981–1989. *New York State Journal of Medicine, 93*, 12–15.

Miller, L. C., Jami-Imam, F., Timouri, M., & Wijnker, J. (1995). Trained traditional birth attendants as educators of refugee mothers. *World Health Forum, 16*, 151–156.

Mirsky, J., & Barasch, M. (1993). Adjustment problems among Soviet immigrants at risk, Part 2: Emotional distress among elderly Soviet immigrants during the Gulf War. *Israeli Journal of Psychiatry and Related Sciences, 30*, 233–243.

Mitchell, J., & Mackerras, D. (1995). The traditional humoral food habits of pregnant Vietnamese-Australian women and their effect on birth weight. *Australian Journal of Public Health, 19*, 629–633.

Moghaddam, F. M., Ditto, B., & Taylor, D. M. (1990). Attitudes and attributions related to psychological symptomatology in Indian immigrant women. *Journal of Cross-Cultural Psychology, 21*, 335–350.

Mor, J. M., Alexander, G. R., Kieffer, E. C., & Baruffi, G. (1993). Birth outcomes of Korean women in Hawaii. *Public Health Reports, 108*, 500–505.

Morrell, S., Taylor, R., Slaytor, E., & Ford, P. (1999). Urban and rural suicide differentials in immigrants and the Australian-born, New South Wales, Australia 1985–1994. *Social Science and Medicine, 49*, 81–91.

Morris, R. (1996). The culture of female circumcision. *Advances in Nursing Science, 19*, 43–53.

Moss, N., Baumeister, L., & Biewener, J. (1996). Perspectives of Latina immigrant women on Proposition 187. *Journal—American Medical Women's Association, 51*, 161–165.

Moss, N., Stone, M. C., & Smith, J. B. (1993). Fertility among Central American refugees and immigrants in Belize. *Human Organization, 52*, 186–193.

Mui, A. C. (1996). Depression among elderly Chinese immigrants: An exploratory study. *Social Work, 41*, 633–645.

Munet-Vilaro, F., Folkman, S., & Gregorich, S. (1999). Depressive symptomatology in three Latino groups. *Western Journal of Nursing Research, 21*, 209–224.

Nahas, V., & Nawal, A. (1999). Culture care meanings and experiences of postpartum depression among Jordanian Australian women: A transcultural study. *Journal of Transcultural Nursing, 10*, 37–45.

Nahas, V. L., Hillege, S., & Amasheh, N. (1999). Postpartum depression: The lived experiences of Middle Eastern migrant women in Australia. *Journal of Nurse-Midwifery, 44*, 65–74.

Nedstrand, E., Ekseth, U., Lindgren, R., & Hammar, M. (1995). The climacteric among South-American women, who immigrated to Sweden and age-matched Swedish women. *Maturitas: Journal of the Climacteric & Postmenopause, 21*, 3–6.

Nemoto, T., Aoki, B., Huang, K., Morris, A., Nguyen, H., & Wong, W. (1999). Drug use behaviors among Asian drug users in San Francisco. *Addictive Behaviors, 24*, 823–838.

Newell, A., Sullivan, A., Halai, R., & Boag, F. (1998). Sexually transmitted diseases, cervical cytology and contraception in immigrants and refugees from the former Yugoslavia. *Venereology, 11*, 25–27.

Neysmith, S. M., & Aronson, J. (1997). Working conditions in home care: Negotiating race and class boundaries in gendered work. *International Journal of Health Services, 27*, 479–499.

Nilsson, B., Gustavson-Kadaka, E., Hakulinon, T , Aareleid, T., Rahu, M., Dyba, T., & Rotstein, S. (1997). Cancer survival in Estonian migrants to Sweden. *Journal of Epidemiology Community Health, 51*, 418–423.

Noh, S., Wu, Z., Speechley, M., & Kaspar, V. (1992). Depression in Korean immigrants in Canada II: Correlates of gender, work, and marriage. *Journal of Nervous and Mental Disease, 180*, 578–582.

Nolan, T. E., Espinosa, T. L., & Pastorek, J. G. (1997). Tuberculosis skin testing in pregnancy: Trends in a population. *Journal of Perinatology, 17*, 199–201.

Nwadiora, E., & McAdoo, H. (1996). Acculturative stress among Amerasian refugees: Gender and racial differences. *Adolescence, 31*, 477–487.

O'Connor, C. C., Berry, G., Rohrsheim, R., & Donovan, B. (1996). Sexual health and use of condoms among local and international sex workers in Sydney. *Genitourinary Medicine, 72*, 47–51.

Ogur, B. (1990). Mental health problems of translocated women. *Health Care for Women International, 11*, 43–47.

Oldenburg, C. E. M., Rasmussen, F., & Cotton, N. U. (1997). Ethnic differences in rates of infant mortality and sudden infant death in Sweden, 1978–1990. *European Journal of Public Health, 7*, 88–94.

O'Malley, A. S., Kerner, J., Johnson, A. E., & Mandelblatt, J. (1999). Acculturation and breast cancer screening among Hispanic women in New York City. *American Journal of Public Health, 89*, 219–227.

Omeri, A. (1997). Culture care of Iranian immigrants in New South Wales, Australia: Sharing transcultural nursing knowledge. *Journal of Transcultural Nursing, 8*, 5–16.

Palacios, C., & Sheps, S. (1992). A pilot study assessing the health status of the Hispanic American community living in Vancouver. *Canadian Journal of Public Health, 83*, 346–349.

Pang, K. Y. C. (1990). Hwabyung: The construction of a Korean popular illness among Korean elderly immigrant women in the United States. *Culture, Medicine and Psychiatry, 14*, 495–512.

Pappagallo, S., & Bull, D. L. (1996). Operational problems of an iron supplementation programme for pregnant women: An assessment of UNRWA experience. *Bulletin of the World Health Organization, 74*, 25–33.

Peel, M. R. (1996). Effects on asylum seekers of ill treatment in Zaire. *British Medical Journal, 312*, 293–294.

Peragallo, N. P., Fox, P. G., & Alba, M. L. (1998). Breast care among Latino immigrant women in the U.S. *Health Care for Women International, 19*, 165–172.

Perez-Escamilla, R., Himmelgreen, D., Segura-Millan, S., Gonzalez, A., Ferris, A. M., Damio, G., & Bermudez-Vega, A. (1998). Prenatal and perinatal factors associated with breastfeeding initiation among inner-city Puerto Rican women. *Journal of the American Dietetic Association, 98*, 657–663.

Peterson, G. W., Cobas, J. A., Balcazar, H., & Amling, J. W. (1998). Acculturation and risk behavior among pregnant Mexican American females: A structural equation model. *Sociological Inquiry, 68*, 536–556.

Phipps, E., Cohen, M. H., Sorn, R., & Braitman, L. E. (1999). A pilot study of cancer knowledge and screening behaviors of Vietnamese and Cambodian women. *Health Care of Women International, 20*, 195–207.

Pickwell, S. M., Schimelpfening, S., & Palinkas, L. A. (1994). 'Betelmania' Betel quid chewing by Cambodian women in the United States and its potential health effects. *Western Journal of Medicine, 160*, 326–330.

Ponizovsky, A., Ginath, Y., Durst, R., Wondimeneh, B., Safro, S., Minuchin-Itzigson, S., & Ritsner, M. (1998). Psychological distress among Ethiopian and Russian Jewish immigrants to Israel: A cross-cultural study. *International Journal of Social Psychiatry, 44*, 35–45.

Ponizovsky, A., Safro, S., Ginath, Y., & Ritsner, M. (1997). Suicide ideation among recent immigrants: An epidemiological study. *Israeli Journal of Psychiatry and Related Sciences, 34*, 139–148.

Porsch-Oezcueruemez, M., Bilgin, Y., Wollny, M., Gediz, A., Arat, A., Karatay, E., Akinci, A., Sinterhauf, K., Koch, H., Siegfried, I., von Georgi, R., Brenner, G., Kloer, H. U., & The Giessen Study Group (1999). Prevalence of risk factors of coronary heart disease in Turks living in Germany: The Giessen study. *Atheroscle-rosis, 144*, 185–198.

Raleigh, V. S., & Balarajan, R. (1992). Suicide and self-burning among Indians and West Indians in England and Wales. *British Journal of Psychiatry, 161*, 365–368.

Raleigh, V. S., Bulusu, L., & Balarajan, R. (1990). Suicides among immigrants from the Indian subcontinent. *British Journal of Psychiatry, 156*, 46–50.

Rapp, R. (1997). Communicating about chromosomes: Patient, providers, and cultural assumptions. *Journal—American Medical Women's Association, 52*, 28–32.

Reichman, N. E., & Kenney, G. M. (1998). Prenatal care, birth outcomes and newborn hospitalization costs: Patterns among Hispanics in New Jersey. *Family Planning Perspectives, 30*, 182–187.

Remennick, L. I. (1999a). Breast screening practices among Russian immigrant women in Israel. *Women and Health, 28*, 29–51.

Remennick, L. I. (1999b). Preventive behavior among recent immigrants: Russian-speaking women and cancer screening in Israel. *Social Science and Medicine, 48*, 1669–1684.

Remennick, L. I., Amir, D., Elimelech, Y., & Novikov, Y. (1995). Family planning practices and attitudes among former Soviet new immigrant women in Israel. *Social Science and Medicine, 41*, 569–577.

Remennick, L. I., & Ottenstein-Eisen, N. (1998). Reaction of new Soviet immigrants to primary health care services in Israel. *International Journal of Health Services, 28*, 555–574.

Remis, R. S., Eason, E. L., Palmer, R. W. H., Najjar, M., Leclerc, P., Lebel, F., & Fauvel, M. (1995). HIV infection among women undergoing abortion in Montreal. *Canadian Medical Association Journal, 153*, 1271–1279.

Reubsaet, H., & Ineichen, B. (1996). Afro-Surinamese women in the Netherlands: Sexual education, the initiation of sex, and contraceptive use. *European Journal of Contraception and Reproductive Health Care, 1*, 331–335.

Reynolds, D. L., Evangelista, F., Ward, B. M., Notenboom, R. H., Young, E. R., & D'Cunha, C. O. (1998). Syphilis in an urban community. *Canadian Journal of Public Health, 89*, 248–252.

Rice, P. L., & Naksook, C. (1998a). The experience of pregnancy, labour and birth of Thai women in Australia. *Midwifery, 14*, 74–84.

Rice, P. I.., & Nasook, C. (1998b). Caesarean or vaginal birth: Perceptions and experience of Thai women in Australian hospitals. *Australian and New Zealand Journal of Public Health, 22*, 604–608.

Rice, P. L., Naksook, C., & Watson, L. E. (1999). The experiences of postpartum hospital stay and returning home among Thai mothers in Australia. *Midwifery, 15*, 47–57.

Ritsner, M., & Ponizovsky, A. (1998). Psychological symptoms among an immigrant population: A prevalence study. *Comprehensive Psychiatry, 39*, 21–27.

Ritsner, M., Ponizovsky, A., & Ginath, Y. (1999). The effect of age on gender differences in the psychological distress ratings of immigrants. *Stress Medicine, 15*, 17–25.

Rodriguez, M. A., Bauer, H. M., Flores-Ortis, Y., & Szkupinski-Quiroga, S. (1998). Factors affecting patient-physician communication for abused Latina and Asian immigrant women. *Journal of Family Practice, 47*, 309–311.

Romero, G., Wyatt, G. E., Chin, D., & Rodriguez, C. (1998–99). HIV-related behaviors among recently immigrated and undocumented Latinas. *International Quarterly of Community Health Education, 18*, 89–105.

Rossiter, J. C. (1992a). Attitudes of Vietnamese women to baby feeding practices before and after immigration to Sydney, Australia. *Midwifery, 8*, 103–112.

Rossiter, J. C. (1992b). Maternal-infant health beliefs and infant feeding practice: The perception and experience of immigrant Vietnamese women in Sydney. *Contemporary Nurse, 1*, 75–82.

Rossiter, J. C. (1994). The effect of a culture-specific education program to promote breastfeeding among Vietnamese women in Sydney. *International Journal of Nursing Study, 31*, 369–379.

Rossiter, J. C. (1998). Promoting breastfeeding: The perceptions of Vietnamese mothers in Sydney, Australia. *Journal of Advanced Nursing, 28*, 598–605.

Rothenberg, S. J., Manalo, M., Jiang, J., Khan, F., Cuellar, R., Reyes, S., Sanchez, M., Reynoso, B., Aguilar, A., Diaz, M., Acosta, S., Jauregui, M., & Johnson, C.

(1999). Maternal blood lead level during pregnancy in south central Los Angeles. *Archives of Environmental Health, 54,* 151–157.

Ruskin, P. E., Blumstein, Z., Walter-Ginzburg, A., Fuchs, Z., Lusky, A., Novikov, I., & Modan, B. (1996). Depressive symptoms among community-dwelling oldest-old residents in Israel. *American Association for Geriatric Psychiatry, 4,* 208–217.

Russell, A. Y., Williams, M. S., Farr, P. A., Schwab, A. J., & Plattsmier, S. (1999). The mental health status of young Hispanic women residing along the border: A twin cities comparison. *Women and Health, 28,* 15–32.

Santos, S. J., Bohon, L. M., & Sanchez-Sosa, J. J. (1998). Childhood family relationships, marital and work conflict, and mental health distress in Mexican immigrants. *Journal of Community Psychology, 26,* 491–508.

Schreiber, R., Stern, P. N., & Wilson, C. (1998). The contexts for managing depression and its stigma among Black West Indian Canadian women. *Journal of Advanced Nursing, 27,* 510–517.

Schulmeister, L., & Lifsey, D. S. (1999). Cervical cancer screening knowledge, behaviors, and beliefs of Vietnamese women. *Oncology Nursing Forum, 26*(5), 879–887.

Sherraden, M. S., & Barrera, R. E. (1996a). Prenatal care experiences and birth weight among Mexican immigrant women. *Journal of Medical Systems, 20,* 329–350.

Sherraden, M. S., & Barrera, R. E. (1996b). Maternal support and cultural influences among Mexican immigrant mothers. *Families in Society: The Journal of Contemporary Human Services, 77,* 298–313.

Sherraden, M. S., & Barrera, R. E. (1996c). Poverty, family support, and well-being of infants: Mexican immigrant women and childbearing. *Journal of Sociology and Social Welfare, XXIII,* 27–54.

Shin, K. R. (1993). Factors predicting depression among Korean-American women in New York. *International Journal of Nursing Studies, 30,* 415–423.

Shin, K. R. (1994). Psychosocial predictors of depressive symptoms in Korean-American women in New York City. *Women and Health, 21,* 73–82.

Shin, K. R., & Shin, C. (1999). The lived experience of Korean immigrant women acculturating into the United States. *Health Care for Women International, 20,* 603–617.

Silove, D., Sinnerbrink, I., Field, A., Manicavasagar, V., & Steel, Z. (1997). Anxiety, depression and PTSD in asylum-seekers: Associations with pre-migration trauma and post-migration stressors. *British Journal of Psychiatry, 170,* 351–357.

Singer, S. M., Willms, D. G., Adrien, A., Baxter, J., Brabazon, C., Leaune, V., Godin, G., Maticka-Tyndale, E., & Cappon, P. (1996). Many voices—sociocultural results of the ethnocultural communities facing AIDS study in Canada. *Canadian Journal of Public Health, 87,* S26–S32.

Singh, G. K., & Yu, S. M. (1996). Adverse pregnancy outcomes: Differences between US- and foreign-born women in major US racial and ethnic groups. *American Journal of Public Health, 86,* 837–843.

Small, R., Lumley, J., Yelland, J., & Rice, P. L. (1998). Shared antenatal care fails to rate well with women of non-English-speaking backgrounds. *Medical Journal of Australia, 168,* 15–18.

Small, R., Rice, P. L., Yelland, J., & Lumley, J. (1999). Mothers in a new country: The role of culture and communication in Vietnamese, Turkish and Filipino Women's experiences of giving birth in Australia. *Women and Health, 28,* 77–101.

Spring, M. A., Ross, P. J., Etkin, N. L., & Deinard, A. S. (1995). Sociocultural factors in the use of prenatal care by Hmong women, Minneapolis. *American Journal of Public Health, 85,* 1015–1017.

Stanford, J. L., Herrinton, L. J., Schwartz, S. M., & Weiss, N. S. (1995). Breast cancer incidence in Asian migrants to the United States and their descendants. *Epidemiology, 6*(2), 181–183.

Stehr-Green, J. K. (1992). Tuberculosis in New Zealand, 1985–1990. *New Zealand Medical Journal, 105,* 301–303.

Suarez, L., Roche, R. A., Pulley, L. V., Weiss, N. S., Goldman, D., & Simpson, D. M. (1997). Why a peer intervention program for Mexican-American women failed to modify the secular trend in cancer screening. *American Journal of Preventive Medicine, 13,* 411–417.

Sullivan, J. R., & Shepherd, S. J. (1997). Obstetric outcomes and infant birthweights for Vietnamese-born and Australian-born women in southwestern Sydney. *Australian and New Zealand Journal of Public Health, 21,* 159–162.

Sundquist, J., & Johansson, S. E. (1997). The influence of country of birth on mortality from all causes and cardiovascular disease in Sweden 1979–1993. *International Journal of Epidemiology, 26,* 279–287.

Sundquist, J., Cmelic-Eng, M., & Johansson, S. E. (1999) Body mass index and distribution of body fat in female Bosnian refugees—a study in primary health care. *Public Health, 113,* 89–93.

Swerdlow, A. J., Marmot, M. G., Grulich, A. E., & Head, J. (1995). Cancer mortality in Indian and British ethnic immigrants from the Indian subcontinent to England and Wales. *British Journal of Cancer, 72,* 1312–1319.

Tabora, B. L., & Flaskerud, J. H. (1997). Mental health beliefs, practices, and knowledge of Chinese American immigrant women. *Issues in Mental Health Nursing, 18,* 173–189.

Taylor, V. M., Schwartz, S. M., Jackson, J. C., Kuniyuki, A., Fischer, M., Yasui, Y., Tu, S. P., & Thompson, B. (1999). Cervical cancer screening among Cambodian-American women. *Cancer Epidemiology, Biomarkers & Prevention, 8,* 541–546.

Thompson, J. L. (1991). Exploring gender and culture with Khmer refugee women: Reflections on participatory feminist research. *Advances in Nursing Science, 13,* 30–48.

Thorburn, S., Harvey, S. M., & Beckman, L. J. (1998). Emergency contraceptive pills: An exploratory study of knowledge and perceptions among Mexican women from both sides of the border. *Journal of American Medical Women's Association, 53,* 262–265.

Tran, T. V. (1990). Language acculturation among older Vietnamese refugee adults. *Gerontologist, 30,* 94–99.

Tran, V. T. (1993). Psychological traumas and depression in a sample of Vietnamese people in the United States. *Health and Social Work, 18,* 184–194.

Tudiver, F., & Fuller-Thomson, E. (1999). Who has screening mammography? *Canadian Family Physician, 45,* 1901–1907.

Tuttle, C. R., & Dewey, K. G. (1994). Determinants of infant feeding choices among Southeast Asian immigrants in northern California. *Journal of the American Dietetic Association, 94,* 282–286.

Um, C. C., & Dancy, B. (1999). Relationship between coping strategies and depression among employed Korean immigrant wives. *Issues in Mental Health Nursing, 20,* 485–494.

van de Wijngaart, G. F.(1997). Drug problems among immigrants and refugees in the Netherlands and the Dutch health care and treatment system. *Substance Use & Misuse, 32,* 909–938.

Van der Stuyft, P., Woodward, M., Amstrong, J., & De Muynck, A. (1993). Uptake of preventive health care among Mediterranean migrants in Belgium. *Journal of Epidemiology and Community Health, 47,* 10–13.

Van der Zwaard, J. (1992). Accounting for differences: Dutch training and their views on migrant women. *Social Science Medicine, 35,* 1137–1144.

van Enk, A., Buitendijk, S. E., van der Pal, K. M., van Enk, W. J. J., & Schulpen, T. W. J. (1998). Perinatal death in ethnic minorities in the Netherlands. *Journal of Epidemiology and Community Health, 52,* 735–739.

Vangen, S., Stoltenberg, C., & Schei, B. (1996). Ethnicity and use of obstetrical analgesia: Do Pakistani women receive inadequate pain relief in labour? *Ethnicity and Health, 1,* 161–167.

Vega, W. A., Kolody, B., Aguilar-Gaxiola, S., & Catalano, R. (1999). Gaps in service utilization by Mexican Americans with mental health problems. *American Journal of Psychiatry, 156,* 928–934.

Vega, W. A., Kolody, B., Hwang, J., Noble, A., & Porter, P. A. (1997). Perinatal drug use among immigrant and native-born Latinas. *Substance Use & Misuse, 32*(1), 43–62.

Vega, W. A., Kolody, B., Valle, R., & Weir, J. (1991). Social networks, social support, and their relationship to depression among immigrant Mexican women. *Human Organization, 50,* 154–162.

Wang, Q., Ravn, P., Wang, S., Overgaard, K., Hassager, C., & Christiansen, C. (1996). Bone mineral density in immigrants from southern China to Denmark. A cross-sectional study. *European Journal of Endocrinology, 134,* 163–167.

Wasse, H., Holt, V. L., & Daling, J. R. (1994). Pregnancy risk factors and birth outcomes in Washington state: A comparison of Ethiopian-born and US-born women. *American Journal of Public Health, 84,* 1505–1507.

Webster, R. A., McDonald, R., Lewin, T. J., & Carr, V. J. (1995). Effects of a natural disaster on immigrants and host population. *Journal of Nervous and Mental Disease, 183,* 390–397.

Weijers, R. N. M., Bekedam, D. J., & Oosting, H. (1998). The prevalence of type 2 diabetes and gestational diabetes mellitus in an inner city multi-ethnic population. *European Journal of Epidemiology, 14,* 693–699.

Weitzman, B. C., & Berry, C. A. (1992). Health status and health care utilization among New York City home attendants: An illustration of the needs of working poor, immigrant women. *Women and Health, 19,* 87–105.

Welles, S. L., Levine, P. H., Joseph, E. M., Goberdhan, L. J., Lee, S., Miotti, A., Cervantes, J., Bertoni, M., Jaffe, E., & Dosik, H. (1994). An enhanced surveillance program for adult T-cell leukemia in central Brooklyn. *Leukemia, 8* (Suppl. 1), S111–S115.

Westermeyer, J., & Uecker, J. (1997). Predictors of hostility in a group of relocated refugees. *Cultural Diversity and Mental Health, 3,* 53–60.

Wijesinghe, C. P., & Clancy, D. J. (1991). Schizophrenia in migrants living in the western region of Melbourne. *Australian and New Zealand Journal of Psychiatry, 25,* 350–357.

Williams, R., & Hunt, K. (1997). Psychological distress among British South Asians: The contribution of stressful situations and subcultural differences in the West of Scotland Twenty-07 Study. *Psychological Medicine, 27,* 1173–1181.

Williams, R., Bhopal, R., & Hunt, K. (1993). Health of a Punjabi ethnic minority in Glasgow: A comparison with the general population. *Journal of Epidemiology and Community Health, 47,* 96–102.

Willis, W. O., de Peyster, A., Molgaard, C. A., Walker, C., & MacKendrick, T. (1993). Pregnancy outcome among women exposed to pesticides through work or residence in an agricultural area. *Journal of Occupational Medicine, 35,* 943–949.

Woelz-Stirling, N. A., Kelaher, M., & Manderson, L. (1998). Power and the politics of abuse: Rethinking violence in Filipina-Australian marriages. *Health Care for Women International, 19,* 289–301.

Wrightson, K. J., & Wardle, J. (1997). Cultural variation in health locus of control. *Ethnicity and Health, 2,* 13–20.

Yelibi, S., Valenti, P., Volpe, C., Caprara, A., Dedy, S., & Tape, G. (1993). Sociocultural aspects of AIDS in an urban peripheral area of Abidjan (Cote d'Ivoire). *AIDS Care, 5,* 187–197.

Ying, Y. W. (1990). Explanatory models of major depression and implications for help-seeking among immigrant Chinese-American women. *Culture, Medicine and Psychiatry, 14,* 393–408.

Youngshook, H., Williams, R. D., & Harrison, R. A. (1999). Breast self examination (BSE) among Korean American women: Knowledge, attitudes, & behaviors. *Journal of Cultural Diversity, 6,* 115–123.

Yusu, F., Siedlecky, S., & Byrnes, M. (1993). Family planning practices among Lebanese, Turkish and Vietnamese women in Sydney. *Australian and New Zealand Journal of Obstetrics and Gynaecology, 33,* 8–16.

Zambrana, R. E., Dunkel-Schetter, C., & Scrimshaw, S. (1991). Factors which influence use of prenatal care in low-income racial-ethnic women in Los Angeles county. *Journal of Community Health, 16,* 283–295.

Zambrana, R. E., Scrimshaw, S. C. M., Collins, N., & Dunkel-Schetter, C. (1997). Prenatal health behaviors and psychosocial risk factors in pregnant women of Mexican origin: The role of acculturation. *American Journal of Public Health, 87,* 1022–1026.

Ziegler, R. G., Hoover, R. N., Pike, M. C., Hildesheim, A., Nomura, A. M. Y., West, D. W., Wu-Williams, A. H., Kolonel, L. N., Horn-Ross, P. L., Rosenthal, J. F., & Hyer, M. B. (1993). Migration patterns and breast cancer risk in Asian-American women. *Journal of the National Cancer Institute, 85,* 1819–1827.

Zlotnik, H. (1999). Trends of international migration since 1965: What existing data reveal. *International Migration, 37,* 21–61.

PART IV

Research on Women's Health and Illness Issues

Chapter 8

Women and Stress

CHERYL A. CAHILL

ABSTRACT

This review focused on published research reports that explored the association between stress and women's health and illness. Because of the vastness of the literature, the review was limited to three conceptual areas. The first included those studying the association between stress and illness. Most were correlational in design, thus lacking the power to support assertions of a cause-and-effect relationship. The second focused on studies of the psychophysiology of stress. These studies provide nurse scientists and clinicians with insights into the underlying pathology of stress. When paired with behavioral measures, these studies provide a window into brain mechanisms involved in mind/body interactions. The third conceptual area included those studies of stress reduction therapies to influence health and illness. These studies have yielded a mighty arsenal of interventions that may be used to reduce distress.

Key words: behavior, interventions, neuroendocrine regulation, nursing, psychophysiology, stress

The process of living is the process of reacting to stress.

—Stanley J. Sarnoff

As the process of living has become more complicated and fast paced, human reactions to stress have come under scrutiny by nurses and other clinicians striving to understand the mechanisms of adaptation and health. The purpose of this chapter will be to review the results of research into the role of stress in women's health and illness published between 1997 and Spring 2000. Stress will be defined as a bio-behavioral process involved in recognition, perception, and adaptation to the loss or the threat of loss of homeostasis or well-being. This definition was coined to include the various facets of stress addressed by researchers from a variety of disciplines. The definition is broad as are the research approaches taken by scientists. Literature searches were carried out using OVID to access MEDLINE from 1997 to June 2000 and CINAHL from 1982 to 2000. The search was limited to those published in English with keywords, "stress" and "women." This search yielded more than 1000 citations. The search was further limited to three conceptual areas with particular relevance to the practice of nursing. The first consisted of those studies exploring the association between stress and illness. The second perspective focused on investigations of psychophysiological mechanisms of stress as a way to better understand mechanisms of mind–body interactions. Finally, reports of studies of stress reduction strategies to influence health and illness were reviewed. These perspectives were selected because, in the author's opinion, they are most relevant to the practice of nursing and because they include both basic and applied approaches to knowledge development. A total of 500 articles were retrieved and scanned. Those citations that were reports of research studies relevant to women's health and that addressed the three general areas were reviewed in-depth and are reported here.

STRESS AND ILLNESS IN WOMEN

Selye and other scientists who pioneered investigations of neuroendocrine responses to stress postulated that exposure over time would increase wear and tear of living and culminate in disease. These early postulations seemed to be supported by studies that demonstrated an association between reported stressful life events and disease occurrence. Ex post facto studies are inherently dicey because the degree to which those selected for study are representative of the general population is not known. That is, even though a significant number of persons with a particular disease or symptom report having a significant number of daily stresses, there is no way to know whether all persons with similar numbers of daily life stresses experience that disease or symptom. Despite the limitation of the methodology, it has been widely applied to the question of whether stress is associated with disease. The consensus seems to be that such an association exists, however, new approaches to answer this important question have been developed that may suggest otherwise.

Johansen and Olsen (1997) examined the incidence of cancer and deaths in a sample of parents of children diagnosed with cancer between 1943 and 1992. They argued that cancer in a child is a significant stressor and that, if stress were associated with the development of cancer and/or premature death due to other causes, then the parents of such a child would be most vulnerable. Danish parents (11,231) were studied. The incidence of cancer diagnoses among the parents of cancer victims was not significantly different from the incidence of cancers in the general population. Similarly, the number of deaths reported from non-malignant causes were not significantly different from the overall population. The authors concluded that these results did not support the hypothesis that psychological stress and development of malignancies or death from non-malignant causes are associated. One limitation of this study is that the general health status of surviving parents was not evaluated. Parents may be cancer-free and alive, but are they more or less well than the national average?

Leserman and colleagues (Leserman, Li, Hu, & Drossman, 1998) examined the impact of four different stressors on health outcomes. The four stressors were sexual and physical abuse history, lifetime losses and traumas, turmoil in childhood family, and recent stressful life events. Two hundred thirty-nine women were referred to the study from a gastrointestinal clinic. Poor health status was measured by amount of pain, symptoms, bed disability days, physician visits, functional disability, and psychological distress. Exposure to these stressors accounted for 32% of the variance in overall health status. Further, women who reported high scores on one of the stressors also reported having experienced at least one of the other stressors. The authors argued that these data support an association between life stressors and health status, however, since the participants in this study were referred from the same clinic, caution is warranted in generalizing these results to broader populations. The authors advised clinicians to evaluate patients for multiple stressors when patients report one. Further, they noted that, in this sample, social support did not seem to buffer the negative effects of these four stressors.

The advantages of selecting healthy, but stressed, participants in studies to evaluate the impact of stress on health status and disease are compelling. To that end, Scanlan and colleagues (Scanlan, Vitaliano, Ochs, Savage, & Borson, 1998) compared caregiver spouses of persons with Alzheimer's disease to age- and gender-matched spouses of non-demented controls. Caregiver hassles, and depressed mood were used as markers of psychological stress/distress. The purpose of the study was to determine the relationship of gender, psychological stress/distress, absolute count and percentage of CD4 and CD8 cell counts over a 15- to 18-month period of time. CD4 and CD8 cell counts were used as markers of immune function modulated by exposure to stress hormones. The study results suggest that immune markers were associated with markers of psychological stress/distress, but primarily in the male caregivers. Gender differences are difficult to interpret in this study because results were not consistent. At baseline, CD4 and CD8 counts were lower in caregiver men than in control men. Levels of CD8 cells were correlated with reported hassles in men but not in women. Perhaps the instruments did not effectively measure some aspect of caregiver stress that is specific to males. For example, a husband taking care of a wife may be experiencing anxiety because the wife had been the primary caregiver. What is more interesting is whether or not the subtle, but statistically different, changes in CD4 levels impacted overall long-term health. Longitudinal studies would be needed to determine the consequences of these differences in these participants.

Another aspect of vulnerability to the effects of stress on health is individual personality characteristics. Rief, Shaw, and Fichter (1998) studied the psychobiological process of stress in persons with somatization syndrome. Persons with somatization syndrome characteristically develop physical complaints in response to psychological stress. Heart rate, finger pulse volume, electrodermal activity, electromyography, salivary cortisol levels, subjective well-being, selective attention and memory for illness-related words were measured in a group of patients and a control group at rest and during a mental stress task. The patient group demonstrated higher resting salivary cortisol levels and heart rate with lower finger pulse volume than the control group at baseline that was measured upon awakening. During the mental stress task, the patient group reported a higher level of distress and demonstrated higher heart rates than the control group. Repeated exposure to the testing situation resulted in habituation to the situation by the control subjects that was not observed in the patient subjects. There were no observed differences in the attention or memory capabilities in the two groups. Although the authors were most interested in relating these findings to the causal mechanisms of somatization syndrome, there may be implications for understanding the role of stress in disease. Persons with a style, be it psychologically or personality driven, that translates stress into physiological manifestations and maintains them may be at greater risk for stress induced illnesses. This would seem to be an important aspect of stress research that requires more investigation.

Psychological temperament has been associated with early childhood relationships. A study by Russek and Schwartz (1997) examined the relationship between feelings of parental warmth reported by participants in the Harvard Mastery of Stress Study and their health status 35 years later. Ninety-one percent of those who perceived that their relationship with their mother was not warm were diagnosed with health problems including coronary artery disease, alcoholism, hypertension, and ulcer in middle age. Thirty-five percent of those with similar estimates of their relationship with their father had similar diagnoses at middle age. All of the participants in this study were men. The authors argue that these data support the long-term effects of early childhood relationships on health and the significance of the parent-child relationship. In the next section of the chapter, the Stress Diathesis Model of Depression will be fully discussed, however, at this juncture it may be important to note that loss of a parent, particularly a mother, in childhood has been associated with greater risk for at least one major depressive episode. The question of long-term health effects of early childhood relationships and loss points up the importance of considering the type of data to be included in electronic databases. The introduction of the computer as a tool to gather and store medical data throughout an individual's life has given life to the notion that data from large numbers of patients may be merged into a huge data set. This data set could be a valuable tool in understanding the natural history of many diseases and provide insight about ways to prevent and better treat illnesses. Current medical records contain a wealth of information about the physiological status and function of a person, but very little psychosocial data make it to the record. Some consideration must be given to the types of psychosocial records to be included in this grand database.

The studies detailed above reveal statistical associations between incidences of stress, often self-reported, and incidences of disease. While the strength of the reported associations is compelling, they do not demonstrate cause and effect mechanisms that regulate the relationship. Understanding of the causal mechanisms is essential as a basis of interventions to modify risk, prevent disease, and/or treat the root causes. In the next section, research focused on the development of models to explain the mechanistic association between stress responses and disease will be reviewed.

PSYCHONEUROENDOCRINE MECHANISMS OF STRESS

In order to understand the role of stress as a contributing factor in the development of disease, the physiological impact of the process must be understood. Stress must be viewed as a psychophysiologic process designed to maintain homeostasis during threat and/or assault. Acute stress is a rather elegant dynamic and usually short-lived neuroendocrine response designed to prepare an organism for fight or flight. For modern women and men, however, these responses are usually inappropriate for the types of stressors encountered. Epidemiologists report that their studies indicate that women and men differentially respond to life stressors. These differences may be attributable to sex hormones. Several lines of evidence point toward interaction between stress axis and gonadal axis that may effect fertility and mood states in some women. In this section, psychoneuroendocine mechanisms of stress will be detailed. Evidence to support the association between physiologic stress responses and behavior will be discussed. The argument for studies of stress hormones as proxies of central nervous system activity will be reviewed. A critical element of that discussion will be a review of studies that support the Stress Diathesis Model of Depression. The body of work that supports the Stress Diathesis Model of Depression forms a paradigmatic template that may be useful in the study of other models of stress related phenomena such as premenstrual mood changes.

The defining characteristic of the physiological stress response is arousal of the neuroendocrine stress axis. The stress axis consists of limbic and diencephalon structures of the brain, the hypothalamus, the pituitary gland, the adrenal gland, and the autonomic nervous system. Any threat to or loss of homeostasis or well-being results in a cascade of responses from each of these structures. The diencephalon and limbic structures process information from the internal and external environment to detect threats or changes in homeostasis or well-being. The threat or actual loss of homeostasis or well-being is referred to as a stressor. The hypothalamus responds by secreting corticotrophin-releasing hormone (CRH), which in turn stimulates secretion of adrenocorticotropin hormone (ACTH) from the anterior pituitary gland. At the adrenal cortex, ACTH stimulates secretion of cortisol. This neuroendocrine cascade is self-limited through feedback mechanisms. At the hypothalamus, increases in CRH and ACTH inhibit further secretion of CRH. Similarly, critical levels of ACTH and cortisol inhibit further production of ACTH by the anterior pituitary. The hippocampus contains glucocorticoid receptors that appear to have a regulatory effect on cortisol secretion by inhibiting hypothalamic secretion of CRH (Feldman & Weidenfeld, 1999). The hippocampus also contains mineral corticoid steroids. The precise role of these receptors in regulating the stress response is not well understood, but the data suggest that the hippocampus is part of a direct central nervous system pathway or a "rapid feedback loop" regulating the neuroendocrine mechanisms of stress. In general, responses mediated by neuronal pathways are more rapid than those mediated by increases or decreases in hormone concentrations. Arousal of the autonomic nervous system regulates cardiovascular, respiratory and neurological responses including heightened vigilance commonly associated with acute arousal. These responses are short-lived and have been described as classic fight or flight preparations.

Investigations of neuroendocrine responses to stressors have been proposed as a way of better understanding brain function and related behavior.

This perspective is rooted in the observation that endocrine organs active during stress responses share developmental genetic origins with brain structures that regulate behavior. Experiments that cause changes in endocrine activity, therefore, induce concomitant changes in some activities. The argument is further supported by observations that these same experiments induce changes in behavior regulated by specific brain structures. For example, rats exposed to stressors exhibit analgesia and simultaneous changes in plasma levels of CRH, ACTH, and immunoreactive beta-endorphin (β-END). Concomitant increases in concentrations of endorphins were measured in brain areas known to regulate pain perception. Further, if the animals were treated with opiate antagonists prior to the stress event, analgesia did not occur (Akil, Madden, Patrick, & Barchas, 1976; MacLennan, Drugan, Hyson, Maier, & Barchas, 1982; Olson, Olson, & Kastin, 1997). These data suggest that some forms of stress-induced analgesia are opiate mediated, but for the purposes of this discussion these findings are important because they demonstrate that neuroendocrine stress responses induce measurable behavioral changes that can be associated with specific central nervous system events and structures.

The experimental paradigm of analgesia induced by acute stress paved the way for a variety of investigations, but of particular interest were studies in rodents to characterize neuroendocrine responses to chronic stress. Paradoxically, chronic exposure to stressors did not lead to enhanced analgesia. Some investigators even reported hyperalgesia with chronic stress paradigms. Chronic stress is characterized by slight elevations of basal plasma levels of cortisol, an adrenal hormone secreted in response to elevations of ACTH. Behavioral changes were noted in these animals as well, including learned helplessness, anorexia and reduced activity. These behaviors were reminiscent of behaviors associated with altered mood and mood disorders particularly depression. Once associations between behavior and neuroendocrine changes were well characterized in animal models, scientists used studies of hormonal and behavioral changes as a "Window into the Brain."

As study of the neuroendocrine response to acute and chronic stress progressed over the past several decades, a paradigmatic model of stress as a component of the underlying etiology of Major Mood Disorder has evolved. The Stress Diathesis Model of Depression is based on the observation that individuals with recurring depression often report at least one major life stressor prior to the first depressive episode (Anisman & Zacharo, 1982). In vulnerable populations, repeated exposure to stress results in failure to cope and persistent thoughts of inadequacy and guilt commonly associated with depression. The stress axis continues in a state of chronic arousal. The Stress Diathesis Model has been useful in the development of paradigms to study the relationship between behavioral changes and physiological stress axis regulatory mechanisms. Several lines of investigation have demonstrated an association between depression and dysregulation of the stress axis. One group of studies involved studies of baseline levels of stress hormones in depressed and control subjects. The second group of studies involved exploration of the responses of the neuroendocrine stress axis to manipulation directed at discovering altered feed back or feed forward mechanisms. Pharmacological manipulations include administration of dexamethasone (DEX) and corticosterone, synthetic agonists of cortisol, as well as cortisol and CRH. When these studies were carried out in normal control populations, they elucidated the regulatory mechanisms that operate during stress axis arousal. Responses to the same tests in depressed individuals or others with chronic arousal of the stress axis differentiated regulatory mechanisms during chronic stress.

The feedforward and feedback loops of the neuroendocrine response to stress have been widely studied in depression. Depressed individuals have chronically elevated plasma levels of cortisol, suggesting that usual feed back mechanisms are ineffective in attenuating the neuroendocrine stress response resulting in chronic arousal. In order to demonstrate the nature of the dysregulation and in an attempt to pinpoint the site of dysfunction, studies of stress axis responses to manipulation with selected hormones and drugs have been carried out. To identify the nature of the stress axis dysregulation, dexamethasone (DEX), a synthetic form of cortisol was administered to depressed and control subjects. Plasma levels of cortisol were then monitored for the next 24 hours. If the inhibitory feedback loops were intact, usual circadian increases would be inhibited. Approximately 60% of the depressed subjects demonstrated an escape from suppression characterized by increased plasma cortisol levels at about 4:00 p.m. when DEX was administered at midnight (Anisman & Zacharo, 1982; Yehuda, 1997). This finding suggests a failure in the usual feedback inhibitory mechanisms regulating cortisol secretion in depressed individuals and that adrenal axis dysregulation associated with depression involved the adrenal cortex. Additional studies that included measurement of ACTH and β-END demonstrated that the inhibitory effects at the level of the pituitary were also compromised. Young and others have reported that the intravenous administration of CRH to depressed subjects indicates that the hippocampal feedback loop is very important in differentiating the neuroendocrine response in depressed individuals from that in non-depressed subjects. Nondepressed control subjects demonstrated rapid response to CRH by rapid decreases on plasma β-LPH/β-END peptides, whereas depressed subjects demonstrated no response. These data suggest that the site of dysregulation is in the fast feedback loop of the hypothalamus. Manipulation of the stress axis, therefore, demonstrated that depression includes stress axis dysregulation and that the sites of dysregulation include the hippocampus in the CNS.

Stress hormones respond to manipulations of central nervous system (CNS) monoamine systems. Infusion of monoamine agonists and antagonists and related responses of selected hormones have been used as indicators of neurotransmitter receptor activation in psychiatric patients. These data and data associated with therapeutic effects of psychotropic drugs that influence monoamine transmitter activity form the foundation of biological approaches to treat affective disorders. Meltzer (1987) and others administered low doses of serotonin agonists to unmedicated depressed patients, manic patients, and normal persons. The cortisol response of both patient groups was enhanced, illustrating the interactive relationship between the stress axis and CNS monoamine neurotransmitter systems. The effects of CNS adrenergic mechanisms have been differentiated from peripheral effects. High doses of catecholamines administered into the CNS have reduced ACTH and cortisol response to stress (Van Loon, 1973). Norepinephrine has been shown to inhibit CRH and peripheral injection of epinephrine increases ACTH and cortisol levels. In depressed patients, there is evidence to support hyporesponsivity of both stimulatory and inhibitory mechanisms of stress axis regulation. Seiver (Seiver, Coccaro, & Davis, 1987) and others have suggested that this reaction could explain the lack of any change in ACTH levels in response to amphetamine administration. Initially, hormonal responses to noradrenergic manipulations were seen as possible biological markers of CNS disturbances in specific neurotransmitter systems. Cumulative results have been inconclusive, probably because of the remarkable interaction and interreaction between and among multiple systems. In addition to the effects of monoamine systems of the CNS on the stress axis, glucocorticosteroids have an effect on peripheral catecholamine function.

Anecdotal accounts suggest a high incidence of menstrual cycle irregularity among depressed women. A few investigators have considered the influence of the menstrual cycle on DEX tests in depressed women with mixed results. Administration of the DEX suppression test in one study failed to uncover any dysregulatory mechanisms (Haskett, Steiner, & Carrol, 1984). Some of the original investigators, however, have since reported different results in another sample of women (Tandon, Akser, & Greden, 1985; Tandon, Haskett, Cardona, Aleser, & Greden, 1990). They have reported that the results of the DEX test in women with major depressive disorders vary across the menstrual cycle. The lowest post DEX levels were observed during menses while the highest (least suppressed levels) occurred during week 2 or the periovulatory phase of the cycle. Luteal and premenstrual post DEX levels were lower than midcycle levels. Concurrent measures of depression levels with the Hamilton Rating Scale for Depression demonstrated an inverse relationship between depression and responsivity of cortisol post DEX. This group of 25 hospitalized women had fewer symptoms during the middle of the cycle with marked exacerbation in the late luteal phase (Tandon et al., 1985). These studies suggest that chronic arousal of the stress axis is modulated by the gonadal axis vis a vis menstrual cycle phase. These data are further evidence of the close association among the neuroendocrine stress axis, the gonadal axis and mood.

Another group of studies was focused on the development of animal models of stress axis changes similar to those observed in depression by exposing animals to repeated episodes of inescapable physical stressors. In these studies, rats were exposed to intermittent electrical shock through the floor of a cage. The intensity, frequency, and duration of the shock were determined for each session by the investigator. These paradigms permitted exploration of biological regulatory mechanisms of hormone synthesis, processing, and release at the cellular and intracellular level in animals. These studies identified the nature of stress axis regulation in chronic stress and were used to define changes observed in depression as similar to chronic stress conditions. They have led to better understanding of the physiological mechanisms of stress axis regulation in healthy people and have contributed to the development of treatments of depression.

Animal models have been used to demonstrate anatomical interactions between serotonergic pathways of the brain and the stress and gonadal axes (Austin, Rhodes, & Lewis, 1997). Establishment of these connections has led to experimental manipulations of serotonin and other monoamine pathways by administration of steroidal hormones, exposure of animals to stress, and behaviors including exercise. Establishment of these pathways and validation of behavioral and pharmaceutical manipulations of concurrent monoamine and stress axis arousal have led to human studies designed to characterize responses in normal and pathological conditions such as depression. Since direct measurements of serotonin or other neurotransmitters in intact brains are not possible, these studies rely on changes in peripheral levels of stress and gonadal axis hormones. Therefore, plasma levels of β-END/β-LPH, ACTH, prolactin, cortisol, epinephrine, norepinephrine, and progesterone are proxy measures of central nervous system monoamine neurotransmitter activity. Demonstration of concurrence between peripheral measures of proxy hormones in humans and CNS monoamine activity in animals was the basis for the development of drugs to treat depression and other affective disorders. Combination therapy with these drugs and psychotherapy is the "state of the science and art" in treating depression (Block, 2000; Groenink, Mos, Van der Gugten, & Oliver, 1996; Risch, 1997).

Although changes in stress axis regulation have been associated with depression, the question remains as to whether or not these changes always cause mood changes like those associated with depression. Studies of patients with Cushing's Disease, which is characterized by hypercortisolemia, suggest that there is an association with altered mood states (Sonino & Fava, 1998; Sonino, Fava, Raffi, Boscaro, & Fallo, 1998). Yet, the question remains whether HPA axis dysregulation is always present when mood changes occur. Because both depression and Cushing's disease are chronic, there is no way of knowing whether or not the HPA axis was ever functioning normally in these individuals. The ideal experiment would include observations of the HPA axis when the individual is asymptomatic.

The study of premenstrual symptoms (PS) provides a natural experiment that permits examination of the relationships among stress axis arousal, gonadal axis changes, and behavior. Several investigators have reported a relationship between the number of stressful daily life events experienced by women and the number and severity of PS reported during the late luteal phase of the cycle (Taylor, Woods, Lentz, Mitchell, & Lee, 1971). Life events reported by women are often ones that, at other times of the cycle, would be considered a nuisance rather than distressing. These data suggest that women with PS may be differentially sensitive to changes in their environments. Although a link has been made between stress and the severity of PS, this perspective has not been used widely to explore the biobehavioral basis of PS. Thus, an alternative hypothesis is that stress axis psychophysiology may be used to differentiate women with specific type, severity, and patterns of PS. The neuroendocrine stress axis has been shown to interact with the gonadal axis to modulate female reproductive function and hormones of the gonadal axis influence the stress axis. This reciprocal relationship between the two axes may be involved in the neuroendocrine mechanisms underlying some types of PS.

The stress axis and the gonadal axis interact at several neuroendocrine sites. The hypothalamic/pituitary/ovarian or gonadal axis regulates the menstrual cycle. Like the stress axis, neuronal input from the diencephalon and limbic structures in the brain participate in its regulation. In the nonhuman primate and presumably in women, the basal medial hypothalamus serves as a "transducer," integrating signals from the brain and the endocrine system to regulate menstrual cycles. Maintenance of cyclicity, menstruation, and fertility is achieved by precise secretory patterns of gonadotropin releasing hormone (GnRH). GnRH is secreted from the hypothalamus in an oscillating pattern. The frequency and amplitude of the oscillation determines the amount of LH or FSH secreted from the anterior pituitary. The amounts of progesterone and estrogen present influence the frequency of the oscillation. For example, during the luteal phase of the menstrual cycle, progesterone levels are high and GnRH and LH oscillating patterns of secretion are slow. LH pulses occur approximately every 5 to 6 hours, as contrasted to the follicular phase when progesterone is low and pulses occur about every hour. In addition to the effects of ovarian hormones, GnRH secretory patterns can be altered by opioid secretion from neurons arising in the arcuate nucleus and terminating in the hypothalamus. Since endorphin levels increase with arousal of the stress axis, this site of interaction may be an important aspect of the mechanisms underlying premenstrual symptom occurrence and severity.

Basal levels of cortisol were reported to be significantly different during the luteal phase of women with two distinct patterns of PMS (Cahill, 1998). In this study only women with symptom types that were similar to those of depression were studied. Three patterns of symptoms were identified. The first group consisted of few or no symptoms reported throughout the menstrual cycle and were referred to as the Low Symptom Group (LS). These data were used as control data. The other two patterns were distinctly different. The first premenstrual symptom (PMS) pattern consisted of low symptoms during the follicular phase with significant increases in symptoms during the luteal phase. The second pattern was characterized by moderate symptom severity in the follicular phase and severe symptom severity in the luteal phase and was referred to as the premenstrual magnification pattern (PMM). Cortisol levels for all groups were in the normal range. Those collected from women in the low symptom group clustered around the midrange of normal while those from the PMS group clustered toward the lower end during the luteal phase. The values for women who reported moderate symptoms throughout the cycle clustered around the high end during the luteal phase only. There were no statistical differences in cortisol during the follicular phase. These data suggest that the occurrence and severity of symptoms effected cortisol levels. The findings are consistent with a link between stress axis regulation and depressed mood.

Woods and her colleagues have explored stress as a factor in premenstrual symptom occurrence and severity as well. In 1971 Taylor and colleagues (Taylor et al., 1971) reported that " . . . perception of stress appears to increase perimenstrual symptom severity" (p. 115). Subsequently, Woods and her group used techniques developed for use with biofeedback interventions to control arousal and found that women with PMS and PMM patterns of symptoms demonstrated higher levels of arousal, but not low symptom women (Woods, Lentz, Mitchell, & Kogan, 1994). In a study of urinary stress hormone levels, this group of investigators reported increases in stress hormones consistent with arousal (Woods, Lentz, Mitchell, Shaver, & Heitkemper, 1998). Thus, the simple observation that often a major life stressor precedes the onset of recurring depression has led to a substantial body of work supporting the Stress Diathesis Model of Depression. Supporting paradigms progress from initial demonstrations of differences in basal levels of stress hormones to demonstrations of differences in stress axis regulation and finally to the development of animal models of stress axis mechanisms as a way of understanding underlying functional, cellular and subcellular changes in chronic arousal of the stress axis like those associated with depression. These paradigms have been shown to be valid ways to study the stress axis and to further understanding of the interface between behavior and biology. Investigation of the linkage between stress axis function, perceived stress and premenstrual symptoms is a new line of investigation. If this paradigmatic template used to delineate the relationships between stress and depression were applied to PS, a logical next step would be to explore regulation of the axis through behavioral and pharmacological manipulations in women with PS.

STRESS REDUCTION THERAPIES

Despite the lack of a clear and absolute picture of how stress exposure causes illness or exacerbates symptoms, it seems prudent to develop and test interventions to reduce stress and distress associated with modern life. Robert Sapolsky reported that chronic exposure to elevated stress hormones leads to brain atrophy in animals and in humans (Sapolsky, 1996). It appears the hippocampus is particularly vulnerable to atrophy (Yehuda, 1997). Chronic exposure to elevated glucocorticoids associated with Cushing's disease and aging have been associated with increased functional loss of short-term memory (McEwen et al., 1997). In the rodent, repeated stress causes atrophy of dendrites in the CA3 region of the hippocampus. Acute as well as chronic stress suppresses neurogenesis of dentate gyrus granule neurons. McEwen points out that, in humans, hippocampal atrophy is associated with performance on several tasks associated with spatial learning and memory (McEwen, 1999a). A causal relationship between exposure to stress and dementia and other neurologic deficits has not been clearly determined. Not all individuals who are exposed to chronic stress develop cognitive deficits (McEwen, 1999b), but interventions that limit the duration and or the intensity of the stress response seem to be important aspects of nursing care.

Cancer therapy may be particularly stressful. Therapy is usually initiated very quickly after diagnosis leaving little time to cope with the news. Few patients are familiar with environments for therapy and many fear discomforts with therapy. Fuller and associates (Faller, Bulzebruck, Drings, & Lang, 1999) investigated the relationship between coping style and survival of lung cancer after 7 to 8 years. Only 11 of the original 103 patients diagnosed survived. In this group there was an association between coping ability and survival.

The study is clearly limited if not flawed because no data on coping ability were available for those patients who did not survive. Given the virulence of lung cancer, it may not be a particularly good model for this type of retrospective study.

Batey and colleagues (Batey et al., 2000) implemented a Stress Management Intervention as part of a multi-site clinical trial to prevent hypertension. Despite overall significant reductions in diastolic blood pressure for both the treatment group and control group, significant differences were not observed between groups. Secondary analysis of data collected from a subgroup of highly adherent subjects resulted in identification of minimally greater reduction in diastolic pressure in the treatment group. The authors concluded that the minimal positive effect on blood pressure suggested that this program was not sufficiently efficacious to support it. Subjects in this study were healthy. Application of this type of therapy may have greater efficacy with persons at risk for hypertension.

Cardiovascular reactivity was shown to be greater among older persons during a stress task (Uchino, Uno, Holt-Lunstad, & Flinders, 1999). Cardiovascular reactivity was measured by systolic blood pressure. Age-related increased cardiac output and total vascular resistance during stress drove cardiovascular reactivity. There were no detectable differences between men and women in this sample. These data suggest that stress reduction therapies may be effective in reducing hypertension in older people.

Exercise has been encouraged as an effective treatment to improve many aspects of health. Brownley et al. (Brownley, West, Hinderliter, & Light, 1996) investigated the effects of aerobic exercise on blood pressure responses to daily stresses in a men and women. Eleven participants had elevated resting blood pressure and 20 were normotensive. Hourly mean blood pressure was calculated for two 24-hour periods. One 24-hour period was after a 20-minute treatment of aerobic exercise on a bicycle ergometer. The second 24-hour period followed a no-exercise day. Blood pressure was lower during the five hours after the exercise treatment. Overall, blood pressure was lower during work hours on the day of the exercise treatment. The authors conclude that exercise may confirm some degree of protection from transient changes in blood pressure associated with work stress. Yet, no differences in heart rate were noted.

The effects of a program that combined stress management and exercise in a group of 45 (19 men and 5 women) patients in a cardiac rehabilitation program were explored in a (Turner, Linden, van der Wal, & Schamberger, 1995). Subjects were stratified by gender and randomly assigned to the exercise only program or the exercise and stress management treatment. Subjects in the combined therapy group demonstrated reduced blood pressure response to a psychological stress challenge. Gender differences in response to treatments could not be determined because of the few women in the study.

The PMS Symptom Management Program has been designed by Taylor (1999). This package of non-pharmacological strategies was given to 91 women with severe PMS. The strategies involved self-monitoring, personal choice, self-regulation, and self/environmental modification and were combined with peer support and professional guidance. Taylor reports that PMS severity was reduced by 75% after 18 months of treatment. Symptom distress and depression were reduced and self-esteem and well-being increased. Stress as such was not directly measured, although one could argue that symptom severity, mood, well-being, and esteem are influenced by stress. Further, the strategies used are classically associated with stress reduction measures.

Community-based stress management programs have been implemented. Presumably, stress management will reduce stress and thereby diminish the risk of stress-induced illnesses. Hostick et al. (Hostick, Newell, & Ward, 1997) reported that participants in a such a program reported increased effectiveness in stress management at 3 and 6 months after a 2-day workshop. Interventions that effectively enhance an individual's ability to manage stress should contribute to reduced incidence and severity of stress-induced illness or symptoms.

RECOMMENDATIONS FOR FUTURE RESEARCH

Stress is an important component of the body of science striving to better understand human health and wellness. Studies designed to demonstrate associations between stress and illness will be enhanced through the use of new technologies. Completion of the human genome map will be a boon to investigations of the genetic basis of many diseases. Phenotyping of illnesses is a major element of the process and is similar in some ways to ex post facto studies. Individuals diagnosed with or related to persons with specific diseases are studied to document multiple characteristics of the disease and the individual. Statistical analysis of the strength of relationships among these variables and genetic mutations demonstrate the probability of a genetic basis for illness development. Whether or not genetic predisposition can be modified to prevent disease remains to be explored. Although genetic defects like those associated with Down syndrome, cystic fibrosis and the like will require gene manipulation therapies, genetic predisposition is likely to be amenable to therapies to prevent or delay the onset of disease. In-depth evaluation of persons with genetic predisposition to a particular disease but who do not develop it could reveal those life style elements that delay or prevent onset.

The introduction of the computer as a tool to gather and store medical data throughout an individual's life has given impetus to the notion that data from large numbers of patients may be merged into a large data set. This data set could be a valuable tool in understanding the natural history of many diseases and provide insight about ways to prevent and better treat illnesses. These large databases could be used to explore associations between specific antecedent events and the occurrence of an illness. Rather than selecting individuals with a specific disease, the scientist would be able to select individuals who experienced certain events. For example, an association between exposure to influenza during the 1916 epidemic and Parkinson's disease was noted because many who developed Parkinson's in the 1930s and beyond reported having had the flu. But not everyone who had the flu developed influenza. With a computerized longitudinal database, scientists could determine if the victims shared other experiences as well as the flu.

Current medical records contain a wealth of information about the physiological status and function of a person, but very little psychosocial data make it to the record. Consideration must be given to the types of records to be included in this grand database. Stress, a culprit that may contribute to disease with an irrefutable psychological component, provides investigators with a powerful argument for inclusion of specific psychosocial data in any health database. Individual responses to and perceptions of situations may be key to understanding the individual differences in both long-term and short-term responses to stress. Adequately coping with a stressor has long been considered to be effective in insulating the individual from long-term health effects. Large databases with measures of coping effectiveness and duration of perceived stress levels would provide data necessary to support this conclusion. Nurse scientists and clinicians must advocate for inclusion of this data now. If history is a teacher, we know that more effort is required to change standard practices than to introduce elements during an on-going change process.

Practice that is based on intervention studies is the most efficient way to deliver care. Sound interventions are based on clear understanding of the mechanisms regulating function. Investigations of the relationship between stress and physiological function that further explicate these mechanisms will be important. As nurses, we have a unique perspective that recognizes the intrinsic importance of the mind in health. Better understanding of stress requires a better understanding of the mind as a regulator of physiology *and* the body as a regulator of mind. Melding research expertise in studies of human behavior with expertise in biological research will lead to new paradigms to address mind body interaction. This holistic model will provide the basis for new interventions to mitigate stress and its effect on health.

As understanding of the mechanisms of stress and the impact on health increases, interventions with a higher probability of effectiveness may be designed. Intervention studies that examine predictability and efficiency will be needed. Traditional clinical trial design may replace quasi-experimental designs. Increasing the predictability of interventions increases efficiency. Increased efficiency is needed given the shortage of professional nurses. If an intervention effectively treats 80% of those who receive it, the professional nurse is freed to spend additional time and individualize care for the 20% who are non-responders.

SUMMARY

Stress is an enormously important focus of inquiry. As clinicians, nurses recognize the importance of understanding the etiology of disease and the need for effective interventions to prevent and control illness. As scientists, nurses recognize that effective interventions are based on sound understanding of mechanisms that regulated physiologic function. As caregivers, nurses recognize the importance of the mind and soul in human health. Stress research contributes the necessary knowledge base for effective care within these three domains and thus is an element of every nurse's practice.

In this chapter, three perspectives of research were explored. Progress in understanding stress and adaptation focuses in four paradigmatic domains. The first includes studies designed to demonstrate correlational associations between stress and illness. Most of these studies are ex post facto, thus lacking the power to argue for a cause-and-effect association. The second focuses on determining physiological mechanisms of stress. These studies often involve animal models. Although the animal model provides scientists the opportunity to characterize physiologic manifestations of stress including molecular intracellular mechanisms, they provide only limited behavioral data. To demonstrate associations between physiologic changes and human behavior, however, scientists use the physiological data about the stress axis as a window into the brain—the third paradigm. The last paradigm has yielded an arsenal of interventions designed to reduce distress and/or eliminate stressors.

A significant gap in understanding stress is associated with understanding the workings of the human mind. For one person the same situation is exhilarating and exciting, whereas for another it may be fraught with fear. The internal workings of the mind are said by some to be incomprehensible. For this author, consideration of the human mind is at the cusp between philosophy and science.

Since the purpose of this paper was to review the science, the philosophy of mind will be left to another author.

REFERENCES

Akil, H., Madden, J., Patrick, R., & Barchas, D. D. (1976). Stress induced increase in endogenous opiate peptides: Concurrent analgesia and its partial reversal by naloxone. In H. W. Kosterlitz (Ed.), *Opiates and endogenous opioid peptides.* Amsterdam: Elsevier/North Holland Press.

Anisman, H., & Zacharo, R. M. (1982). Depression: The predisposing influence of stress. *Behavioral and Brain Sciences, 5,* 89–137.

Austin, M. C., Rhodes, J. L., & Lewis, D. A. (1997). Differential distribution of corticotropin-releasing hormone immunoreactive axons in monoaminergic nuclei of the human brainstem. *Neuropsychopharmacology, 17,* 326–341.

Batey, D. M., Kaufmann, P. G., Raczynski, J. M., Hollis, J. F., Murphy, J. K., Rosner, B., Corrigan, S. A., Rappaport, N. B., Danielson, E. M., Lasser, N. L., & Kuhn, C. M. (2000). Stress management intervention for primary prevention of hypertension: Detailed results from Phase I of Trials of Hypertension Prevention (TOHP-I). *Annals of Epidemiology, 10,* 45–58.

Block, S. D. (2000). Assessing and managing depression in the terminally ill patient. ACP-ASIM End-of-Life Care Consensus Panel. American College of Physicians—American Society of Internal Medicine. *Annals of Internal Medicine, 132,* 209–218.

Brownley, K. A., West, S. G., Hinderliter, A. L., & Light, K. C. (1996). Acute aerobic exercise reduces ambulatory blood pressure in borderline hypertensive men and women. *American Journal of Hypertension, 9,* 200–206.

Cahill, C. A. (1998). Differences in cortisol, a stress hormone, in women with turmoil-type premenstrual symptoms. *Nursing Research, 47,* 278–284.

Faller, H., Bulzebruck, H., Drings, P., & Lang, H. (1999). Coping, distress, and survival among patients with lung cancer. *Archives of General Psychiatry, 56,* 756–762.

Feldman, S., & Weidenfeld, J. (1999). Glucocorticoid receptor antagonists in the hippocampus modify the negative feedback following neural stimuli. *Brain Research, 821,* 33–37.

Groenink, L., Mos, J., Van der Gugten, J., & Olivier, B. (1996). The 5-HT1A receptor is not involved in emotional stress-induced rises in stress hormones. *Pharmacology, Biochemistry, and Behavior, 55,* 303–308.

Haskett, R., Steiner, M., & Carrol, B. S. (1984). Dexamethasone suppression test and the menstrual cycle. *Journal of Affective Disorders, 6,* 191.

Hostick, T., Newell, R., & Ward, T. (1997). Evaluation of stress prevention and management workshops in the community. *Journal of Clinical Nursing, 6,* 139–145.

Johansen, C., & Olsen, J. H. (1997). Psychological stress, cancer incidence and mortality from non-malignant diseases. *British Journal of Cancer, 75,* 144–148.

Leserman, J., Li, Z., Hu, Y. J., & Drossman, D. A. (1998). How multiple types of stressors impact on health. *Psychosomatic Medicine, 60,* 175–181.

MacLennan, A. J., Drugan, R. C., Hyson, R. L., Maier, S., Madden, J., & Barchas, J. D. (1982). Corticosterone: A critical factor in an opioid form of stress-induced analgesia. *Science, 215,* 1530–1532.

McEwen, B. S. (1999a). Stress and hippocampal plasticity. *Annual Review of Neuroscience, 22,* 105–122.

McEwen, B. S. (1999b). Stress and the aging hippocampus. *Frontiers in Neuroendocrinology, 20,* 49–70.

McEwen, B. S., Conrad, C. D., Kuroda, Y., Frankfurt, M., Magarinos, A. M., & McKittrick, C. (1997). Prevention of stress-induced morphological and cognitive consequences. *European Neuropsychopharmacology, 7*(Suppl. 3), S323–S328.

Meltzer, H. Y. (Ed.). (1987). *An overview of hormones and monamine receptors.* New York: Raven Press.

Olson, G. A., Olson, R. D., & Kastin, A. J. (1997). Endogenous opiates: 1996. *Peptides, 18,* 1651–1688.

Rief, W., Shaw, R., & Fichter, M. M. (1998). Elevated levels of psychophysiological arousal and cortisol in patients with somatization syndrome. *Psychosomatic Medicine, 60,* 198–203.

Risch, S. C. (1997). Recent advances in depression research: From stress to molecular biology and brain imaging. *Journal of Clinical Psychiatry, 58*(Suppl. 5), 3–6.

Russek, L. G., & Schwartz, G. E. (1997). Feelings of parental caring predict health status in midlife: A 35-year follow-up of the Harvard Mastery of Stress Study. *Journal of Behavioral Medicine, 20,* 1–13.

Sapolsky, R. M. (1996). Why stress is bad for your brain. *Science, 273,* 749–750.

Scanlan, J. M., Vitaliano, P. P., Ochs, H., Savage, M. V., & Borson, S. (1998). CD4 and CD8 counts are associated with interactions of gender and psychosocial stress. *Psychosomatic Medicine, 60,* 644–653.

Server, L. J., Coccaro, E. F., & Davis, K. L. (1987). Hormonal response to noradrenergic stimulation in depression. In U. Halbreich (Ed.), *Hormones and depression* (pp. 161–193). New York: Raven Press.

Simpson, J. B. (1988). *Simpson's contemporary quotations* [Available: www.bartleby.com/63/ (2000, March 10)].

Sonino, N., & Fava, G. A. (1998). Psychosomatic aspects of Cushing's disease. *Psychotherapy & Psychosomatics, 67,* 140–146.

Sonino, N., Fava, G. A., Raffi, A. R., Boscaro, M., & Fallo, F. (1998). Clinical correlates of major depression in Cushing's disease. *Psychopathology, 31,* 302–306.

Tandon, R., Akser, K., & Greden, J. F. (1985). *Effects of menstrual cycle on the dexamethasone suppression test.* Paper presented at the 40th Annual Meeting of the Society of Biological Psychiatry, Dallas.

Tandon, R., Haskett, R. F., Cardona, D., Aleser, K., & Greden, J. F. (1990). Menstrual cycle effects on dexamethasone suppression test in major depression. *Biological Psychiatry, 28,* 485–488.

Taylor, D. (1999). Effectiveness of professional–peer group treatment: Symptom management for women with PMS. *Research in Nursing & Health, 22,* 496–511.

Taylor, D. L., Woods, N. F., Lentz, M. J., Mitchell, E. S., & Lee, K. A. (1991). Perimenstrual negative affect: Development and testing of an exploratory model. In D. L. Taylor & N. F. Woods (Eds.), *Menstruation, health and wellness* (pp. 103–117). New York: Hemisphere.

Turner, L., Linden, W., van der Wal, R., & Schamberger, W. (1995). Stress management for patients with heart disease: A pilot study. *Heart & Lung: Journal of Critical Care, 24,* 145–153.

Uchino, B. N., Uno, D., Holt-Lunstad, J., & Flinders, J. B. (1999). Age-related differences in cardiovascular reactivity during acute psychological stress in men and women. *Journals of Gerontology, Series B, Psychological Sciences & Social Sciences, 54,* P339–P346.

Van Loon, G. R. (1973). Catecholamines and ACTH secretion. In W. F. Ganong & L. Martin (Eds.), *Frontiers in neuroendocrinology* (pp. 209–247). New York: Oxford Press.

Woods, N. F., Lentz, M. J., Mitchell, E. S., & Kogan, H. (1994). Arousal and stress response across the menstrual cycle in women with three perimenstrual symptom patterns. *Research in Nursing and Health, 17,* 99–110.

Woods, N. F., Lentz, M. J., Mitchell, E. S., Shaver, J., & Heitkemper, M. (1998). Luteal phase ovarian steroids, stress arousal, premenses perceived stress, and premenstrual symptoms. *Research in Nursing and Health, 21,* 129–142.

Yehuda, R. (1997). Stress and glucocorticoid [letter; comment]. *Science, 275,* 1662–1663.

Young, E., & Korszun, A. (1998). Psychoneuroendocrinology of depression. Hypothalamic-pituitary-gonadal axis. *Psychiatric Clinics of North America, 21,* 309–323.

Chapter 9

Sleep and Fatigue

KATHRYN A. LEE

ABSTRACT

This chapter provides a review and synthesis of research on women's sleep and fatigue from a nursing perspective. Most of the research involves four primary issues for women: menstrual cycles, childbearing, chronic mental or physical illness, and oncology. Research with healthy women focused on diurnal fluctuations in fatigue and relationships to sleep, without regard for exercise or level of daytime activity. Research on chronic illness and cancer fatigue focused on general fatigue and its impact on activity, without regard for sleep or therapeutic use of rest and naps. A comparison of these two areas highlights gaps in nursing knowledge about sleep and fatigue. Further research is needed to understand relationships between nonrestorative sleep, fatigue, and symptoms related to poor quality of life. From a synthesis of these studies, nonpharmacologic interventions that could be prove useful in promoting a higher quality of life for those with either acute or chronic fatigue are then proposed.

Key words: activity, energy, fatigue, insomnia, rest, sleep, women

INTRODUCTION: METHODS OF RESEARCH RETRIEVAL

This chapter reviews nursing research related to women's sleep and fatigue published through 1999. Studies include those in which a nurse-scientist was the primary author, and research questions addressed gender differences or women-specific issues related to sleep or fatigue. Computer searches of Cumulative Index to Nursing and Allied Health Literature (CINAHL), MEDLINE, and PsychINFO were conducted using the following nine key words: gender, women, sleep, fatigue, energy, insomnia, tiredness, rest, activity. A manual search was also conducted with specific sleep and women's health journals. A list of past and currently funded NIH grants from the National Institute of Nursing Research was also examined for computer searches by potential nurse authors. A total of 90 English language citations were found for inclusion in this review.

CONCEPTUAL FRAMEWORK AND DEFINITIONS

To complete a review and synthesis of research on women's sleep and fatigue from a nursing perspective, it is first necessary to define these two phenomena and discuss how they are conceptually related. Why these two phenomena require review and synthesis specifically from a women's health perspective will also be discussed.

A nursing definition for fatigue has always included components of both physical and mental activity, and always assumes fatigue to be a symptom perceived by the individual. There is general acceptance of the North American Nursing Diagnosis Association (NANDA) definition that fatigue is a "self-recognized state in which an individual experiences an overwhelming sustained sense of exhaustion and decreased capacity for physical and mental work that is not relieved by rest" (Carpenito, 1995, p. 379). Some nurse researchers take issue with this definition, however, because it assumes a pathologic or chronic illness perspective, is difficult to distinguish from a definition of depression, and fails to consider normal daily fluctuations in fatigue or consider fatigue as a protective, healthy human response to physical or mental exertion (Cahill, 1999; Lee, Lentz, Taylor, Mitchell, & Woods, 1994; Piper, 1993; Tack, 1990).

The NANDA definition also fails to consider the effect of activity on fatigue. Current nursing research is demonstrating that activity, rather than rest, should be prescribed to relieve fatigue. Therefore, many nurse researchers who work with chronically fatigued patients have extended the definition of fatigue from "relieved by rest" to include "relieved by activity" (Graydon, Bubela, Irvine, & Vincent, 1995; Neuberger et al., 1997; Winningham et al., 1994; van Servellen, Sarna, & Jablonski, 1998; Schwartz, 1998) and include both rest and activity, or the balance between them, in their research (Piper, Lindsey, & Dodd, 1987).

According to many dictionary definitions, fatigue is not limited to a state of exhaustion, but includes less severe forms. The entire range of fatigue, from mild tiredness to overwhelming exhaustion, is discussed by Ream and Richardson (1996) in their concept analysis. An appropriate definition should encompass this entire range to be useful to researchers who study acute or chronic aspects of fatigue. Nurse researchers have also suggested that an aspect of "unpleasantness" or discomfort be incorporated in the definition of fatigue as part of the experience of this symptom (Milligan, Lenz, Parks, Pugh, & Kitzman, 1996).

As defined by NANDA, fatigue is limited to that which is unrelieved by rest, without considering inadequate or nontherapeutic rest. With the vague nature in which rest is incorporated into the definition, we turn to dictionaries where rest is defined as: "a period of inactivity," "absence of motion," or "refreshment as produced by sleep." Sleep, in turn, can be defined as a "period of diminished responsiveness to external stimuli" that alternates with wakefulness or alertness (Lee, 1999, p. 724). These definitions, however, assume that rest and sleep are restorative. If rest or sleep is inadequate or not therapeutic, the fatigue that should be relieved by sleep on a diurnal basis may become chronic. In a study of battered women living in shelters with other women and their children, the number of recorded awakenings was high, and this type of nontherapeutic rest was related to perception of fatigue severity in the morning; 40% of the 50 women woke up very fatigued (Humphreys, Lee, Neylan, & Marmar, 1999).

To understand how fatigue is influenced by rest and sleep, it must be made clear that it is not merely *quantity* that makes rest or sleep restorative; nor is it a linear relationship, since too much rest can also be fatiguing. Researchers and clinicians should also not assume that individuals can accurately perceive the quantity and quality of their own rest or sleep. A discussion of the function of sleep is beyond the scope of this chapter and was recently reviewed by other nurse researchers (Shaver & Giblin, 1989; Floyd, 1999; Richardson, 1996). Perception of fatigue is influenced by the *quality* of rest or sleep, and how often it is interrupted by internal physiologic variables (such as apneic events, urinary frequency, pain, or night sweats) or external environmental variables (such as noise or light). Interrupted sleep, whatever the source, results in fatigue regardless of whether the individual is aware of the interruptions and regardless of the cause (Martin, Wraith, Deary, & Douglas, 1997). Furthermore, self-perception of sleep is not often highly correlated with objective measures (Elek, Hudson, & Fleck, 1997; Franck et al., 1999). As Evans and Rogers (1994) suggest, perception of sleep quality is influenced by how we adapt to worsening sleep quality over time, whether it be from age, chronic illness, or childbearing and child-rearing. In reality, a bed partner often provides a more valid description of someone's sleep.

In addition to the balance between rest and activity to be considered in the definition of fatigue, there is also a need to consider the balance between energy demands and resources (Cahill, 1999). Lee and colleagues (1994) define fatigue as a perception of severity along a continuum from tired to exhausted that results from the balance between resources and demands placed on women by their internal (physiologic) and external (social) environments. From the earlier work of Lazarus and Folkman (1984) on stress and coping and person–environment interactions, they further developed the concept of a balance of coping resources and stressful demands, and proposed that fatigue could be a useful indicator of that balance in women's lives. To provide empirical data for this model, a community-based random sample of 262 healthy menstruating women was used in a secondary analysis of the Seattle Women's Health Study (Woods, 1987). There were far more internal (including illness, menstrual cycle phase, depression, anxiety, low self-esteem, and poor sleep) than external correlates of fatigue. Rather than income, employment, or children, the only external demand related to fatigue was number of stressful life events. These findings were supported by a subsequent study in which Libbus and colleagues (1995) also found that internal demands (depression, exercise, sleep and rest) were significant predictors of fatigue in their convenience sample of 155 women with persistent fatigue.

Aaronson and colleagues (1999) built from previous nursing research and utilized a self-monitoring and self-regulating framework to redefine fatigue. They incorporate the concept of "balance" from earlier research, avoid the use of "exhaustion" and "rest" in their definition, and define fatigue as an "awareness of a decreased capacity for physical and/or mental activity due to an imbalance in the availability, utilization, and/or restoration of resources needed to perform activity" (p. 46). They then discuss five components of fatigue that are important to quantify for research, regardless of the population of interest: (1) amount of fatigue; (2) distress or degree of unpleasantness associated with fatigue; (3) effects of fatigue on activities of daily living; (4) key biological parameters associated with fatigue; and (5) other correlates of fatigue, such as sleep, depression, or stress.

For the purpose of this review, studies were limited primarily to nursing research focused on fatigue or sleep with either women as the targeted sample, or addressing questions about gender differences. Most of the research concerns four primary issues: menstrual cycles, childbearing, chronic mental or physical illness, and oncology. Recent nursing research involves sleep and fatigue issues for women as caregivers. Although only one publication was found (Teel & Press, 1999), this will become an area of expanding knowledge based on current funding from the National Institute of Nursing Research.

SLEEP AND FATIGUE IN HEALTHY POPULATIONS OF WOMEN

Women across many age groups, and in many national surveys, report less sleep and more fatigue than men in the general population (Chen, 1986; Hagnell, Grasbeck, Ojesjo, & Otterback, 1993). In a recent U.S. poll of over 1000 women between 30 and 60 years of age, 48% complained of sleep problems compared to 38% of men, and 22% of women complained of daytime sleepiness that interfered with activities compared to 15% of men (National Sleep Foundation, 1998). The high prevalence for women has led researchers to examine specific and salient aspects of women's lives that may be the source of the problem. This section reviews literature on healthy women's sleep and fatigue related to adolescence, menstrual cycles, and menopause.

Young Women

Very little nursing research on sleep and fatigue has been done in populations of young adolescents. Lee, McEnany, and Weekes (1998) surveyed adolescents about self-reported sleep patterns on school days and weekends. On school days, girls reported less sleep, awakening earlier, and falling asleep on the way home from school compared to boys. There was also a relationship between self-reported caffeine consumption and disturbed sleep. From this one study, using only a self-report measure, less sleep is already a health issue for young women. As they mature and acquire adult health habits, issues of adequate sleep and exercise, use of over the-counter stimulants, and caffeinated beverages become critical for nurses who work with communities of young women.

Menstrual Cycles and Menopausal Transition

Women who ovulate experience fluctuations in gonadal hormone levels, particularly estrogen and progesterone. In fact, progesterone is known to be a soporific, sleep-inducing hormone that also raises core body temperature (Lee, 1988). Sleep deprivation has an effect on core body temperature (Landis, Savage, Lentz, & Brengelmann, 1997), but very little research has been done to describe sleep or fatigue patterns during the menstrual cycle. In a rodent model, estrus and changes in gonadal hormones significantly influenced circadian rhythms for activity and temperature (Labyak & Lee, 1995). In ovulating women, Lee and colleagues (1990) found an earlier onset of the first rapid-eye-movement sleep after ovulation, and the seven women with premenstrual negative affect symptoms had significantly less deep sleep (delta sleep, stages 3–4) than the six asymptomatic women. A significant relationship between fatigue and phase of the menstrual cycle was also found in a secondary analysis of the Seattle Women's Health Study, discussed earlier, but more research is needed to help explain the symptom experience of menstruating women. Sleep and fatigue research related to the menstrual cycle is scant in the nursing literature, but also rare in other disciplines. Recent reviews can be found in the medical literature (Driver & Baker, 1998; Manber & Armitage, 1999).

Sleep problems and fatigue are common among adult women. There may be a difference in the reasons for these complaints across the life span, but there does not appear to be a difference in prevalence based on findings from a secondary analysis of 266 employed midlife women (Lee & Taylor, 1996). The purpose of the original study was to survey employed women and describe their sleep and fatigue in relation to various shift schedules. Lee (1992) studied 760 nurses working at least 32 hours per week and found that poor sleep and fatigue was common, with younger women having awakenings for child care responsibilities and older women awakening due to hot flashes and night sweats.

Clark and colleagues (1995) studied 23 midlife women (ages 40 to 54) who specifically complained of sleep problems. Measures of depression and hormone levels were included, but there was no assessment of fatigue. They found a high prevalence of periodic leg movements, a condition in which muscle contractions occur during sleep. These contractions disrupt sleep by causing partial awakenings that may never be consciously perceived. This is a condition in which bed partners are likely to be awakened and may provide a more valid description of a subject's sleep than the subject herself.

Shaver, Giblin, Lentz, and Lee (1988) studied women between 40 and 59 years of age in a sleep laboratory with polysomnography, a well-accepted methodology for measurement of sleep stages (recording electroencephalography, electrooculography, and electromyography) for two consecutive nights. They found that sleep was most interrupted for women with hot flashes. Further results from that sample indicate a strong relationship between sleep disruption and psychological symptom distress (Paulsen & Shaver, 1991; Shaver, Giblin, & Paulsen, 1991; Shaver & Paulsen, 1993). A comprehensive review of menopausal sleep research and hormone replacement therapy can be found in a recent medical review on the topic (Krystal, Edinger, Wohlgemuth, & Marsh, 1998).

Pregnancy

Sleep and fatigue during pregnancy and postpartum are well-documented concerns for new mothers. In the National Sleep Foundation's (1998) Women and Sleep Poll, 55 of the 1012 women (5%) were pregnant or recently pregnant, and 79% complained of disturbed sleep. A recent interdisciplinary review of sleep and pregnancy can be found in the medical literature (Lee, 1998). What is synthesized here are nursing research findings related to both sleep and fatigue.

Elek, Hudson, and Fleck (1997) recognized the need to assess fluctuations in fatigue during pregnancy. They studied 24 nulliparous couples for four consecutive mornings and evenings (Saturday to Tuesday) each month during the last trimester of pregnancy. As the delivery date approached, perception of fatigue severity increased for women but did not change for their male partners. These findings have relevance to the concept of "restorative sleep" discussed earlier, since they found less difference between evening and morning fatigue for the mothers after a night of sleep, but the same difference in fatigue was maintained over time for the fathers. Fatigue and sleep were not correlated, but sleep, assessed by diary and wrist actigraphy, was operationalized as 90-minute cycles, and there was low agreement ($r = .55$) between the two measures. Wrist actigraphy is a valid and reliable method for assessing continuity of sleep and is minimally invasive but lacks the ability to determine amounts of deep sleep thought to be the most restorative, and rationale for using 90-minute cycles of sleep time was not strong. Number of objective awakenings, or percentage of time spent awake during the time in bed trying to sleep (sleep efficiency), may be more valid indicators of sleep quality and quantity in future research.

Elek and colleagues' (1997) study involved nulliparous women, and interesting contrasts emerge when both nulliparas and multiparas are studied. Lee and colleagues studied fatigue and sleep during pregnancy and postpartum. In a protocol similar to Coble and colleagues' (1994) study of women with and without a history of affective disorder, sleep was monitored for two consecutive nights at seven time points with polysomnography in the home setting. Fatigue was evident as early as 11–12 weeks of pregnancy, but was highest in primiparas at 1-month postpartum (Lee & Zaffke, 1999). Perception of fatigue severity did not return to prepregnancy values for primiparas, even by the third month. Higher fatigue severity was correlated with lower hemoglobin and serum ferritin, as well as younger age and more disturbed sleep. As in other research findings, fatigue was unrelated to external social demands and role responsibilities.

Sleep disturbance was also present at 11–12 weeks gestation, regardless of parity (Lee, Zaffke, & McEnany, 2000). The amount of deep sleep decreased and wake time increased from pre-pregnancy levels and remained stable during each trimester for both nulliparas and multiparas. As pregnancy progressed, it was the 24 nulliparas who had even more disturbed sleep than the 18 multiparas. Their participation in household chores, as a measure of functional status, was also significantly less than multiparas (Waters & Lee, 1996).

Like the midlife transition, the transition from pregnancy to postpartum has a similar prevalence of disturbed sleep, but reasons for the disturbances differ. Baratte-Beebe and Lee (1999) conducted a secondary analysis of diary data from 25 women during pregnancy and found that the need to urinate was a major reason for awakening, even in first trimester. Awakenings during the third trimester were due to joint pain, muscle aches, and noises from bed partner, children, and pets.

Labor and Delivery

Evans and colleagues (1998) studied sleep quality during the week prior to onset of labor in relation to labor and delivery outcomes. No association was found, perhaps because there was so little variance in outcome measures, but also of concern was the measure of sleep quality. Sleep quality was estimated with the 15-item Verran and Snyder-Halpern Sleep Scale, a self-report instrument often used in nursing research, but its three subscales (sleep effectiveness, sleep disturbance, and sleep supplementation) had questionable validity in this sample.

Pugh (1990) enlisted a convenience sample of 100 primiparas for a study of fatigue during labor. Fatigue was already high on admission, but significantly increased during labor. On admission, the factors associated with fatigue included state and trait anxiety, amount of sleep, and medications. Those who reported stronger contractions had higher fatigue, and there was a relationship between length of labor and fatigue assessed within 24 hours of delivery. Even at two weeks postpartum, Troy and Dalgas-Pelish (1997) found that those with longer labors were still more fatigued. Pugh (1990) also noted that those who used intense breathing during labor also had high fatigue. This led to secondary analysis of 56 primiparas during the latent and active phases of labor (Pugh, Milligan, Gray, & Strickland, 1998). Because of differences in fatigue, they recommend postponing patterned breathing until the active phase of labor.

Mayberry and colleagues (1999) found that the number of minutes spent pushing during labor was associated with perception of fatigue severity at one hour after delivery, and women with a cesarean delivery had more severe and longer lasting fatigue than the women who delivered vaginally. The effects of prior fatigue and sleep were not examined in this study but remain an important area for future research related to perinatal outcomes.

Postpartum

Tribotti and colleagues (1988) surveyed 231 primiparas and multiparas within 72 hours after a vaginal or cesarean birth and found that, overall, 66% complained of sleep disturbance. The disturbance was more prevalent among the cesarean birth mothers (73%) than the vaginal birth mothers (57%). Sleep disturbance in the hospital setting may be the major reason for women's satisfaction with early hospital discharge (Keefe, 1988). Lentz and Killien (1991) found that women were awake between 5 and 30 times during the 32 observations made every 15 minutes in the hospital between 11:00 P.M. and 7:00 A.M. Those who were awake more often also felt the most tired and the least rested.

As sleep disturbed and fatigued as women are in the immediate postpartum period, it continues well into the first month postpartum (Lee & Zaffke, 1999; Lee, Zaffke, & McEnany, 2000; Graef, McGhee, Rozychki, Fescina-Jones, Clark, Thompson, & Brooten, 1988). Wambach (1998) also found that fatigue peaked during the first month, but, contrary to earlier studies (Milligan, 1989; Troy & Dalgas-Pelish, 1997), the fatigue was associated with breastfeeding problems. Quillin (1997) reported that the 32 breastfeeding mothers had more fatigue and slept less, according to their sleep logs, than the 12 bottle-feeding mothers. More importantly, she noted that their perception of a good night's sleep was dependent on continuity of sleep, rather than the actual amount of sleep.

The relationship between fatigue and type of infant feeding remains unclear, as does the relationship between age and fatigue. Wambach (1998) and Troy and Dalgas-Pelish (1997) found higher fatigue levels in older mothers, in contrast to Gardner (1991) and Lee and Zaffke (1999) in which fatigue was inversely related to age. These conflicting findings support the notion that fatigue is more likely based on multiple factors in a woman's life, rather than a single factor such as type of infant feeding, length of labor, or age alone.

Concerns about sleep and fatigue do not resolve during the typical postpartum recovery period of 6 weeks when most women return to work or maternity leave is terminated. Parks, Lenz, Milligan, and Han (1999) analyzed data from a community-based sample of 229 mothers between 1–18 months postpartum using two fatigue subscales (physical and mental) with questionable internal consistency reliability in this sample (Cronbach alpha coefficients < .72). Nevertheless, the majority (52%) were categorized as persistently fatigued and more (34%) were physically fatigued than mentally fatigued (11%).

Troy (1999) found that women were just as fatigued 14–19 months postpartum as they were at 6 weeks. She introduces employment as a variable, noting that 89% of her sample was working at the second time point. Lee and DeJoseph (1992) did a secondary analysis of 24 pregnant women and 29 postpartum women (up to 15 months) who were employed at least 32 hours per week. They completed the 21-item General Sleep Disturbance Scale (GSDS) and a 100 mm visual analogue line for fatigue during the past week. Fatigue was related to GSDS ($r = .60$), and the postpartum group was only slightly more fatigued (68.5 ± 31.7 mm) than the pregnant group (64.7 ± 32.1 mm). The small effect size (0.11 *S.D.* units) for the difference between these two groups supports Troy's (1999) findings that fatigue does not improve with time, regardless of employment. Although the fatigue scores did not differ, GSDS scores were significantly higher in the pregnant group (62.8 ± 24.9) compared to postpartum group (56.2 ± 22.2), and the effect size was moderate (0.28 *S.D.* units).

Walker and Best (1991) confirmed Troy's (1999) findings when they compared homemakers ($n = 70$) with full-time employed new mothers ($n = 78$). Homemakers had lower stress scores and their major source of stress was fatigue and sleep disturbance. For employed mothers, fatigue and sleep disturbance was the third major stressor, after conflicts with returning to work and lack of time.

Night awakenings are unavoidable for pregnant women and new mothers. Research into ways in which these awakenings can be reduced to a minimal number or duration need to be considered. Ways in which naps might be used as restorative sleep periods to minimize daytime fatigue should also be considered.

SLEEP AND FATIGUE IN CHRONIC ILLNESS

Depression

Nonpharmacologic approaches to treatment of depression are appealing alternatives for women diagnosed with major depression, particularly for those who experience adverse side effects of medication. There are two strategies of interest to nurse researchers that involve manipulation of sleep and circadian rhythms: partial sleep deprivation and phototherapy.

Rapid-eye-movement (REM) sleep typically occurs about 90 minutes after falling asleep and occupies most of the second half of sleep. In persons with major depression, however, REM sleep occurs earlier after sleep onset and is a much higher proportion of total sleep time than seen in the general population. In an effort to reduce REM sleep time for women with major depression, McEnany and Lee (1994) tested the effects of late partial sleep deprivation in 18 women. After two consecutive nights in which they were only allowed to sleep from 10:00 P.M. to 2:00 A.M., 12 (67%) responded to the sleep deprivation, and only two (11%) responded to placebo. They felt positive about continuing to use partial sleep deprivation periodically to control their depressive symptoms.

Since the first REM period is earlier and early morning awakening is a frequent complaint of depressed subjects, McEnany and Lee (1997) hypothesized that phototherapy would shift (phase delay) their early rhythm patterns and thus improve sleep and depressive symptoms. Women with major depression were randomized to either 1 hour of 2500 lux in the morning or placebo. Beck Depression Inventory scores for the 13 women in the placebo group did not change, whereas 56% (9 of 16) improved with phototherapy. These findings need to be replicated but begin to provide psychiatric nurses with nonpharmacologic alternatives for assisting women to manage their depression.

Pulmonary Disease

Women and men with chronic obstructive pulmonary disease (COPD) have been studied to learn more about their symptom experience and functional performance. Leidy and Traver (1995) found fatigue to be the best indicator of performance for women while dyspnea was the best indicator for men. Gift and Shepard (1999) assessed fatigue and other symptoms in 48 women and 56 men with severe COPD. With the global fatigue measure (Medical Outcomes Study, SF-36) used in this study, both men and women reported moderate fatigue, however, the women were younger, had poorer lung function, and had more symptom distress than the men. Dyspnea and physical symptoms predicted 67% of the variance in fatigue scores for women. Research in this area could be enhanced with measures to assess the influence of rest and sleep on fatigue.

Cardiac Disease

Most patients scheduled for coronary artery bypass surgery are fatigued before the surgery is performed (King & Parrinello, 1988). Sleep disturbance is prevalent during the three weeks after surgery, and their greatest fatigue is one week after surgery. Pain and discomfort in the hospital are primary reasons for their disturbed sleep (Simpson, Lee, & Cameron, 1996). Redeker and colleagues (1994, 1995, 1996) found that women with stronger circadian wake/ sleep rhythms one week after surgery, as assessed by wrist actigraphy, had shorter hospital stays and better health outcomes. They also found that, over the next six months, nap time decreased while the amount of night-time sleep stayed consistent. These studies make a very important contribution to nursing knowledge and further research on how perception of fatigue is influenced by reduced nap time over time. Reasons for nighttime awakenings at home would add further to nursing knowledge about symptom management for this population of women.

Sleep and fatigue are also related variables in women with heart failure. Friedman and King (1995) found sleep disturbance to be the next most bothersome symptom, after fatigue, in this population. Redeker, Tamburri, and Howland (1998) studied adults with myocardial infarction. From diary reports, the 23 men had more sleep disturbances than the 10 women. But the women, who were slightly older, had longer awakenings (11.96 ± 7.22) than men (8.68 ± 4.4) and more disturbed sleep according to wrist actigraphy data. Although the difference was not statistically significant in this small sample ($p = .06$), the effect size was large (0.61 $S.D.$ units), indicating significance for clinical practice, since 73% of the 10 women had longer awake times than the average male participant.

Human Immunodeficiency Virus

Most research on HIV-infected women involves larger components of health, such as quality of life (Sowell, Seals, Moneyham, Demi, Cohen, & Brake, 1997) rather than sleep or fatigue. Semple and colleagues (1993) interviewed HIV-infected women and found that fatigue and disturbed sleep were their primary complaints. Phillips (1999) recently reviewed HIV and drug treatment, and discussed their effects on sleep. Van Servellen, Sarna, and Jablonski (1998) interviewed HIV-infected women and found that fatigue was their most common symptom (97.6%), followed by pain and diarrhea. Most (59%) used rest or sleep and decrease activity to manage their fatigue, but 9% (4 women) used exercise.

Cohen and colleagues (1996) surveyed 30 men and 20 women infected with HIV about sleep and found that they averaged 3–12 hours (7.2 ± 2.3 hr). Most (66%) had difficulty falling asleep, which was more common for the women than the men. They reported up to 10 awakenings (2.5 ± 2.0), with

70% awakening more than once, primarily for trips to the bathroom. More women (40%) reported feeling very tired in the morning compared to men (13%). In a study of 100 HIV-infected women, wrist actigraphy was used to estimate quantity and quality of sleep over a 48-hour period, and fatigue severity was assessed morning and evening. Lower CD4 cell count was related to more daytime sleep, higher evening fatigue, and higher morning fatigue. Morning fatigue was related to more awake time during the night (Lee, Portillo, & Miramontes, 1999).

Musculoskeletal Disease

Sleep and fatigue are major concerns for anyone living with chronic pain such as that associated with rheumatoid arthritis (RA) or fibromyalgia (FM). Crosby (1988, 1991) was the first to study persons with arthritis in a sleep laboratory. After surveying 100 people with RA, she noted that disturbed sleep was a major contributing factor to their fatigue. After inviting over 75 subjects to participate in a sleep study, 15 self-selected for one night of polysomnography; 11 were women, but results were not gender-specific. Five of the 15 experienced an exacerbation of their disease during the study. Sleep was significantly more disrupted in RA subjects compared to controls, and those with a current flare had twice the awakenings compared to controls and RA nonflare subjects. Fatigue was correlated with joint pain and sleep disturbance, but severity of fatigue did not differ between the three groups, either because it was measured with one item asking about current fatigue that evening, or because the control group was employed and had worked that day while only a few RA subjects were employed.

After developing a valid and reliable instrument for assessing fatigue in arthritis patients, Belza (1995) was able to document a higher level of fatigue in persons with RA compared to healthy controls. The RA group also had a higher prevalence of self-reported sleep problems, but there was no group difference in depressive symptoms. Fatigue was present in half of the RA group on most days or every day in the past week; it interfered with their activity, and it was related to sleep disturbance and low hematocrit. There was no difference in fatigue between men and women with RA, whereas there was a gender difference for the control group, with women experiencing significantly more fatigue than the men.

Neuberger and colleagues (1994, 1997) surveyed 100 people (78% women) with RA or osteoarthritis to ascertain their perceptions of benefits and barriers to exercise. They found that, during the past week, 46% had not done any range of motion exercise and 76% had not done any strengthening exercises. They then initiated a 12-week aerobics program with 25 RA patients. There was no change in sedimentation rate or joint count, but fatigue decreased, pain decreased, and grip strength increased, even three weeks after the program officially ended. When categorized by level of participation in the aerobics program (low, medium, and high), there was a dose-related decrease in fatigue.

Schaefer conducted studies (1995a, 1995b) on sleep and fatigue in women with FM and documented a relationship between fatigue and sleep problems, particularly awakenings during the night. She also found that the time reportedly spent asleep was not a good indicator of sleep quality. Using polysomnography, Shaver and colleagues (1997) studied 11 women with FM, and compared to healthy controls, those with FM had poorer sleep quality, with more fragmented sleep, and higher symptom distress. This group of researchers then conducted an intriguing experiment. They recruited 12 healthy women and deprived them of deep sleep (delta stages 3-4) for 3 nights in the laboratory. Every time delta waves appeared on the polysomnogram, a tone was emitted to cause a brief nonperceived arousal. This was in an effort to replicate a specific type of sleep (alpha-delta) often seen with FM patients. After 3 nights of delta sleep deprivation, pain threshold was increased, and fatigue scores increased on the Profile of Mood States without any change in tension, depression, anger, or confusion subscale scores (Lentz, Landis, Rothermel, & Shaver, 1999).

SLEEP AND FATIGUE IN WOMEN WITH CANCER

Fatigue is a major concern for nurses who care for patients with cancer. That concern is reflected in many review articles (Irvine, Vincent, Bubela, Thompson, & Graydon, 1991; Nail & King, 1987; Winningham et al., 1994). Fatigue and sleep problems also cause the greatest distress and are by far the most common complaints from cancer patients across many studies (Blesch et al., 1991; Knobf, 1986; Irvine, Vincent, Graydon, & Bubela, 1998; Rhodes, Watson, & Hanson, 1988; Larson, Lindsey, Dodd, Brecht, & Packer, 1993; Degner & Sloan, 1995; King, Nail, Kreamer, Strohl, & Johnson, 1985). Cimprich (1999) reported that the four most frequent symptoms experienced by newly diagnosed women with breast cancer included mood state disturbance (90%), insomnia (88%), fatigue (77%), and loss of concentration (65%). The fatigue was described as mental, rather than physical, and there was no difference by type of surgery, but, as with some groups of pregnant and postpartum women, it was younger women who experienced more symptom distress than older women.

Review articles by oncology nurses also raise issues of factors that can influence fatigue, and therefore any interpretation of research findings for clinical practice. These factors include how and when fatigue is measured (Pickard-Holley, 1991; Winningham et al., 1994), type of cancer (Faithfull, 1991), pain medication (Cimprich, 1999; Miaskowski & Lee, 1999), and whether treatment involves surgery, chemotherapy, radiation, or combinations (Simms, Rhodes, & Madsen, 1993; Woo, Dibble, Piper, Keating, & Weiss, 1998; Ehlke, 1988; Cimprich, 1992). For women who experience cancer, like community-based samples of healthy women, social factors are also related to fatigue (Jamar, 1989).

Sleep disturbance is as frequent a concern for cancer patients as fatigue, yet sleep research involving women is rare. With earlier technology for objective measures of sleep limited to polysomnography, recruitment for these studies would be as difficult as Neuberger's earlier experience in recruiting patients with arthritis, but even self-report studies focused on sleep are rare. Lamb (1982) was the first to study sleep patterns of patients with malignancy. Using an investigator-developed questionnaire, she found higher anxiety but no difference in sleep problems compared to patients hospitalized for other conditions.

With the advent of less invasive objective measures of sleep, researchers can now begin to incorporate objective sleep parameters in their studies of cancer patients and fatigue. Berger and Farr (1999) used wrist actigraphy to study 72 women receiving chemotherapy after surgery for Stage I-II breast cancer and found that fatigue was related to more awakening at night, being less active during the day, and taking more naps. By the end of the third cycle of chemotherapy, there was a "fatigue rebound" where they slept more and had higher fatigue.

In patients receiving radiation for bone metastasis, Miaskowski and Lee (1999) monitored 12 men and 12 women for 48 hours using wrist actigraphy. The sample was too small to test for gender differences, but sleep disturbance was related to dose of radiation received and sleep was disrupted primarily by pain or need to urinate. There was a positive relationship between pain and fatigue, but pain scores did not change from evening to morning, while fatigue severity was lower in the morning. Findings indicate that sleep was somewhat restorative and reduced fatigue, but pain management should be a major focus of intervention to relieve fatigue and sleep disturbance for those with painful bone metastasis.

REST OR EXERCISE? INTERVENTIONS TO RELIEVE FATIGUE

With the exception of Neuberger and colleagues' (1997) research with RA patients, it is primarily oncology nurses who have studied the role of exercise in relief of fatigue. Yet women with cancer rarely report increasing their activity as a strategy to reduce fatigue (Dodd, 1984; Irvine & colleagues, 1998). Richardson and Ream (1997) surveyed over 100 patients with various types of cancer and different chemotherapy regimens. They found that most (89%) complained of fatigue and categorized self-care strategies according to components of the Piper Fatigue Framework (1993). The top two strategies were modifying activity patterns (84%) and altering sleep/wake patterns (37%), however, neither was reported as very effective. In contrast, Graydon and colleagues (1995) found that sleep and exercise were the most effective strategies for reducing fatigue.

MacVicar and Winningham (1986) argue that exercise not only improves functional capacity, but also improves mental health and well-being. They demonstrated these findings in women with breast cancer after a 10-week aerobic exercise program. When Young-McCaughan and Sexton (1991) surveyed women with breast cancer, those who exercised regularly ($n = 42$) had a higher quality of life than those ($n = 20$) who did not. Exercise does not need to be intensive. Mock and colleagues (1997) enrolled 45 women in a walking program after breast cancer surgery and found that the most frequent and intense symptom was fatigue, but anxiety and difficulty sleeping were also present. Those who participated in the walking program had less fatigue and better sleep than controls.

Schwartz (1998) recruited 219 cancer patients from advertisements in sports magazines. As in other studies, fatigue was prevalent (69%) but worse for those who had received chemotherapy compared to radiation or surgery. Because they were recruited from sports magazines, it was not surprising that almost all (90%) used a combination of exercise and rest to reduce their fatigue, but this is the first study to address the time of day when fatigue is worse. Although 14% reported no pattern to their fatigue, 30% had their worse fatigue in the evening, 22% were worse in the afternoon, and only 7% were worse in the morning. This study needs to be replicated, but findings indicate that, for most persons living with cancer, sleep is restorative and they are less fatigued after a night of sleep. The optimal amount of exercise, the best time of day for exercise, and patients who best respond to exercise are important areas for further research.

SUMMARY AND FUTURE DIRECTIONS FOR NURSING RESEARCH

Whether acute or chronic, fatigue is a major concern for women because it interferes with self-care, causes distress, and reduces quality of life (Rhodes,

Watson, & Hanson, 1988). Much new knowledge can be gained from using a full range of fatigue severity in research questions, from mild and less distressing fatigue to utter exhaustion that causes great distress and limitations in self-care.

Although not a focus of this review, measurement issues can be summarized with three key points. First, sleep measures include both subjective and objective options, and researchers should not necessarily expect a strong correlation between these options, but validity and reliability should be established for the population in which they are being used. Second, because fatigue is a subjective perception, objective measures are rarely used in nursing research. Aaronson and colleagues (1999) discussed strengths and limitations of many fatigue self-report instruments and make an appeal for the use of biomarkers, such as hemoglobin or immune factors. Third, researchers must differentiate between measures of "fatigue" and "sleepiness," both with diurnal fluctuations, and "depression," which is more likely a steady state. To the extent that symptoms of depression overlap with fatigue and sleep problems, results should be cautiously interpreted and multicollinearity between these concepts should be assessed.

A review of the research on healthy women indicates that fatigue is primarily a result of nonrestorative sleep or inadequate rest. The prevalence of sleep disturbance and fatigue remains fairly constant over the childbearing years, but reasons for awakenings vary and require a greater understanding prior to initiating interventions. More research is also needed to understand relationships between nonrestorative sleep, fatigue, and perimenstrual symptoms as well as menopausal symptoms of nocturnal hot flashes and night sweats. For pregnant women, sleep problems and fatigue occur early in pregnancy and continue after birth for different reasons. Of note was the finding that those with cesarean births had longer lasting fatigue. They may labor longer prior to a surgical decision or the effects of surgery may compound the normal postpartum fatigue experience.

Scant research exists on sleep and fatigue in women experiencing surgical procedures such as hysterectomy. Yet, women who have had coronary bypass surgery are already fatigued prior to surgery. Research on some types of chronic illness is substantial, while little exists for other chronic conditions prevalent in women, such as diabetes, chronic fatigue syndrome, or depression.

Rather than focusing on rest, nurses working with chronic illness and cancer populations are examining the role of exercise in relieving fatigue. As in illness populations, healthy women who experience fatigue could benefit from research on exercise as a variable. The role of exercise in promoting restorative sleep, as a possible mechanism for its effectiveness in reducing fatigue, also needs to be studied in health and illness. Many sleep researchers have documented that exercise improves sleep, particularly restorative deep sleep (King, Oman, Brassington, Bliwise, & Haskell, 1997; Youngstedt, O'Connor, & Dishman, 1997), but effects on fatigue, well-being, or immune function are not considered.

Exercise as an intervention to relieve fatigue is a critical area for future research, but researchers should not diminish the importance of strategic rest periods and restorative aspects of sleep. In order to effectively intervene with women who experience acute or chronic episodes of fatigue, more research is needed on circadian rhythms and understanding the best times of day for suggesting a nap or rest period, the appropriate length of rest periods, and the strategic use of sleep.

The review of literature from healthy women and women with health problems provides interesting comparisons of factors that influence fatigue and sleep in similar ways. Research with healthy women focused on diurnal fluctuations in fatigue and relationships to sleep, without regard for exercise or levels of activity. Research on chronic illness and cancer fatigue has focused on general fatigue and its impact on activity, without regard for sleep or therapeutic use of rest and naps. A comparison of these two areas highlights gaps in nursing knowledge about fatigue and nonpharmacologic interventions that could be tested to minimize fatigue and promote a higher quality of life for those with either acute or chronic fatigue.

REFERENCES

Aaronson, L. S., Teel, C. S., Cassmeyer, V., Neuberger, G. B., Pallikkathayil, L., Pierce, J., Press, A. N., Williams, P. D., & Wingate, A. (1999). Defining and measuring fatigue. *Image: Journal of Nursing Scholarship, 31*, 45–50.

Affonso, D. D., Lovett, S., Paul, S. M., & Sheptak, S. (1990). A standardized interview that differentiates pregnancy and postpartum symptoms from perinatal clinical depression. *Birth, 17*, 121–130.

Baratte-Beebe, K. R., & Lee, K. A. (1999). Sources of mid-sleep awakenings in childbearing women. *Clinical Nursing Research, 8*, 386–397.

Belza, B. L. (1995). Comparison of self-reported fatigue in rheumatoid arthritis and controls. *Journal of Rheumatology, 22*, 639–643.

Berger, A. M. &, Farr, L. (1999). The influence of daytime inactivity and nighttime restlessness on cancer-related fatigue. *Oncology Nursing Forum, 26*, 1663–1671.

Blesch, K. S., Paice, J. A., Wickham, R., Harte, N., Schnoor, D. K., Purl, S., Rehwalt, M., Kopp, P. L., Manson, S., Coveny, S. B., McHale, M., & Cahill, M. (1991). Correlates of fatigue in people with breast or lung cancer. *Oncology Nursing Forum, 18*, 81–87.

Carpenito, L. J. (1995). *Nursing diagnosis: Application to clinical practice.* Philadelphia: Lippincott.

Cahill, C. A. (1999). Differential diagnosis of fatigue in women. *Journal of Obstetric, Gynecologic, and Neonatal Nursing, 28,* 81–86.

Chen, M. K. (1986). The epidemiology of self-perceived fatigue among adults. *Preventive Medicine, 15,* 74–81.

Cimprich, B. (1992). Attentional fatigue following breast cancer surgery. *Research in Nursing & Health, 15,* 199–207.

Cimprich, B. (1999). Pretreatment symptom distress in women newly diagnosed with breast cancer. *Cancer Nursing, 22,* 185–194.

Clark, A. J., Flowers, J., Boots, L., & Shettar, S. (1995). Sleep disturbance in midlife women. *Journal of Advanced Nursing, 22,* 562–568.

Coble, P. A., Reynolds, C. F., Kupfer, D. J., Houck, P. R., Day, N. L., & Giles, D. E. (1994). Childbearing in women with and without a history of affective disorder. II. Electroencephalographic sleep. *Comprehensive Psychiatry, 35,* 215–224.

Cohen, F. L., Ferrans, C. E., Vizgirda, V., Kunkle, V., & Cloninger, L. (1996). Sleep in men and women infected with human immunodeficiency virus. *Holistic Nurse Practitioner, 10*(4), 33–43.

Crosby, L. J. (1988). Stress factors, emotional stress and rheumatoid arthritis disease activity. *Journal of Advanced Nursing, 13,* 452–461.

Crosby, L. J. (1991). Factors which contribute to fatigue associated with rheumatoid arthritis. *Journal of Advanced Nursing, 16,* 974–981.

Degner, L. F., & Sloan, J. A. (1995). Symptom distress in newly diagnosed ambulatory cancer patients and as a predictor of survival in lung cancer. *Journal of Pain and Symptom Management, 10,* 423–431.

Dodd, M. (1984). Measuring informational intervention for chemotherapy knowledge and self-care behavior. *Research in Nursing & Health, 7,* 43–50.

Driver, H. S., & Baker, F. C. (1998). Menstrual factors in sleep. *Sleep Medicine Reviews, 2,* 213–229.

Ehlke, G. (1988). Symptom distress in breast cancer patients receiving chemotherapy in the outpatient setting. *Oncology Nursing Forum, 15,* 343–346.

Elek, S. M., Hudson, D. B., & Fleck, M. O. (1997). Expectant parents' experience with fatigue and sleep during pregnancy. *Birth, 24,* 49–54.

Evans, B. D., & Rogers, A. E. (1994). 24-hour sleep/wake patterns in healthy elderly persons. *Applied Nursing Research, 7,* 75–83.

Evans, M. L., Dick, M. J., Shields, D. R., Shook, D. M., & Smith, M. B. (1998). Postpartum sleep in the hospital. *Clinical Nursing Research, 7,* 379–389.

Faithfull, S. (1991). Patients' experiences following cranial radiotherapy: A study of the somnolence syndrome. *Journal of Advanced Nursing, 16,* 939–946.

Floyd, J. A. (1999). Sleep promotion in adults. In J. J. Fitzpatrick (Ed.), *Annual review of nursing research* (Vol. 17, pp. 27–56). New York: Springer Publishing Co.

Franck, L. S., Johnson, L. M., Lee, K., Hepner, C., Lamber, L., Passeri, M., Manio, E., Dorenbaum, A., & Wara, D. (1999). Sleep disturbances in children with HIV infection. *Pediatrics On-Line, 104*(5), e62.

Friedman, M. M., & King, M. B. (1995). Correlates of fatigue in older women with heart failure. *Heart & Lung, 24,* 512–518.

Gardner, D. L. (1991) Fatigue in postpartum women. *Applied Nursing Research,* *4*(2), 57–62.

Gift, A. G., & Shepard, C. E. (1999). Fatigue and other symptoms in patients with chronic obstructive pulmonary disease: Do women and men differ? *Journal of Obstetric, Gynecologic, and Neonatal Nursing, 28,* 201–208.

Graef, P., McGhee, K., Rozychki, J., Fescina-Jones, D., Clark, J. A., Thompson, J., & Brooten, D. (1988). Postpartum concerns of breastfeeding mothers. *Journal of Nurse Midwifery, 33*(2), 62–66.

Graydon, J. E., Bubela, N., Irvine, D., & Vincent, L. (1995). Fatigue-reducing strategies used by patients receiving treatment for cancer. *Cancer Nursing, 18,* 23–28.

Hagnell, O., Grasbeck, A., Ojesjo, L., & Otterbeck, L. (1993). Mental tiredness in the Lundby study: Incidence and course over 25 years. *Acta Psychiatrica Scandinavica, 88,* 316–321.

Humphreys, J., Lee, K. A., Neylan, T., & Marmar, C. (1999). Sleep patterns of sheltered battered women. *Image: Journal of Nursing Scholarship, 31,* 139–143.

Irvine, D. M., Vincent, L., Graydon, J. E., & Bubela, N. (1998). Fatigue in women with breast cancer receiving radiation therapy. *Cancer Nursing, 21,* 127–135.

Irvine, D. M., Vincent, L., Bubela, N., Thompson, L., & Graydon, J. (1991). A critical appraisal of the research literature investigating fatigue in the individual with cancer. *Cancer Nursing, 14,* 188–199.

Jamar, S. C. (1989). Fatigue in women receiving chemotherapy for ovarian cancer. In S. G. Funk, E. M. Tornquist, M. T. Champagne, L. A. Copp, & P. A. Wiese (Eds.), *Key aspects of comfort: Management of pain, fatigues, and nausea* (pp. 224–228). New York: Springer Publishing Co.

Keefe, M. R. (1988). The impact of infant rooming-in on maternal sleep at night. *Journal of Obstetric, Gynecologic, and Neonatal Nursing, 17,* 122–126.

King, A. C., Oman, R. F., Brassington, G. S., Bliwise, D. L., & Haskell, W. L. (1997). Moderate-intensity exercise and self-rated quality of sleep in older adults. *Journal of the American Medical Association, 277,* 32–37.

King, K. B., & Parrinello, K. A. (1988). Patient perceptions of recovery from coronary artery bypass grafting after discharge from the hospital. *Heart & Lung, 17,* 708–715.

King, K. B., Nail, L. M., Kreamer, K., Strohl, R. A., & Johnson, J. (1985). Patients' descriptions of the experience of receiving radiation therapy. *Oncology Nursing Forum, 12,* 55–61.

Knobf, M. T. (1986). Physical and psychologic distress associated with adjuvant chemotherapy in women with breast cancer. *Journal of Clinical Oncology, 4,* 678–684.

Krystal, A. D., Edinger, J., Wohlgemuth, W., & Marsh, G. R. (1998). Sleep in perimenopausal and post-menopausal women. *Sleep Medicine Reviews, 2,* 243–253.

Labyak, S. E., & Lee, T. M. (1995). Estrus- and steroid-induced changes in circadian rhythms in a diurnal rodent, octodon degus. *Physiology & Behavior, 58,* 573–585.

Lamb, M. A. (1982). The sleeping patterns of patients with malignant and nonmalignant diseases. *Cancer Nursing, 5,* 389–396.

Landis, C. A., Savage, M. V., Lentz, M. J., & Brengelmann, G. L. (1997). Sleep deprivation alters body temperature dynamics to mild cooling and heating not sweating threshold in women. *Sleep, 21,* 101–108.

Larson, P. J., Lindsey, A. M., Dodd, M. J., Brecht, M., & Packer, A. (1993). Influence of age on problems experienced by patients with lung cancer undergoing radiation therapy. *Oncology Nursing Forum, 20,* 473–480.

Lazarus, R. S., & Folkman, S. (1984). *Stress, appraisal, and coping.* New York: Springer Publishing Co.

Lee, K. A. (1988). Circadian temperature rhythms in relation to menstrual cycle phase. *Journal of Biological Rhythms, 3,* 255–263.

Lee, K. (1992). Self-reported sleep disturbances in employed women. *Sleep, 15,* 493–498.

Lee, K. A. (1998). Alterations in sleep during pregnancy and postpartum: A review of 30 years of research. *Sleep Medicine Reviews, 4,* 231–242.

Lee, K. A. (1999). Rest and sleep. In C. A. Lindeman & M. McAthie (Eds.), *Fundamentals of contemporary nursing practice* (pp. 723–744). Philadelphia: Saunders.

Lee, K. A., & DeJoseph, J. (1992). Sleep disturbance, vitality, and fatigue among a select group of employed childbearing women. *Birth, 19,* 208–213.

Lee, K. A., Lentz, M. J., Taylor, D., Mitchell, E. S., & Woods, N. F. (1994). Fatigue as a response to environmental demands in women's lives. *Image: Journal of Nursing Scholarship, 26,* 149–154.

Lee, K. A., McEnany, G., & Weekes, D. (1998). Gender differences in sleep patterns for early adolescents. *Journal of Adolescent Health, 24,* 16–20.

Lee, K. A., Portillo, C. J., & Miramontes, H. (1999). The fatigue experience for women with Human Immunodeficiency Virus. *Journal of Obstetric, Gynecologic, and Neonatal Nursing, 28,* 193–200.

Lee, K. A., Shaver, J., Giblin, E., & Woods, N. F. (1990). Sleep patterns related to menstrual cycle phase and premenstrual affective symptoms. *Sleep, 13,* 403–409.

Lee, K. A., & Taylor, D. L. (1996). Is there a generic midlife woman? The health and symptom experience of midlife women. *Menopause: Journal of North American Menopause Society, 3,* 154–164.

Lee, K. A., & Zaffke, M. E. (1999). Longitudinal changes in fatigue and energy during pregnancy and the postpartum period. *Journal of Obstetric, Gynecologic, and Neonatal Nursing, 28,* 183–191.

Lee, K. A., Zaffke, M. E., & McEnany, G. (2000) Parity and sleep patterns during and after pregnancy. *Obstetrics & Gynecology, 95,* 14–18.

Leidy, N. K., & Traver, G. A. (1995). Psychophysiologic factors contributing to functional performance in people with COPD: Are there gender differences? *Research in Nursing & Health, 18,* 535–546.

Lentz, M. J., & Killien, M. G. (1991). Are you sleeping? Sleep patterns during postpartum hospitalization. *Journal of Perinatal Neonatal Nursing, 4*(4), 30–38.

Libbus, K., Baker, J. L., Osgood, J. M., Phillips, T. C., & Valentine, D. M. (1995). Persistent fatigue in well women. *Women and Health, 23,* 57–72.

MacVicar, M. G., & Winningham, M. L. (1986). Promoting the functional capacity of cancer patients. *Cancer Bulletin, 38,* 235–239.

Manber, R., & Armitage, R. (1999). Sex, steroids, and sleep: A review. *Sleep, 22,* 540–555.

Martin, S. E., Wraith, P. K., Deary, I. J., & Douglas, N. J. (1997). The effect of nonvisible sleep fragmentation on daytime function. *American Journal of Respiratory Critical Care Medicine, 155,* 1596–1601.

Mayberry, L. J., Gennaro, S., Strange, L., Williams, M., & De, A. (1999). Maternal fatigue: Implications of second stage labor nursing care. *Journal of Obstetric, Gynecologic, and Neonatal Nursing, 28,* 175–181.

McEnany, G. W., & Lee, K. A. (1994). Effects of late partial sleep deprivation in women with major depression. *Sleep Research, 23,* 203.

McEnany, G. W., & Lee, K. A. (1997). Effects of phototherapy in women with nonseasonal/non-bipolar major depression. *Sleep Research, 26,* 294.

Miaskowski, C., & Lee, K. (1999). Pain, fatigue, and sleep disturbances in oncology outpatients receiving radiation therapy for bone metastasis: A pilot study. *Journal of Pain and Symptom Management, 17,* 320–332.

Milligan, R. (1989). Maternal fatigue during the first three months of the postpartum period. *Dissertation Abstracts International, 50,* 07–B.

Milligan, R., Lenz, E. R., Parks, P. L., Pugh, L. C., & Kitzman, H. (1996). Postpartum fatigue: Clarifying a concept. *Scholarly Inquiry for Nursing Practice: An International Journal, 10,* 279–291.

Mock, V., Dow, K. D., Meares, C. J., Grimm, P. M., Dienemann, J. A., Haisfield-Wolfe, M. E., Quitasol, W., Mitchell, S., Chakravarthy, A., & Gage, I. (1997). Effects of exercise on fatigue, physical functioning, and emotional distress during radiation therapy for breast cancer. *Oncology Nursing Forum, 24,* 991–1000.

Nail, L. M., & King, K. B. (1987). Fatigue. *Seminars in Oncology Nursing, 3,* 257–262.

National Sleep Foundation. (1998). *Women and Sleep Poll, and Omnibus Sleep in America Poll.* Washington, D.C. (www.sleepfoundation.org)

Neuberger, G. B., Press, A. N., Lindsley, H. B., Hinton, R., Cagle, P. E., Carlson, K., Scott, S., Dahl, J., & Kramer, B. (1997). Effects of exercise on fatigue, aerobic fitness, and disease activity measures in persons with rheumatoid arthritis. *Research in Nursing & Health, 20,* 195–204.

Neuberger, G. B., Kasal, S., Vogel Smith, K., Hassanein, R., & DeViney, S. (1994). Determinants of exercise and aerobic fitness in outpatients with arthritis. *Nursing Research, 43,* 11–17.

Parks, P. L., Lenz, E. R., Milligan, R. A., & Hae-Ra, H. (1999). What happens when fatigue lingers for 18 months after delivery. *Journal of Obstetric, Gynecologic, and Neonatal Nursing, 28,* 87–93.

Paulsen, V., & Shaver, J. (1991). Stress, support, psychological states and sleep. *Social Science & Medicine, 32,* 1237–1243.

Phillips, K. D. (1999). Physiological and pharmacological factors of insomnia in HIV disease. *Journal of the Association of Nurses in AIDS Care, 10*(5), 93–97.

Pickard-Holley, S. (1991). Fatigue in cancer patients. *Cancer Nursing, 14,* 13–19.

Piper, B. F. (1993). Fatigue. In V. Carrier-Kohlman, A. M. Lindsey, & C. M. West (Eds.), *Pathophysiological phenomena in nursing: Human responses to illness* (pp. 279–302). Philadelphia: Saunders.

Piper, B. F., Lindsey, A. M., & Dodd, M. J. (1987). Fatigue mechanisms in cancer: Developing nursing theory. *Oncology Nursing Forum, 14,* 17–23.

Pugh, L. C. (1990). Psychophysiological correlates of fatigue during childbirth. University of Maryland, Baltimore, Dissertation Abstracts (DA 9014660).

Pugh, L. C., Milligan, R. A., Gray, S., & Strickland, O. L. (1998). First stage labor management: An examination of patterned breathing and fatigue. *Birth, 25,* 241–245.

Quillin, S. I. M. (1997). Infant and mother sleep patterns during 4th postpartum week. *Issues in Comprehensive Pediatric Nursing, 20,* 115–123.

Ream, E., & Richardson, A. (1996). Fatigue: A concept analysis. *International Journal of Nursing Studies, 33,* 519–529.

Redeker, N. S., Mason, D. J., Wykpisz, E., & Glica, B. W. (1995a). Women's patterns of activity over 6 months after coronary artery bypass surgery. *Heart & Lung, 24,* 502–511.

Redeker, N. S., Mason, D. J., Wykpisz, E., & Glica, B. (1995b). Sleep patterns in women after coronary artery bypass surgery. *Applied Nursing Research, 9,* 115–122.

Redeker, N. S., Mason, D. J., Wykpisz, E., Glica, B. W., & Miner, C. (1994). First postoperative week activity patterns and recovery in women after coronary artery bypass surgery. *Nursing Research, 43,* 168–173.

Redeker, N. S., Tamburri, L., & Howland, C. L. (1998). Prehospital correlates of sleep in patients hospitalized with cardiac disease. *Research in Nursing & Health, 21,* 27–37.

Rhodes, V. A., Watson, P. M., & Hanson, B. M. (1988). Patients' descriptions of the influence of tiredness and weakness on self-care abilities. *Cancer Nursing, 11,* 186–194.

Richardson, A., & Ream, E. K. (1997). Self-care behaviors initiated by chemotherapy patients in response to fatigue. *International Journal of Nursing Studies, 34*(1), 35–43.

Richardson, P. (1996). Sleep in pregnancy. *Holistic Nursing Practice, 10*(4), 20–26.

Schaefer, K. M. (1995a). Sleep disturbances and fatigue in women with fibromyalgia and chronic fatigue syndrome. *Journal of Obstetric, Gynecologic, and Neonatal Nursing, 24,* 229–233.

Schaefer, K. M. (1995b). Struggling to maintain balance: A study of women living with fibromyalgia. *Journal of Advanced Nursing, 21,* 95–102.

Schwartz, A. L. (1998). Patterns of exercise and fatigue in physically active cancer survivors. *Oncology Nursing Forum, 25,* 485–491.

Semple, S. J., Patterson, T. L., Temoshok, L. R., McCutchan, J. A., Straits-Troster, K. A., Chandler, J. L., & Grant, I. (1993). Identification of psychobiological stressors among HIV-positive women. *Women and Health, 20*(4), 15–36.

Shaver, J., Giblin, E., Lentz, M., & Lee, K. (1988). Sleep patterns and stability in perimenopausal women. *Sleep, 11,* 556–561.

Shaver, J., & Paulsen, V. (1993). Sleep quality, psychological distress and somatic symptoms in menopausal women. *Journal of Family Practice Research, 13,* 373–384.

Shaver, J. L. F., & Giblin, E. C. (1989). Sleep. In J. J. Fitzpatrick (Ed.), *Annual review of nursing research* (Vol. 7, pp. 71–93). New York: Springer Publishing Co.

Shaver, J. L. F., Giblin, E., & Paulsen, V. (1991). Sleep quality subtypes in midlife women. *Sleep, 14*(1), 18–23.

Shaver, J. L. F., Lentz, M., Landis, C. A., Heitkemper, M. M., Buchwald, D. S., & Woods, N. F. (1997). Sleep, psychological distress, and stress arousal in women with fibromyalgia. *Research in Nursing & Health, 20,* 247–257.

Simms, S. G., Rhodes, V. A., & Madsen, R. W. (1993). Comparison of prochlorperazine and lorazepam antiemetic regimens in the control of postchemotherapy symptoms. *Nursing Research, 42,* 234–239.

Simpson, T., Lee, E. R., & Cameron, C. (1996). Relationship among sleep dimensions and factors that impair sleep after cardiac surgery. *Research in Nursing & Health, 19,* 213–223.

Sowell, R. L., Seals, B. F., Moneyham, L., Demi, A., Cohen, L., & Brake, S. (1997). Quality of life in HIV-infected women in the south-eastern United States. *AIDS Care, 9,* 501–512.

Tack, B. (1990). Fatigue in rheumatoid arthritis: Conditions, Strategies, and Consequences. *Arthritis Care and Research, 3*(2), 65–70.

Teel, C. S., & Press, A. N. (1999). Fatigue among elders in caregiving and noncaregiving roles. *Western Journal of Nursing Research, 21,* 498–520.

Tribotti, S., Lyons, N., Blackburn, S., Stein, M., & Withers, J. (1988). Nursing diagnoses for the postpartum woman. *Journal of Obstetric, Gynecologic, and Neonatal Nursing, 17,* 410–416.

Troy, N. W. (1999). A comparison of fatigue and energy levels at 6 weeks and 14 to 19 months postpartum. *Clinical Nursing Research, 8,* 135–152.

Troy, N. W., & Dalgas-Pelish, P. (1997). The natural evolution of postpartum fatigue among a group of primiparous women. *Clinical Nursing Research, 6,* 126–141.

van Servellen, G., Sarna, L., & Jablonski, K. J. (1998). Women with HIV: Living with symptoms. *Western Journal of Nursing Research, 20,* 448–464.

Walker, L. O., & Best, M. A. (1991). Well-being of mothers with infant children: A preliminary comparison of employed women and homemakers. *Women and Health, 17,* 71–78.

Wambach, K. A. (1998). Maternal fatigue in breastfeeding primiparae during the first nine weeks postpartum. *Journal of Human Lactation, 14,* 219–229.

Waters, M., & Lee, K. (1996). Differences between primigravidae and multigravidae mothers in sleep disturbances, fatigue, and functional status. *Journal of Nurse-Midwifery, 41,* 364–367.

Winningham, M. L., Nail, L. M., Burke, M. B., Brophy, L., Cimprich, B., Jones, L. S., Rickard-Holley, S., Rhodes, V., St. Pierre, B., Beck, S., Glass, E. C., Mock, V. L., Mooney, K. H., & Piper, B. (1994). Fatigue and the cancer experience: The state of the knowledge. *Oncology Nursing Forum, 21,* 23–36.

Woo, B., Dibble, S. L., Piper, B. F., Keating, S. B., & Weiss, M. C. (1998). Differences in fatigue by treatment methods in women with breast cancer. *Oncology Nursing Forum, 25,* 915–920.

Woods, N. F. (1987). Women's health: The menstrual cycle. Premenstrual symptoms: Another look. *Public Health Reports Supplement, 107,* 106–112.

Young-McCaughan, S., & Sexton, D. L. (1991). A retrospective investigation of the relationship between aerobic exercise and quality of life in women with breast cancer. *Oncology Nursing Forum, 18,* 751–757.

Youngstedt, S. D., O'Connor, P. J., & Dishman, R. K. (1997). The effects of acute exercise on sleep: A quantitative synthesis. *Sleep, 20,* 203–214.

Chapter 10

Intimate Partner Violence Against Women

Janice Humphreys, Barbara Parker, and Jacquelyn C. Campbell

ABSTRACT

Intimate partner violence against women has received considerable attention from nurse-researchers over the past 10 years. Although the amount and sophistication of both quantitative and qualitative research have changed over time, nursing research on intimate partner violence against women has not lost its perspective; nurse-researchers have continued to address women survivors' full range of human responses to violence. Research into violence during pregnancy and battered women's psychological responses to abuse have received considerable attention. Research into violence during pregnancy and battered women's psychological responses to abuse have received considerable attention. Research into violence during pregnancy accounts for fully 20% of all the reviewed nursing research. The largely qualitative research into women's psychological responses to violence is particularly rich and remarkably similar across multiple studies. International studies on intimate partner violence are beginning to appear in the literature and research that addresses the unique experience of ethnically diverse women is occurring with greater frequency. The purpose of this chapter is to review nursing research on intimate partner violence against women in the past decade. Future directions for nursing research, practice, and education are included.

Key words: abuse, battering, nursing, pregnancy, research, violence, women

Intimate partner violence against women has received considerable attention from nurse-researchers over the past 10 years. The original review of nursing research on abused women and their children identified less than 60 databased reports (Campbell & Parker, 1992). Nurse-researchers continue to be concerned with women survivors' full range of human responses to violence.

DEFINITION OF TERMS

"Intimate partner violence," "woman abuse," and "woman battering" are used interchangeably in this chapter. Intimate partner violence, abuse, and battering are defined here as repeated physical and/or sexual assault by an intimate partner within the context of coercive control (Campbell & Humphreys, 1993). Research reviewed in this chapter is limited to violence committed against women by their intimate partner, most often men.

METHODS OF RETRIEVAL

This chapter is limited to a review of nursing research reported in English published from 1990 through 1999. Studies reviewed included those in which the investigators addressed intimate partner violence against women as a significant study variable either at the outset or as an outcome variable of the research. The children of abused women will not directly be considered in this chapter, however, battered women's responses and experiences as mothers will be addressed.

A computer search using Medline/Healthstar and Psycinfo databases covering 1990 to 1999 was conducted. First and second author names, credentials, and affiliations were examined to determine professional background. It was not always clear whether the authors were nurses or other health professionals. This was particularly the case for international studies. When in doubt, attempts were made to contact the authors themselves for clarification of educational preparation. Analysis of the study's purposes, content, and references determined its inclusion in this review of nursing research. Additionally, review of the reference lists of cited articles and examination of reviews by other authors were included in the search. One hundred twenty-five studies met the criteria for this review.

OVERVIEW OF NURSING RESEARCH

There has been a substantial increase in the number and complexity of nursing research on intimate partner violence against women in the past decade. Both qualitative and quantitative methods have been used to study this phenomenon. Qualitative methods have elucidated battered women's experiences of and responses to violence in greater depth. Quantitative methods have grown increasingly sophisticated and explored predictors as well as long-term outcomes of violence. There is beginning intervention research that seeks to ameliorate battered women's responses or to prevent future episodes of violence.

Research into violence during pregnancy and battered women's psychological responses to abuse have received considerable attention. Research into violence during pregnancy accounts for 20% of all the reviewed nursing research. The largely qualitative research into women's psychological responses to violence is particularly rich and remarkably similar across multiple studies. International studies on intimate partner violence are beginning to appear in the literature and research which addresses the unique experience of ethnically diverse women are occurring with greater frequency.

The conceptual bases for nursing research of intimate partner violence have varied with the majority of studies still largely atheoretical. Nursing research has been guided by social cognitive learning theory (Gagan, 1998), Gordon's functional health patterns (Carlson-Catalano, 1998), survivor-group prototype (Dimmitt & Davila, 1995), Compensatory Model of Helping (Dickson & Tutty, 1998), symptom management (Humphreys, Lee, Neylan, Marmar, 1999a, 1999b; Humphreys, 2000), empowerment (Parker, McFarlane, Soeken, Silva, & Reel, 1999), and advocacy models (McFarlane & Wiist, 1997). Several researchers have used Orem's framework to guide their work (Campbell, Kub, Belknap, & Templin, 1997; Campbell & Soeken, 1999a; Humphreys, 1995a; Renker, 1999).

PREVALENCE AND RISK FACTORS

In recent reviews of U.S. and Canadian population-based surveys (1985–98), between 8% and 14% of women of all ages report physical assault in the prior year by a husband, boyfriend or ex-partner (Jones et al., 1999; Dekeseredy & MacLeod, 1997). The one nursing population-based study from Ratner (1993, 1995) found a past year prevalence of 11% in Alberta, Canada, with abuse associated with women being younger, separated or divorced, low combined partner income, and male partner unemployment, similar to U.S. national statistics (Bachman & Saltzman, 1995).

In health care setting sample investigations overall, annual prevalence has varied between 4% and 44%, with the lower percentages in middle class, well-educated samples and the higher in poorer women (Dearwater et al.,

1998; Page-Adams & Dersch, 1998; Jones et al., 1999; Quillian, 1996). The range of lifetime prevalence found among these samples, however, has been much narrower (33%–39%), suggesting that economic and educational resources do *not* necessarily keep women from being abused, but rather make it more possible for them to escape or end the violence against them. In other words, poverty may be less a risk factor for a woman being abused by a male partner in the first place than for her becoming trapped in an abusive relationship. The far higher prevalence of lifetime than past year prevalence supports findings in longitudinal studies (e.g., Campbell, Miller, Cardwell, & Belknap, 1994) that the majority of abused women eventually leave the abusive relationship or manage to make the violence end.

Two large scale ($N = 3,455$ and $1,138$, respectively) nursing investigations (Dearwater et al., 1998; Jones et al., 1999) of health care setting samples (emergency department [ED] and health maintenance organization [HMO]) found the prevalence of abuse within the ranges identified previously; both found significant risk factors of separated and divorced marital status, low income, low education and minority ethnicity. In multivariate (controlled) analyses, education persisted as a risk factor for the HMO women, and young age, low income and ending the relationship in the last year for the ED sample. That women continue to be at risk for physical assault, stalking, and harassment after they leave the abusive relationship has been supported by other nursing research (Campbell, Rose, Kub, & Nedd, 1998; McFarlane, Campbell et al., 1999; Merritt-Gray & Wuest, 1995). In both of the large health care setting samples, the risk associated with minority ethnicity was lowered considerably when controlling for education and income; in the ED sample the risk became nonsignificant (Dearwater et al., 1998; Jones et al., 1999).

Primary Prevention

Although few primary prevention interventions have been tested in any discipline, it is clear that opinions in the United States about abuse over the past 10 years have changed dramatically. Perhaps partly as the result of a public service announcement campaign initiated by the interdisciplinary Family Violence Prevention Fund (FVPF), population-based survey found that, in 1995 as compared to 1992, significantly more Americans thought that domestic violence is an important problem and reported that they would do something if they saw or heard a woman being abused (Kline, Campbell, Soler, & Ghez, 1997). The results were similar across ethnic groups (African American, Latino, Asian American, Caucasian) and supported by ethnic group specific focus group data at both points in time. There were, however, significant gender differences in almost all measures with women indicating that domestic violence was more important and suggesting they were more likely to take action as compared to men.

WOMEN'S RESPONSES TO BATTERING

Nursing research continues to address women's physical and psychological responses to intimate partner violence, laying important groundwork for clinical intervention. In addition, nursing research has examined the psychological processes of resisting abuse as well as the affect of being a mother on battered women.

Physical Responses

Ratner's (1993, 1995) random sample telephone survey of 406 married (including common-law) adult female residents of Alberta, Canada is one of the few large sample, controlled nursing investigations of women's physical and mental health effects of intimate partner violence. Abused women in that sample (response rate 78.7%) were significantly more likely than those not abused to have visited an emergency department, to have been hospitalized, and to have been in contact with public health nurses, psychiatrists, and psychologists in the prior year, a finding supported by Gerlock (1999). Frequency of headaches and backaches in this study as well as others (Eby, Campbell, Sullivan, Davidson, 1995; Rodriguez, 1989) were also associated with abuse, suggesting the possibility of back and head injuries.

In the only known study specifically investigating neurological outcomes from abuse, Diaz-Olavarrieta and associates (1999) found that of 1106 Mexican women with chronic neurological problems, those with functional (vs. structural) diagnoses were most likely to experience abuse (31.4%), with 9% reporting loss of consciousness from the violence.

In emergency department settings, both Vavaro and Lasko (1993) and Campbell, Pliska, Taylor, and Sheridan (1994) corroborated findings from other studies that the majority of injuries to known battered women seeking care in the ED are to the face, head, back, and neck; that contusions, soft tissue, and multiple site injuries are the most common types of injury; that many women were not referred to any services for the abuse; and that more than half had a negative ED experience. In two large scale ED investigations either led by a nurse-researcher (Dearwater et al., 1998) or with a nurse-researcher on the team (Abbott, Johnson, Koziol-McLain, & Lowenstein,

1995), a relatively low proportion (2.2%–2.6%) of women actually presented to the ED with trauma directly from the abuse, but a much higher prevalence (14.4%) of women in the ED said they had been assaulted by a partner or ex-partner in the prior year. The findings of these studies support the premise that battered women present in emergency and other health care settings with a wide variety of physical and mental health problems and demographic characteristics, and therefore support the need to conduct routine universal screening of women for battering in health care settings (FVPF, 1999).

Several studies have sought to describe sheltered, battered women's physical symptoms (Eby, Campbell, Sullivan, & Davidson, 1995; Wang & McKinney, 1997). Humphreys, Lee, Neylan, and Marmar (1999a) conducted the first descriptive study of ethnically diverse, sheltered, battered women's ($N = 50$) subjective and objective sleep patterns and resulting daytime fatigue. Seventy percent of the participants reported poor (subjective) sleep and 34% had sleep efficiency indices (objective sleep quality) of 80% or less (very poor). Twenty-eight percent of the women went to bed very fatigued and 40% woke up feeling equally fatigued. Pilot testing of an educational intervention directed toward improving sleep and reducing distress in sheltered, battered women is currently underway.

Psychological Responses

Ratner (1993) found that the abused women were significantly more depressed, had more physical symptoms of stress, more anxiety and insomnia, and exhibited more social dysfunction than those not abused, with physical violence having a stronger effect than psychological abuse in all aspects. Physically abused women were eight times more likely to be alcohol dependent. Most of these findings have been documented elsewhere (e.g., Martin et al., 1998), but the findings are seldom from population-based samples.

Campbell and associates (Campbell, Kub, Belknap, & Templin, 1997), using the Beck Depression Inventory, found 39% of a volunteer community sample of primarily African American battered women ($N = 164$) qualified for a psychiatric diagnosis of major depression. Stress, self-care agency, childhood physical violence, and relationship physical violence were significant predictors (in descending order of magnitude) of depressive symptoms by multiple regression analysis, explaining a total of 44% of the variance. Non-physical relationship (emotional and sexual) abuse, childhood or adolescent sexual abuse, tangible resources (education, occupation, income), and ethnicity were *not* significant predictors of depressive symptoms.

Silva and colleagues (1997) sought to describe the relationship between symptoms of posttraumatic stress disorder (PTSD) and severity of abuse in an ethnically stratified cohort of 131 abused women in a primary care setting. Symptoms of PTSD were significantly correlated to severity of abuse, regardless of ethnicity. This study was limited, however, by its cross-sectional design and the failure to measure other nonabuse sources of trauma. Humphreys, Lee, Neylan, and Marmar (1999b) caution researchers and clinicians alike not to limit their operational definitions of trauma to battering alone. In a survey of 50 ethnically diverse, sheltered, battered women, they note that participants reported lifetime exposure to an average of eight traumatic events, many unrelated to battering and likely associated with low socioeconomic status.

Humphreys (2000) examined the relationship between spiritual beliefs and psychological distress in sheltered, battered women ($N = 50$). Sheltered, battered women were found to place a high value upon their spiritual beliefs and used a variety of spiritual practices to aid them. Her findings suggest that among sheltered, battered women spirituality may be associated with greater internal resources that buffer distressing feelings and serve to calm the mind. This and other studies (Farrell, 1996) provide support of spirituality as a means of reducing distress through greater connection to oneself and higher powers.

Battered Women As Active Resisters to Abuse

Starting with Landenburger's (1989) important grounded theory study of the process of entrapment in and recovery from an abusive relationship, several different nursing studies have addressed, both qualitatively and quantitatively, women's processes of leaving or otherwise dealing with abuse. Campbell, in two separate longitudinal studies, found that the majority (67% and 56% in the two samples) of both African American (40% and 80% sample proportions) and Anglo battered women in community-based samples either left the abusive relationship or managed to make the violence end (Campbell, Miller, et al., 1994; Campbell & Soeken, 1999c). Using discriminant function analysis, the first study found no predictive factors for continuing relationship violence for either the battered ($n = 51$) or nonbattered (but having serious relationship problems) comparison group ($n = 65$). The second study followed 141 battered women over time and found that both physical and mental health status generally improved during the process of women becoming violence free (Campbell & Soeken, 1999c), and that self-care agency (or women's ability to take care of themselves) was important in protecting women from deleterious health outcomes (Campbell & Soeken, 1999b). The findings of Dimmitt (1995; Champion, 1996) of differences in self-concept in abused and nonabused rural Mexican American and non-Hispanic White women and Torres' (1991) findings of differences in American ($n = 25$) and Mexican American ($n = 25$) women's perceptions and attitudes about wife abuse support the need to further examine the process of resistance and recovery in ethnically diverse women.

Several studies using qualitative data have further explicated the process of leaving and recovery from violence. Curnow (1997), using Walker's (1979) cycle of violence, conceptualized battered women's helpseeking as a manifestation of the process of leaving the abusive situation. Merritt-Gray and Wuest (1995; 1999) and others (Belknap, 1999; Newman, 1993; Landenburger, 1989; Ulrich, 1991) found the same process of first diminishing or silencing of self and then reclaiming the self. Draucker (1997) found similar themes of first "restriction" and then "resolve" in the responses of sexual abuse survivors who had been abused by familial (including partner) and nonfamilial perpetrators. Similarly, Langford (1996), used grounded theory to describe how battered women develop sophisticated knowledge of impending violence (such as specific changes in their partner's eyes, speech, tone of voice) and response strategies to avoid their partner's abuse temporarily, if not permanently. Clarke, Pendry, and Kim (1997) demonstrate that homelessness was an adaptive response in their theory of abused women's freedom-seeking behavior. In the only prospective analysis using qualitative data, Campbell, Rose and associates' (1998) patterns of responses also demonstrated resistance and resourcefulness, with active problem solving.

Moss and associates (1997) and Rose and associates (2000) also explicated the complex role of social support for women's process of dealing with abuse. In their sample they found that primarily African American communities were not always supportive of their leaving the abusive relationship or naming the abuser to outsiders (e.g., the police, professionals), but extended families and religious beliefs were extremely important in supporting healthy decisions.

Wuest and Merritt-Gray's (1999) work has been particularly important in its exploration of a phase of "not going back" when women have to "claim and maintain territory" by getting to a safe place, learning to use resources and gaining control. They also have to go through a process of "relentless justifying" to others and to themselves, a process similar to Belknap's (1999) description of addressing the moral conflicts in decision making or negotiating with self (Campbell, Rose, Kub, & Nedd, 1998).

An important component of all of these studies describing battered women's responses to abuse is the description of the women's strengths and abilities, or "creativity within severely limited options" (Langford, 1996), a perspective not always pursued in research from other disciplines. Also notable is the expansion of research limited by primarily White, middle-class samples (Belknap, 1999; Landenburger, 1989; Merritt-Gray & Wuest, 1995; Ulrich, 1991) to studies of ethnically diverse groups of women (Campbell et al., 1998; Langford, 1999; Moss et al., 1997).

BATTERED WOMEN AS MOTHERS

Researchers (Belknap, 1999; Henderson, 1990; Newman, 1993; Ulrich, 1991) note that a critical factor for many abused women in the process of leaving a violent relationship is the well-being of their children. Ericksen and Henderson (1998) used phenomenology to examine abused women's ($N = 10$) perceptions of their children's experiences while living with their mothers during and after leaving an abusive relationship. Researchers noted that, although all the women had left the abusive relationship, they were in no way free of abuse. Participants reported being inadequately prepared to meet their children's enormous, unmet needs. They described themselves as being too tired, stressed, and over-whelmed to deal with their children, and they found communication with them difficult.

Humphreys (1995a) described sheltered, battered women's dependent-care on behalf of their children. The participants in her qualitative research described deliberate, creative, and diverse actions directed toward protecting their children. In a subsequent study Humphreys (1995b) used ethnography to describe battered women's worries about their children and their responses to those worries. In this study, sheltered, battered women acknowledged the needs of their children much like those described by Ericksen and Henderson (1998). During their time in the battered women's shelter, however, mothers also described their creative efforts on behalf of their children. Both of these studies suggest that research with battered women should also consider the responsibilities of motherhood as a significant factor in their own responses and actions.

INTERNATIONAL RESEARCH

Nursing research on intimate partner violence has begun to investigate international aspects of the issue. Counts, Brown, and Campbell (1999) edited a text using primary ethnographic evidence collected from 14 different societies worldwide, representing a range of geographic locations, industrialization, household arrangements, and degree of spousal violence. The evidence from the primary data support feminist (or patriarchal) theoretical premises, how-ever, all forms of violence against women could *not* be considered aspects of the same phenomenon. They conclude that the status of women is a complex, multifaceted phenomenon that may have a curvilinear rather than direct relationship with wife battering. The review also demonstrated the importance of societal influences on individual couples. Wife *beating* (occasional, non-escalating, without serious or permanent injury, and seen as ordinary by most members of the culture) was differentiated from wife *battering* (continuing, usually escalating, potentially injurious pattern of physical violence within a context of coercive control). Factors found that discouraged the escalation of wife *beating* to *battering* across societies included community level sanctions against battering and sanctuary for beaten wives enacted in culturally specific and appropriate forms. In an investigation using in-depth interviews of key informants from a legal clinic providing such sanctuary and a small sample of battered women in Nicaragua, Wessel and Campbell (1997) describe the importance of historical context as well as societal norms in both the occurrence and facilitation of battering.

In a survey of 150 Pakistani women seeking health care in Karachi, 34% reported being physically abused and 15% reported being abused while pregnant (Fikree & Bhatti, 1999). Similar to studies in the U.S., 73% of the abused Pakistani women were also found to be anxious and depressed. Keenan, El-Hadad, and Balian (1998) used qualitative content analysis of descriptive narratives ($N = 60$) to analyze the cultural context of domestic violence in low-income Moslem and Christian-Armenian families living in Lebanon. Contextual factors for violence included unmet gender role expectations, conflict with husband's relatives, and alcohol abuse. Family stressors were emotional, financial, and work. Women described using three types of conflict management; negotiation, taking initiative, and passive resignation. These studies validate the need for community level sanctions and culturally specific and appropriate support.

BATTERING DURING PREGNANCY

Abuse during pregnancy has been a topic of a significant amount of nursing research. Early research focused on establishing the rate of abuse during pregnancy including rates in specific ethnic groups. Subsequent research established the effects of abuse during pregnancy on maternal and infant health and predictors of abuse in pregnancy. Later research validated previous findings, included new variables, and tested beginning nursing interventions.

Incidence

Early prospective surveys of pregnant women in public prenatal facilities ($N = 1,203$) found 18% of African American, 17% Caucasian women, and

13% first generation Mexican American were abused while they were pregnant (McFarlane, Parker, & Soeken, 1996a; McFarlane, Parker, Soeken, Silva, & Reed, 1999) Abuse in the year prior to the pregnancy was a major predictor of abuse during pregnancy, with 55% of women who were abused while pregnant reporting prior abuse. When the same data set was analyzed by age, the investigators found that 22% of the adolescents reported abuse during pregnancy compared to 16% of the adults (Parker, 1993; Parker et al., 1994). Rates in the year prior to pregnancy were 32% for teens and 24% for adults. Curry, Doyle, and Gilhooley (1998) found similar rates of 38% of teens and 23% of adults. Both Curry (1998; Curry & Harvey, 1998) and Parker, McFarlane, and Soeken (1994; McFarlane, Parker, & Soeken, 1996a) found a relationship between abuse and subsequent low birth weight of the infant, validating the original work documenting this relationship by Bullock and McFarlane (1989).

Several other nursing studies examined rates of abuse in specific populations of pregnant women. Kershner, Long, and Anderson's (1998) descriptive study employed a self-administered questionnaire to survey 1693 women (83% response rate) using eight medical clinics and 17 WIC sites in west-central Minnesota. The survey instrument was given to a sample of 94% percent Caucasian and 4% Native American women. Using the Abuse Assessment Screen (AAS), 21% of respondents reported abuse in the past 12 months of which 89% was perpetrated by a current or former intimate partner.

Mattson and Rodriguez (1999) surveyed 450 pregnant Latina women to determine prevalence and type of abuse, level of acculturation to the American community, and self-esteem. Additionally, a focus group discussion was held in each site to elicit women's feedback on perceptions about the causes of violence and interventions that might help decrease violence. Based on the AAS, 6.2% indicated abuse during the past year. Self-esteem for abused women was significantly lower than for non-abused women ($p < .05$), and acculturation scores for abused women were significantly higher, although the level was not indicated. Focus group data indicated that the women felt that alcohol intake by the abuser was the factor most likely to contribute to abuse.

A different approach to the study of abuse in pregnancy was undertaken by Sampselle et al. (1992) who used a two-item written questionnaire given on the first prenatal visit to compare the amounts of reported abuse between women who choose to obtain prenatal care from a certified nurse midwife or a physician. They found a much lower rate of reported abuse than any other study, however, Sampselle was able to determine that women who selected a nurse midwife for care had a higher reported rate of past abuse. As this was a relatively affluent population, the study provides further evidence that abuse is not restricted to women in lower socioeconomic classes.

Curry and Harvey (1998) in a study of 403 pregnant women found that 17% reported being abused. They also noted that abused women reported more stress, less support from partner, less support from others, and lower self-esteem than nonabused women. Regression analysis of data from abused women revealed six variables that were significant predictors of infant birth weight: age, education, number of prenatal visits, stress due to abuse, stress due to recent loss of a loved one, and stress due to problems with friends.

Campbell, Torres, et al. (1999) used a multi-site case control design with a sample of 1004 women to determine the relative risk of low birth weight (LBW) associated with intimate partner abuse. Women were purposively recruited to represent six different ethnic groups (African American, Anglo American, Cuban and Central American, Mexican American, and Puerto Rican). They were interviewed during the first 72 hours after delivery, with abuse determined by the written Index of Spouse Abuse (ISA) and a modification of the AAS. Puerto Rican women reported the highest prevalence of abuse during pregnancy of all ethnic groups, a significantly greater proportion than the other three Latina groups (Torres et al., in press). The Mexican American, Cuban, and Central American women also reported a lower prevalence of abuse during pregnancy than African American and Anglo women. More acculturation was associated with more physical abuse during pregnancy as were several of the indicators of cultural norms, such as belief in wife/mother role supremacy for women and cultural group belief in the acceptability of men hitting women.

In the same study, multiple logistic regression model analyses were conducted for term and preterm infants controlling for other complications of pregnancy. Physical and nonphysical abuse were both significant risk factors for LBW for the term but not the preterm infants on a bivariate analysis, but the risk estimates became nonsignificant in the adjusted models, suggesting a confounding or mediating effect of other abuse-related maternal health problems (notably low weight gain and poor obstetrical history).

Interrelationships Between Physical Abuse and Substance Abuse

Curry (1998) conducted a prospective study of the interrelationship between abuse during pregnancy, substance use, and psychosocial stress during pregnancy. A total of 1937 English-speaking women receiving care at one of six prenatal clinics in a large city in the northwestern United States participated in the study. Twenty-seven percent of the participants reported abuse, and 14% reported stress related to abuse. African American women reported the highest rates of abuse, but the lowest rates of stress related to abuse. Abused White women were more likely to report smoking or alcohol/drug use than nonabused women, but there was no association between substance use and partner abuse for African American, Hispanic, Asian or "other" ethnicity women. Abused women from all ethnic groups reported significantly more stress, less social support, and lower self esteem than did nonabused women ($p < .05$). Similarly, Campbell, Poland, et al. (1992) found that violence during pregnancy was positively related to drug and alcohol abuse and inversely related to social support during pregnancy in a post partum sample of 900 primarily poor, urban African American women. McFarlane, Parker, and Soeken (1996b) also found that significantly more abused African American and Caucasian pregnant women smoked and used alcohol/illicit drugs during pregnancy than non-abused women. They report that, as a triad, smoking, physical abuse, and alcohol/illicit drug use were significantly related to birthweight (F [3,1040] = 30.19, $p < 0.001$).

Pregnancy Complications and Comorbidities

A number of studies have repeatedly validated the relationship between abuse in pregnancy and delayed entry into prenatal care. Parker, McFarlane, Soeken, Torres, and Campbell (1993) first documented that abused women were twice as likely to begin prenatal care during the third trimester than nonabused women. Abused African American women were twice as likely to begin care during the third trimester, and abused Hispanic women were at a threefold risk of not starting care until the final trimester. Taggart and Mattson (1996) found that abused women sought prenatal care 6.5 weeks later than the non-abused women. Almost 14% of the abused women stated that they had delayed care because of injuries. Long and Curry (1998) noted that domestic violence was identified by Native American women as a significant impediment to obtaining prenatal care.

In Attala's (1994) survey of 400 women participating in the Women, Infants, and Children (WIC) supplemental food program, however, with 31% experiencing some physical abuse, there was no relationship between a history of physical abuse and delay in seeking prenatal care. Even though no statistically significant relationship was found between abuse and delay in seeking prenatal care, 25% of women had begun prenatal care after the first trimester.

In the previously cited study Curry (1998) and colleagues (Curry, Perrin, & Wall, 1998) found that abused adult women were significantly more likely to have unplanned pregnancies and to begin care after 20 weeks than nonabused women. Abused women were also more likely to have poorer, past obstetric histories and to use tobacco, alcohol, and other drugs.

In a focus group with sheltered women, Campbell, Pugh, Campbell, and Visscher (1995) described the relationship of abuse to pregnancy intention, pregnancy resolution (abortion, adoption, unwanted infant, wanted infant), and the decision-making process leading to the pregnancy and its resolution. Thematic analysis revealed five major themes: (1) male-partner control; (2) relentless abuse; (3) lack of consistency and jealousy in the partner's relationship with the woman and with offspring; (4) definition of manhood; and (5) health problems. Although limited by the non-representativeness of the sample (only women in shelters), the study suggested several theoretical links between unintended pregnancy and abuse deserving further investigation. It also provided support for the findings of another qualitative study (Campbell, Oliver, et al., 1993) which noted that severe abuse during pregnancy can be motivated by the husband's (unfounded) suspicion that the baby does not belong to him.

Interventions

Building on previous research documenting the relationship between abuse and low birth weight, Parker et al. (1999) tested an intervention to prevent further abuse to pregnant women. This prospective, ethnically stratified cohort design included 199 pregnant African American, Hispanic, and Caucasian pregnant women who presented for care in prenatal public health clinics. All of the women had experienced abuse within the prior 12 months according to the AAS and were still in a relationship with the abuser. Women who received a nursing intervention designed to provide them with information on the cycle of violence, a danger assessment, the options available to them, safety planning, and resource referrals in an empowering manner had significantly lower scores for both physical and non-physical abuse (as measured by the ISA) at six and 12 months postintervention. The difference in group scores remained significant when ethnicity and age (teen vs. adult) were included in the analysis and women in the intervention group used significantly more safety behaviors than did the comparison group. These findings suggest that, regardless of age and ethnicity, basic information about woman abuse, resources, and safety planning can affect positive outcomes for battered women.

McFarlane et al. (1998) further examined the changes in 15 specific safety behaviors of the women in this same study group across five visits. Safety behaviors included such actions as hiding money or keys, asking a neighbor to call the police, and gathering important papers. Eleven of the 15 behaviors showed a significant change from visit one to visit two. Three additional behaviors changed significantly by visit three, and the fourth (removing weapons from the home) increased significantly by visit four. There were no significant differences between ethnic groups. In a related analysis McFarlane and colleagues (McFarlane, Soeken, Reel, Parker, & Silva, 1997) report that women's use of resources (police, shelters) was related to the severity of the abuse and not to being in the intervention vs. control group. This research demonstrated the effectiveness of empowering interventions with women of different ethnic backgrounds across the childbearing years.

A different intervention approached was explored by McFarlane and Wiist (1997). This advocacy model was one of three strategies in a three-year, longitudinal experimental study to examine the effectiveness of three different abuse prevention services. The authors evaluated the effectiveness of lay advocates ("mentor mothers") in establishing and maintaining contact with pregnant abused women throughout their pregnancy. The records of the first 100 women enrolled in the mentor mother program to deliver were reviewed in this evaluation. Ninety-six percent of the women self-identified as Hispanic and 70% spoke only Spanish. The authors reported that mentor mothers made a total of 922 contacts with the women, of which 74% were by telephone. Advocates made a total of 870 referrals for medical services, social services, abuse counseling, food, and other needs. This initial report demonstrates the feasibility of longitudinal research and does not as yet indicate outcomes specific to the abuse.

HEALTH EFFECTS OF INTIMATE PARTNER FORCED SEX

Forty-five percent of physically abused women are also forced to have sex with their intimate partner (Campbell & Soeken, 1999a; Davila & Brackley, 1999; Eby, Campbell, Sullivan, & Davidson, 1995). Other battered women report sexually abusive and controlling acts, such as refusing to use safe sex practices, contraception, or verbal sexual degradation. Many studies across disciplines have reported increased risk of gynecological and reproductive health problems associated with intimate partner violence, but generally forced sex is not measured separately (e.g., Plichta & Abraham, 1996). Yet, it is probably not only the stress from an abusive relationship but also the particular trauma and stress of forced sex that contributes to the high rates of gynecological problems in battered women. Three nursing investigations have particularly investigated the effects of forced sex on women's health (Campbell & Soeken, 1999a; Eby et al., 1995; Golding & Taylor, 1996). Both Campbell and Soeken

(1999a) and Eby and colleagues (1995) used samples (N = 159 & 110 respectively) of relatively poor battered women in the Midwest. In the Campbell and Soeken's (1999a) predominantly African American community sample, sexually assaulted women had significantly higher symptom frequency than those not assaulted. They also reported significantly more gynecological problems, including abdominal pain, urinary problems, decreased sexual desire, and genital irritation. The number of problems remained significant even after adjusting for age, race, tangible resources, and stress, with an adjusted odds ratio for gynecological problems of 2.65 (95% CI: 1.11–6.32). Eby and colleagues (1995) also found that women who were sexually as well as physically abused had more symptoms than those reporting sexual abuse in their half Anglo-American, 42% African American sample from a shelter. They noted moderate to high (.50–.58) correlations between frequency and/or severity of physical and sexual abuse with physical symptoms. Both studies found abdominal cramping or (pelvic) pain and pain on intercourse as two of the most common symptoms. Golding and Taylor (1996) using two survey data sets (N = 1,099 & 2,993) studied the association between sexual assault history and self-reported premenstrual distress. They found that premenstrual distress was more common among women who had been repeatedly sexually assaulted by the same offender as compared to women who had not so been assaulted, even when controlling for depression. In community samples Campbell and Soeken (1999a) and others have noted that women reporting more forced sex experiences also reported significantly greater levels of depression (Weingourt, 1990), less positive physical self-image (Smith 1997a, 1997b), and higher scores for homicide risk as measured by the Danger Assessment instrument than those not sexually assaulted. Weaknesses of both studies included a limited number of gynecologically related items on the health symptom inventory and volunteer convenience samples, but the similarity of findings adds to their credence.

    The Eby and associates (1995) study also demonstrated other implications of forced sex within intimate partner relationships for reproductive health, particularly surrounding contraception and STD/HIV prevention. Population-based studies from other disciplines have established the link of intimate partner violence and unintended pregnancy and STDs including HIV/AIDS (e.g., Gazamararian et al., 1995; Maman, Campbell, Sweat, & Gielen, 2000; Wingood & DiClemente, 1997), but have seldom considered forced sex separately. Several qualitative nursing investigations have illustrated how abuse interacts with the complex social, psychological, and cultural factors involved in decisions and actions to prevent pregnancy or STDs, including HIV/AIDS. Across all studies, male partner control of contraception and pregnancy decisions and aversion to condom use as well as relationship forced sex (but not defined as rape) demonstrated the impossibility of true negotiation of condom use or contraception in violent relationships (Campbell, Pugh, Campbell, & Visscher, 1995; Champion & Shain, 1998; Davila & Brackley, 1999; Lathrup, 1998; Leenerts, 1999; Stevens & Richards, 1998). Although all had small samples, they varied in ethnic background (Anglo, African American, and Latina), sample origin (shelters, STD, and HIV clinics), and methodological approach (grounded theory, case study, focus group, ethnography and pheno-menologic/hermeneutic). This strengthened the validity and generalizability of the shared findings. Additional themes in at least one of the studies included definitions of manhood that include: violence; aversion to condom use; having children and lack of involvement in child care (Campbell, Campbell, et al., 1994; Champion & Shain, 1998); requests for condom use increasing risk of abuse; accusations of infidelity (Davila & Brackley, 1999); self-images of being unlovable and searching for love through sexual relationships that involved needle sharing or repeat STDs; and/or having babies as an inevitable part of life (Lennert, 1999; Champion & Shain, 1998).

Finally, in another aspect of reproductive health, Glander, Moore, Michie-lutte and Parsons (1998) investigated the prevalence of abuse among 486 primarily White (46.5%) and African American (45.9%) young ($M = 25$ years) women seeking outpatient elective termination of pregnancy. Overall, 39.5% reported any history of abuse by the AAS with White women significantly more likely to report abuse than Black women. Abused women were significantly less likely to inform their partner of the pregnancy than nonabused women and less likely to have partner support or involvement in the abortion decision. Limitations to this study included nonrandom sampling with possible bias from the exclusion of women with a male partner present.

BATTERED WOMEN IN THE HEALTH CARE SYSTEM

A significant focus of nursing research has been the identification of battered women in the health care system and determination of how best to assess for intimate partner violence. Investigations of attitudes of nurses toward survivors of violence reveal both disappointing and instructive trends and suggest the need for continued professional development.

Assessment Tools

Over the past decade, nurse-researchers have been involved in the development and use of several instruments to assess intimate partner violence: the Abuse

Assessment Scale (AAS) (Parker & McFarlane, 1991), the Index of Spousal Abuse (ISA) (Hudson & McIntosh, 1981), the Partner Abuse Scale (Hudson, 1990), and the Danger Assessment Scale (©1985, 1988, J. Campbell).

Many of the previously examined studies used the AAS in one form or the other. Originally used to screen pregnant women for intimate partner violence, the five-question instrument has proven successful in both research and clinical practice in diverse settings. Soeken, McFarlane, Parker, and Lominack (1998) report on the test-retest reliability (83–98%) and criterion-related validity (96%) of the five-question AAS in identifying abused pregnant women.

McFarlane (1993; McFarlane, Parker, Soeken, & Bullock, 1992) provides support for the usefulness of a (shortened) two- or three-question AAS in clinical settings. Her study showed that the AAS was as reliable and sensitive to identification of abuse as a different more involved research instrument. In a subsequent study, McFarlane and colleagues (McFarlane, Greenberg, Weltge, & Watson, 1995) demonstrated the effectiveness of a two-question, nurse-administered version of the AAS to detect physical abuse in a ethnically diverse sample ($N = 416$) women coming to ED's with vaginal bleeding. She concluded that two questions, asked in privacy, successfully can identify women who have experienced physical or sexual abuse. Feldhaus and associates (1997) also found a three-question adaptation of the AAS to be sufficiently sensitive in the identification of battered women in a large-scale emergency department investigation.

To assess instrument reliability and validity in the measurement of abuse in different ethnic groups, Doris Campbell and colleagues (1994) conducted a psychometric evaluation of the ISA with a sample of 504 African American women. Campbell found three factors with the African American sample compared with the original two reported by Hudson and McIntosh (1981). The new factor identified with this sample reflected behaviors of an extremely controlling and isolating nature. Campbell interprets this phenomena by using the work of Oliver (1989) which indicates that "when Black males engage in violence against Black females, it is because they have defined the situation as one in which the female's actions constitute a threat to their manhood" (p. 265).

Attala, Hudson, and McSweeney (1994) also conducted a validation study of the new version of the ISA, the Partner Abuse Scale (PAS) with separate physical (PASPH), and nonphysical (PASNP) subscales in a primarily White sample of 90 known abused women in a wife abuse shelter compared with 50 Associate Degree nursing students. Evidence of discriminant validity was modified or mediated by differences in education, ethnicity, income, and number of children between the two groups. Internal consistency reliability of both versions of the instrument were high (> .94) in both samples. Based on the findings, Attala and associates suggested a lower cut score than the original authors of the instrument.

Nursing leadership was shown in the development by Campbell (1992; 1995) of the Danger Assessment Scale (DA). The DA was developed to determine homicide risk for battered women. Several small and intermediate size studies (Campbell, Sharps & Glass, 2001; Campbell, Soeken, et al., 1998; Goodman, Dutton, & Bennett, 2000; McFarlane, Parker & Soeken, 1995) indicate support for instrument reliability and construct validity in diverse samples. In addition to the DA's use for predicting dangerous assault, the instrument has therapeutic utility whereby the woman determines her own degree of risk based on the instrument. Precise prediction of the degree of risk based on any cutoff score remains premature. In addition, it is important to include the calendar portion of this instrument to facilitate the woman's remembrance of abuse and to counteract the minimization of episodes that many battered women demonstrate.

Two other research instruments developed by nurse-researchers are Vavaro's (Vavaro & Lasko, 1993) self-efficacy in battered women and Sheridan's (Campbell et al., 1993) HARASS instrument. Both have initial support for reliability and validity, are undergoing further development, and hold promise for future investigations. The HARASS instrument has been used in a large multicity study of intimate partner femicide and attempted femicide. Results thus far suggest that stalking and harassment are important precursors of lethality in battering relationships (McFarlane, Campbell, et al., 1999).

Emergency Departments

Clinicians have long noted that battered women frequently present to EDs. Pakieser, Lenaghan, and Muelleman (1998) conducted a study to determine where women actually sought help when abused. Women, ages 19 to 65, were recruited when they came to 10 EDs in two cities. Of the 4448 women who completed the questionnaire, 37% acknowledged physical abuse by a partner at some time, 10% reported current abuse, and 4% indicated that their visit to the ED was due to abuse. When asked to identify helping resources, the three most common resources identified by women were family and friends, police, and the ED.

Muelleman, Lenaghan, and Pakieser (1998) identified diagnoses, apart from battering injuries, that were more common among women who were living in physically abusive relationships versus women who were not. Six percent of the women seen in 10 EDs in two cities were identified as abused.

Women in abusive relationships were more likely to be diagnosed with urinary tract infections, neck pain, vaginitis, foot wound, suicide attempt, and finger fracture, however, these represented only 20% of the diagnoses for battered women.

Although EDs may be seen as a resource by abused women, their reception from staff and professionals in the ED has been reported as less than ideal. Campbell, Pliska, Taylor, and Sheridan (1994) surveyed battered women ($n = 74$) and battered women's advocates ($n = 49$) to determine their perceptions of treatment of battered women in EDs. Half of the battered women reported negative experiences in EDs such as feeling humiliated, being blamed for their abuse, having abuse minimized, being given insufficient referrals, and not being identified as battered women. These participants also felt that their insurance status (Medicaid) negatively affected their treatment, and 28.6% of the women of color believed that racism had affected their treatment in the ED. Advocates for battered women recommended that ED staff have more education and training about battered women, facilitate referrals to advocates or shelters, give more information to battered women, and improve skill and sensitivity in conducting patient interviews.

Grunfeld, Ritmiller, Mackay, Cowan, and Hotch (1994) studied the effectiveness of a single question by the ED triage nurse about the history of intimate partner violence in identifying abused women. They noted that 6% of the women in their sample ($N = 252$) disclosed abuse, however, they also noted that the environmental layout of the ED often prevented even the asking of a single question.

Other Health Care Settings

Nursing research in non-ED settings has begun to describe the quality and complexity of care needed by women experiencing intimate partner violence and advanced nursing practice in battered women's shelters.

Gagan (1998) conducted a cross-sectional descriptive study using both domestic violence and control case study vignettes to determine diagnosis and intervention performance accuracy, variables that influence this performance accuracy, and barriers that impede performance accuracy of adult nurse practitioners (ANP) and family nurse practitioners (FNP). In this sample of advanced practice nurses (APN) ($N = 118$), accuracy in diagnosis and treatment of domestic violence was correlated with taking college courses containing relevant content, having a professional interest in woman abuse, and fewer years of experience. Perceived barriers included time constraint, client reluctance, and insufficient referral resources.

Dickson and Tutty (1996) surveyed 125 public health nurses to determine their knowledge, comfort, and skill in intervening abused women. In this sample, a high frequency (81%) of thoughts, feelings, and interventions that would facilitate abused women feeling helped were noted, however, while the nurses believed that addressing abuse was within their professional role, 55% were unsure of what to say to initiate the topic. The authors urge further education about family violence in basic nursing programs.

Carlson-Catalano (1998) described the complexity of nursing care required of eight rural Appalachian battered women. After interviewing participants on two occasions, using Gordon's (1994) functional health patterns, she identified 53 nursing diagnoses and 52 nursing interventions. Of these, 24 nursing diagnoses and 26 nursing interventions were applicable to all eight participants.

Attala and Warmington (1996) conducted a study to evaluate battered women's shelter-based health care services provided by APNs, concluding that clients (96%) identified strongly positive responses to health services provided to themselves and their children. In a further evaluation of APN practice in battered women's shelters, Attala, McSweeney, Mueller, Bragg, and Hubertz (1999) analyzed the content of written communications among the APNs providing battered women's shelter-based health care. Three communication themes were identified: (1) nursing assessments, (2) nursing interventions, and (3) program operations.

These study findings describe the complex and individualized care needed by women experiencing intimate partner violence. They also demonstrate that, with appropriate education and support, nurses are able to provide needed care to battered women and shelter and nonshelter settings.

Nursing Attitudes, Education, and Helpfulness Toward Battered Women

In a well-designed study, Tilden and associates (1994) surveyed a random sample of three groups of professionals from six disciplines (dentists/dental hygienists, nurses/physicians, and psychologists/social workers) about their basic professional educational content on child, spouse and elder abuse, with response rates ranging from 69%–83%. Participants with more education on the topic were more likely to consider abuse in their patients. Spouse abuse was the most frequently assessed and elder abuse the least assessed across groups. Nurses were in the middle range of disciplines (below psychologists and social workers, above the dental professions, and about the same as physicians) in rates of identification and educational content except for elder abuse (where they were the highest). The majority of nurses (86.7%) saw themselves as having as much responsibility in terms of family violence as other clinical problems but, like the other professionals, had little confidence in the effectiveness of current family violence laws. In a later extension of this research (Limandri & Tilden, 1996), the authors used interviews and surveys to explore nurses' reasoning in the assessment of family violence. The nurses reported that the major advantage for identifying victims of abuse was to provide safety to the victim and prevent further abuse. When asked how they would intervene, 83% of the nurses chose "passive" interventions (make a note in the chart, observe over time) rather than "active" interventions that would require more involvement with the family. Passive interventions are a less optimal choice according to Yam's (1995) findings and earlier nursing research (King & Ryan, 1989).

Using a written questionnaire, Hamilton and Coates (1993) examined the perceived helpfulness and use of professional services by a volunteer clinical sample of 270 Canadian abused women, primarily employed, single parents. Social workers were the professionals from whom help was sought most often for all three types of relationship abuse, with physicians second (emotional abuse) or third (after police for physical and sexual abuse), and nurses in the bottom third of the list of 13 professionals. The helpfulness ratings of nurses were similar to those of physicians, except for sexual abuse where the scores were much lower. Important clinically were the findings that, for all three kinds of abuse, "listened respectfully and took me seriously" and "believed my story" were deemed the *most* helpful responses by professionals. Other helpful responses were "helping me see my strengths" (emotional and sexual), "helping me understand the effects on my children" (emotional and physical), "helping me see I was in danger," and "figure out ways of making my present situation safer" (physical abuse only), with referrals helpful but endorsed by a much smaller number of women. Unhelpful responses to all three kinds of abuse reflected a lack of attentiveness, disbelief, and/or a failure to treat the situation seriously (especially for sexual abuse). The study was limited by its purely descriptive analysis and nonrepresentative although large sample. These and similar findings by Dixon and Tutty (1998), however, offer reassurance to nurses who lack confidence in their ability to assess and intervene with abused women.

According to Yam (1995) 75% of nurses had educational content on child abuse, but in this and other research only 30%–54% reported any content in spouse abuse (Hegge & Condon, 1996; Moore, Zaccaro, & Parsons, 1998; Yam, 1995). In a later report of a survey of baccalaureate nursing programs, however, Woodtli and Breslin (1995) found that almost all of the programs reported content on intimate partner violence, although generally it was in the form of one or two lectures (rather than any direct clinical experience) as part of community health, mental health, or maternal child health courses.

Three other studies suggest other barriers to the provision of nursing care of abused women. Coleman and Stith (1997) surveyed nursing students ($N = 155$) to determine attitudes that influence the provision of care to abused women. They report that gender-role egalitarianism was found to be the best predictor of attitudes toward battered women. Janssen, Basso, and Costanzo (1998) surveyed nurses in a large Canadian hospital to determine the incidence of exposure to domestic violence among all the nursing staff. Among their participants ($N = 198$) 38% indicated that they had had some personal exposure to violence in intimate relationships either in the past or present. Attala, Oetker, and McSweeney (1995) report that a survey of eight basic nursing programs—four Associate Degree and four Baccalaureate Degree—8% of the students ($N = 243$) reported a history of physical abuse and almost 20% reported experiencing non-physical abuse. These findings suggest that nursing education on intimate partner violence should also include opportunities for self-reflection as well as resources and support of currently or formerly battered students.

FUTURE DIRECTIONS

Based upon this review of the nursing research on intimate partner violence against women, the following are offered as suggestions for further research and changes in nursing education and practice:

- Research that involves larger ethnically diverse samples including shelter and community-based samples will aid our understanding of the influence of culture, resources, and socioeconomic factors.
- Longitudinal research that includes comparison groups will provide important information about the experience of living with violence, the process of resisting violence, and factors that contributed to the successful recovery from abuse.
- Research is needed that attends to specific symptom patterns, their underlying dynamics, and the development and testing of clinically useful interventions.
- Research is needed that further explores the interconnections between battered women and their children, including the relationship between abuse of mother and infant health and development.
- There is a continued need for research collaboration between battered women's shelters and other survivor advocacy and community groups (Campbell, Dienemann, et al., 1999).

- Attention to and the development of research safety protocols that protect both battered women and investigators is needed (e.g., Langford, 1999).
- There is critical need for research into appropriate and effective ways that battered women can protect themselves from STDs including AIDS.
- Nursing must continue to advocate for and research the benefits and risks of routine screening for intimate partner violence in all health care settings. Concurrently, practice settings should be evaluated for clinical environment that is conducive to disclosure of abuse.
- Nursing schools need to integrate intimate partner violence content throughout educational programs. Program should include content both on abuse as well as clinical experiences with families experiencing violence.

REFERENCES

Abbott, J., Johnson, R., Koziol-McLain, J. & Lowenstein, S. (1995). Domestic violence against women: Incidence and prevalence in an emergency department population. *Journal of the American Medical Association, 273,* 1763–1767.

Attala, J. M. (1994). Risk identification of abused women participating in a women, infants, and children program. *Health Care for Women International, 15,* 587–597.

Attala, J. M., Hudson, W. W., & McSweeney, M. (1994). A partial validation of two short-form Partner Abuse Scales. *Women and Health, 21*(2-3), 125–139.

Attala, J. M., McSweeney, M., Mueller, A., Bragg, B., & Hubertz, E. (1999). An analysis of nurses' communications in a shelter setting. *Journal of Community Health Nursing, 16,* 29–40.

Attala, J. M., Oetker, D., & McSweeney, M. (1995). Partner abuse against female nursing students. *Journal of Psychosocial Nursing, 33,* 17–24.

Attala, J. M., & Warmington, M. (1996). Clients' evaluation of health care services in a battered women's shelter. *Public Health Nursing, 13,* 269–275.

Bachman, R., & Saltzman, L. E. (1995). *Violence against women: Estimates from the redesigned survey* (Document NCJ-154348). Washington, DC: Bureau of Justice Statistics, National Institute of Justice.

Belknap, R. A. (1999). Why did she do that? Issues of moral conflict in battered women's decision making. *Issues in Mental Health Nursing, 20,* 387–404.

Bullock, L. F., & McFarlane, J. (1989). The birth-weight/battering connection. *American Journal of Nursing, 89,* 1153–1155.

Campbell, D. W., Campbell, J. C., King, C., Parker, B., & Ryan, J. (1994). The reliability and factor structure of the Index of Spouse Abuse with African-American battered women. *Violence and Victims, 9,* 259–274.

Campbell, J., Dienemann, J., Kub, J., Wurmser, T., & Loy, M. (1999). Collaboration as partnership. *Violence Against Women, 5*(10), 1140–1157.

Campbell, J., Miller, P., Cardwell, M., & Belknap, R. (1994). Relationship status of battered women over time. *Journal of Family Violence, 9,* 99–111.

Campbell, J., Rose, L., Kub, J., & Nedd, D. (1998). Voices of strength and resistance: A contextual and longitudinal analysis of women's responses to battering. *Journal of Interpersonal Violence, 13,* 743–762.

Campbell, J. C. (1992). "If I can't have you, no one can": Power and control in homicide of female partners. In J. Radford & D. E. H. Russell (Eds.), *Femicide: The politics of woman killing* (pp. 99–113). New York: Twayne.

Campbell, J. C. (1995). *Assessing dangerousness.* Newbury Park, CA: Sage.

Campbell, J. C., & Humphreys, J. (1993). *Nursing care of survivors of family violence.* St. Louis: Mosby-Yearbook.

Campbell, J. C., Kub, J., Belknap, R. A., & Templin, T. (1997). Predictors of depression in battered women. *Violence Against Women, 3,* 271–293.

Campbell, J. C., Oliver, C., & Bullock, L. (1993). Why battering during pregnancy? *AWHONN'S Clinical Issues, 4*(3), 343–349.

Campbell, J. C., & Parker, B. (1992). Battered women and their children. In J. Fitzpatrick (Ed.), *Annual review of nursing research* (Vol. X, pp. 77–94). New York: Springer Publishing Co.

Campbell, J. C., Pliska, M. J., Taylor, W., & Sheridan, D. (1994). Battered women's experiences in emergency departments: Need for appropriate policy and procedures. *Journal of Emergency Nursing, 20,* 280–288.

Campbell, J. C., Poland, M. L, Waller, J. B., & Ager, J. (1992). Correlates of battering during pregnancy, *Research in Nursing and Health, 15,* 219–226.

Campbell, J. C., Pugh, L. C., Campbell, D., & Visscher, M. (1995). The influence of abuse on pregnancy intention. *Women's Health Issues, 5,* 214–223.

Campbell, J. C., Sharps, P., & Glass, N. E. (2001). Risk Assessment for Intimate Partner Violence. In G. F. Pinard & L. Pagani (Eds.), *Clinical assessment of dangerousness: Empirical contributions* (pp. 136–157). New York: Cambridge University Press.

Campbell, J. C., & Soeken, K. L. (1999a). Forced sex and intimate partner violence: Effects on women's risk and women's health. *Journal of Interpersonal Violence, 5,* 1017–1035.

Campbell, J. C., & Soeken, K. L. (1999b). Women's responses to battering over time: An analysis of change. *Journal of Interpersonal Violence, 14,* 21–40.

Campbell, J. C., & Soeken, K. L. (1999c). Women's responses to battering: A test of the model. *Research in Nursing and Health, 22,* 49–58.

Campbell, J. C., Soeken, K. L., McFarlane, J., & Parker, B. (1998). Risk factors for femicide among pregnant and nonpregnant battered women. In J. C. Campbell (Ed.), *Empowering survivors of abuse: Health care for battered women and their children* (pp. 90–97). Thousand Oaks, CA: Sage.

Campbell, J. C., Torres, S., Ryan, J., King, C., Campbell, D., Stallings, R., & Fuchs, S. (1999). Physical and nonphysical abuse and other risk factors for low birthweight among term and preterm babies: A multiethnic case control study. *American Journal of Epidemiology, 150*, 714–726.

Campbell, J. C., & Weber, N. (2000). An empirical test of a selfcare model of women's responses to battering. *Nursing Science Quarterly, 13*, 45–53.

Carlson-Catalano, J. (1998). Nursing diagnoses and interventions for post-acute-phase battered women. *Nursing diagnosis, 9*, 101–110.

Champion, J. D. (1996). Woman abuse, assimilation, and self-concept in a rural Mexican American Community. *Hispanic Journal of Behavioral Sciences, 18*, 508–521.

Champion, J. D., & Shain, R. N. (1998). The context of sexually transmitted disease: Life histories of woman abuse. *Issues in Mental Health Nursing, 19*, 463–479.

Clarke, P. N., Pendry, N. C., & Kim, Y. S. (1997). Patterns of violence in homeless women. *Western Journal of Nursing Research, 19*, 490–500.

Coleman, J. U., & Stith, S. M. (1997). Nursing students' attitudes toward victims of domestic violence as predicted by selected individual and relationship variables. *Journal of Family Violence, 12*, 113–138.

Counts, D. C., Brown, J., & Campbell, J. C. (1999). *To have and to hit: Cultural perspectives on the beating of wives.* Chicago: University of Illinois Press.

Curnow, S. A. (1997). The Open Window Phase: Helpseeking and reality behaviors by battered women. *Applied Nursing Research, 10*, 128–135.

Curry, M. A. (1998). The interrelationships between abuse, substance use, and psychosocial stress during pregnancy. *Journal of Obstetrics, Gynecological and Neonatal Nursing, 27*, 692–699.

Curry, M. A., & Harvey, S. M. (1998). Stress related to domestic violence during pregnancy and infant birth weight. In J. C. Campbell (Ed.), *Empowering survivors of abuse: Health care for battered women and their children* (pp. 98–108). Thousand Oaks, CA: Sage.

Curry, M. A., Doyle, B. A., & Gilhooley, J. (1998). Abuse among pregnant adolescents: Differences by developmental age. *MCN: Journal of Maternal Child Nursing, 23*, 144–150.

Curry, M. A., Perrin, N., & Wall, E. (1998). Effects of abuse on maternal complications and birth weight in adult and adolescent women. *Obstetrics & Gynecology, 92*, 530–534.

Davila, Y. R., & Brackley, M. H. (1999). Mexican and Mexican American women in a battered women's shelter: Barriers to condom negotiation for HIV/AIDS prevention. *Issues in Mental Health Nursing, 20*, 333–355.

Dearwater, S. R., Coben, J. H., Nah, G., Campbell, J. C., McLoughlin, E., Glass, N., & Bekemeier, B., (1998). Prevalence of Domestic Violence in Women Treated at Community Hospital Emergency Department. *Journal of the American Medical Association, 480*(5), 433–438.

DeKeseredy, W. S., & MacLeod, L. (1997). *Woman abuse: A sociological story.* Toronto: Harcourt Brace.

Diaz-Olavarrieta, C., Campbell, J., Garcia de la Cadena, C., Paz, F., & Villa, A. R. (1999). Domestic violence against patients with chronic neurologic disorders. *Archives of Neurology, 56*, 681–685.

Dickson, F., & Tutty, L. M. (1996). The role of public health nurses in responding to abuse women. *Public Health Nursing, 13*, 263–268.

Dickson, F., & Tutty, L. M. (1998). The development of a measure of public health nurses' practice responses to women who are abused. *Journal of Nursing Measurement, 6*, 87–103.

Dimmitt, J. H. (1995). Self-concept and woman abuse: A rural and cultural perspective. *Issues in Mental Health Nursing, 16*, 567–581.

Dimmitt, J., & Davila, Y. R. (1995). Group psychotherapy for abused women: A survivor-group prototype. *Applied Nursing Research, 8*, 3–7.

Draucker, C. B. (1997). Impact of violence in the lives of women: Restriction and resolve. *Issues in Mental Health Nursing, 18*, 559–586.

Draucker, C. B., & Madsen, C. (1999). Women dwelling with violence. *Image: Journal of Nursing Scholarship, 31*, 327–332.

Eby, K. K., Campbell, J. C., Sullivan, C. M., & Davidson, W. S. (1995). Health effects of experiences of sexual violence for women with abusive partners. *Health Care for Women International, 16*, 563–576.

Ericksen, J. R., & Henderson, A. D. (1998). Diverging realities: Abuse women and their children. In J. C. Campbell (Ed.), *Empowering survivors of abuse: Health care for battered women and their children* (pp. 138–155). Thousand Oaks, CA: Sage.

Family Violence Prevention Fund. (1999). *Preventing domestic violence: Clinical guidelines on routine screening.* San Francisco, CA: Family Violence Prevention Fund.

Farrell, M. L. (1996). Healing: A qualitative study of women recovering from abusive relationships with men. *Perspectives in Psychiatric Care, 32*, 23–32.

Feldhaus, K. M., Koziol-McLain, J., Amsbury, H. L., Norton, I. M., Lowenstein, S. R., & Abbott, J. T. (1997). Accuracy of 3 brief screening questions for detecting partner violence in the emergency department. *Journal of the American Medical Association, 277*, 1357–1361.

Fikree, F. F., & Bhatti, L. I. (1999). Domestic violence and health of Pakistani women. *International Journal of Gynecology & Obstetrics, 65*, 195–201.

Gagan, M. J. (1998). Correlates of nurse practitioners' diagnostic and intervention performance for domestic violence. *Western Journal of Nursing Research, 20*, 536–553.

Gazmararian, J. A., Adams, M., Saltzman, L., Johnson, C. H., Bruce, F. C., Marks, L., & Zahniser, S. C. (1995). The relationship between intendedness and physical violence in mother's of newborns. *Obstetrics and Gynecology, 85*, 131–138.

Gerlock, A. A. (1999). Health impact of domestic violence. *Issues in Mental Health Nursing, 20*, 373–385.

Glander, S. S., Moore, M. L., Michielutte, R., & Parsons, L. H. (1998). The prevalence of domestic violence among women seeking abortion. *Obstetrics & Gynecology, 91*, 1002–1006.

Golding, J. M., & Taylor, D. L. (1996). Sexual assault history and premenstrual distress in two general population samples. *Journal of Women's Health, 5*, 143–151.

Goodman, L. A., Dutton, M. A., & Bennett, M. (2000). Predicting repeat abuse among arrested batterers: Use of the Danger Assessment scale in the criminal justice system. *Journal of Interpersonal Violence, 15,* 63–74.

Grunfeld, A. F., Ritmiller, S., Mackay, K., Cowan, L., & Hotch, D. (1994). Detecting domestic violence against women in the emergency department: A nursing triage model. *Journal of Emergency Nursing, 20,* 271–274.

Hegge, M., & Condon, B. A. (1996). Nurses' educational needs regarding battered women. *Journal of Nursing Staff Development, 12,* 229–235.

Henderson, A. (1990, June/September). Children of abused women: Their influences on their mother's decisions. *Canada's Mental Health, 38,* 10–13.

Hudson, W. W. (1990). *Partner Abuse Scale: Physical.* Tempe, AZ: Walmyr.

Hudson, W. W., & McIntosh, S. R. (1981). The assessment of spouse abuse: Two quantifiable dimensions. *Journal of Marriage and the Family, 43,* 873–885.

Humphreys, J. (1995a). Dependent-care by battered women: Protecting their children. *Health Care for Women International, 16*(1), 9–20.

Humphreys, J. (1995b). The work of worrying: Battered women and their children. *Scholarly Inquiry for Nursing Practice: An International Journal, 9*(2), 126–145.

Humphreys, J. (2000). Spirituality in sheltered battered women. *Journal of Nursing Scholarship, 32,* 273–278.

Humphreys, J. C., Lee, K. A., Neylan, T. C., & Marmar, C. R. (1999a). Sleep patterns of sheltered battered women. *Image: Journal of Nursing Scholarship, 31,* 139–143.

Humphreys, J. C., Lee, K. A., Neylan, T. C., & Marmar, C. R. (1999b). Trauma history of sheltered battered women. *Issues in Mental Health Nursing, 20,* 319–332.

Janssen, P. A., Basso, M. C., & Costanzo, R. M. (1998). The prevalence of domestic violence among obstetric nurses. *Women's Health Issues, 8,* 317–323.

Jones, A. S., Gielen, A. C., Campbell, J. C., Schollenberger, J., Dienemann, J. A., Kub, J., O'Campo, P. J., & Wynne, E. C. (1999). Annual and lifetime prevalence of partner abuse in a sample of female HMO enrollees. *Women's Health Issues, 9,* 295–305.

Keenan, C. K., El-Hadad, A., & Balian, S. A. (1998). Factors Associated with domestic violence in low-income Lebanese families. *Image: Journal of Nursing Scholarship, 30,* 357–362.

Kershner, M., Long, D., & Anderson, J. E. (1998). Abuse against women in rural Minnesota. *Public Health Nursing, 15,* 422–431.

Klein, E., Campbell, J., Soler, E., & Ghez, M. (1997). *Ending domestic violence: Changing public perceptions.* Newbury Park, CA: Sage.

Landenburger, K. (1989). A process of entrapment in and recovery from an abusive relationship. *Issues in Mental Health Nursing, 10,* 209–227.

Langford, D. R. (1996). Predicting unpredictability: A model of women's processes of predicting battering men's violence. *Scholarly Inquiry for Nursing Practice, 10,* 371–385.

Langford, D. R. (2000). Pearls, pith, and provocation: Developing a safety protocol in qualitative research involving battered women. *Qualitative Health Research, 10,* 133–142.

Lathrop, A. (1998). Pregnancy resulting from rape. *Journal of Obstetrics, Gynecological, and Neonatal Nursing, 2,* 25–30.

Lawson, E. J. (1998). A narrative analysis: A Black woman's perceptions of breast cancer risks and early breast cancer detection. *Cancer Nursing, 21,* 421–429.

Leenerts, M. H. (1999). The disconnected self: Consequences of abuse in a cohort of low-income White women living with HIV/AIDS. *Health Care for Women International 10,* 381–400.

Limandri, B. J., & Tilden, V. P. (1996). Nurses' reasoning in the assessment of family violence. *Image: The Journal of Nursing Scholarship, 28,* 247–252.

Long, C. R., & Curry, M. A. (1998). Living in two worlds: Native American women and prenatal care. *Health Care for Women International, 19,* 205–215.

Maman, S., Campbell, J. C., Sweat, M., & Gielen, A. C. (2000). The intersection of HIV and violence: Directions for future research and interventions. *Social Science and Medicine, 50,* 459–478.

Martin, S. L., Kilgallen, B., Dee, D. L., Dawson, S., & Campbell, J. (1998). Women in a prenatal care/substance abuse treatment program: Links between domestic violence and mental health. *Maternal and Child Health Journal, 2,* 85–94.

Mattson, S., & Rodriguez, E. (1999). Battering in pregnant Latinas. *Issues in Mental Health Nursing, 20,* 405–422.

McFarlane, J. (1993). Abuse during pregnancy: The horror and the hope. *AWHONN's Clinical issues in Perinatal and Women's Health Nursing, 4,* 350–362.

McFarlane, J., Campbell, J. C., Wilt, S., Sachs, C., Ulrich, Y., & Xu, X. (1999). Frequency and type of stalking before attempted and actual intimate partner femicide. *Homicide Studies, 3,* 300–316.

McFarlane, J., Greenberg, L., Weltge, A., & Watson, M. (1995). Identification of abuse in emergency departments: Effectiveness of a two-question screening tool. *Journal of Emergency Nursing, 21,* 391–394.

McFarlane, J., Parker, B., & Soeken, K. (1995). Abuse during pregnancy: Frequency, severity, perpetrator and risk factors of homicide. *Public Health Nursing, 12,* 284–289.

McFarlane, J., Parker, B., & Soeken, K. (1996a). Abuse during pregnancy: Associations with maternal health and infant birth weight. *Nursing Research, 45,* 37–42.

McFarlane, J., Parker, B., & Soeken, K. (1996b). Physical abuse, smoking, and substance use during pregnancy: Prevalence, interrelationships and effects on birthweight. *Journal of Obstetric, Gynecologic and Neonatal Nursing, 25,* 313–320.

McFarlane, J., Parker, B., Soeken, K., & Bullock, L. (1992). Assessing for abuse during pregnancy: Severity and frequency of injuries and associated entry into prenatal care. *Journal of the American Medical Association, 267,* 3176–3178.

McFarlane, J., Parker, B., Soeken, K., Silva, C., & Reed, S. (1999). Severity of abuse before and during pregnancy for African American, Hispanic, and Anglo women. *Journal of Nurse-Midwifery, 44,* 139–144.

McFarlane, J., Soeken, K., Campbell, J., Parker, B., Reel, S., & Silva, C. (1998). Severity of abuse to pregnant women and associated gun access of the perpetrator. *Public Health Nursing, 15,* 201–206.

McFarlane, J., Soeken, K., Reel, S., Parker, B., & Silva, C. (1997). Resource use by abused women following an intervention program: Associated severity of abuse and reports of abuse ending. *Public Health Nursing, 14,* 244–250.

McFarlane, J., & Wiist, W. (1997). Preventing abuse to pregnant women: Implementation of a "Mentor Mother" advocacy model. *Journal of Community Health Nursing, 14,* 237–249.

Merritt-Gray, M., & Wuest, J. (1995). Counteracting abuse and breaking free: The process of leaving revealed through women's voices. *Health Care for Women International, 16,* 399–412.

Moore, M. L., Zaccaro, D., & Parson, L. H. (1998). Attitudes and practices of registered nurses toward women who have experienced abuse/domestic violence. *Journal of Obstetrics, Gynecological, and Neonatal Nursing, 27,* 175–182.

Moss, V. A., Pitula, C. R., Campbell, J. C., & Halstead, L. (1997). The experience of terminating an abusive relationship from an Anglo and African American perspective: A qualitative descriptive study. *Issues in Mental Health Nursing, 18,* 433–454.

Muelleman, R. L., Lenaghan, P. A., & Pakieser, R. A. (1998). Nonbattering presentations to the ED of women in physically abusive relationships. *American Journal of Emergency Medicine, 16,* 128–131.

Newman, K. D. (1993). Giving up: Shelter experiences of battered women. *Public Health Nursing, 10,* 108–113.

Oliver, W. (1989). Sexual conquest and patterns of Black-on-Black violence: A structural-cultural perspective. *Violence and Victims, 4,* 257–274.

Orem, D. (1995). *Nursing concepts of practice* (5th ed.). New York: McGraw Hill.

Page-Adams, D., & Dersch, S. (1998). Assessing physical and nonphysical abuse against women in a hospital setting. In J. C. Campbell (Ed.), *Empowering survivors of abuse: Health care for battered women and their children* (pp. 204–213). Thousand Oaks, CA: Sage.

Pakieser, R. A., Lenaghan, P. A., & Muelleman, R. L. (1998). Battered women: Where they go for help. *Journal of Emergency Nursing, 24,* 16–19.

Parker, B. (1993). Abuse of adolescents: What can we learn from pregnant teenagers? *AWHONN's Clinical issues in Perinatal and Women's Health Nursing, 4,* 363–370.

Parker, B., & McFarlane, J. (1991) Nursing assessment of the battered pregnant woman. *American Journal of Maternal Child Nursing, 16,* 161–164.

Parker, B., McFarlane, J., & Soeken, K. (1994). Abuse during pregnancy: Effects on maternal complications and birthweight in adult and teenage women. *Obstetrics and Gynecology, 84,* 323–328.

Parker, B., McFarlane, J., Soeken, K., Silva, C., & Reel, S. (1999). Testing an intervention to prevent further abuse to pregnant women. *Research in Nursing and Health, 22,* 59–66.

Parker, B., McFarlane, J., Soeken, K., Torres, S., & Campbell, D. (1993). Physical and emotional abuse in pregnancy: A comparison of adult and teenage women. *Nursing Research, 42,* 173–178.

Plichta, S. B., & Abraham, C. (1996). Violence and gynecologic health in women <50 years old. *American Journal of Obstetrics and Gynecology, 174,* 903–907.

Quillian, J. P. (1996). Screening for spousal or partner abuse in a community health setting. *Journal of the American Academy of Nurse Practitioners, 8,* 155–160.

Ratner, P. A. (1993). The incidence of wife abuse and mental health status in abused wives in Edmonton, Alberta. *Canadian Journal of Public Health, 84,* 246–249.

Ratner, P. A. (1995). Indicators of exposure to wife abuse. *Canadian Journal of Nursing Research, 27,* 31–46.

Renker, P. R. (1999). Physical abuse, social support, self-care, and pregnancy outcomes of older adolescents. *Journal of Obstetrics, Gynecological, and Neonatal Nursing, 28,* 377–388.

Rodriguez, R. (1989). Perception of health needs by battered women. *Response, 12,* 22–23.

Rose, L., Campbell, J., & Kub, J. (2000). The role of social support and family relationships in women's responses to battering. *Health Care for Women International, 21,* 27–39.

Sampselle, C. M., Petersen, B. A., Murtland, T. L., & Oakley, D. J. (1992). Prevalence of abuse among pregnant women choosing certified nurse-midwife or physician providers. *Journal of Nurse-Midwifery, 37,* 269–273.

Silva, C., McFarlane, J., Socken, K., Parker, B., & Reel, S. (1997). Symptoms of post-traumatic stress disorder in abused women in a primary care setting. *Journal of Women's Health, 6,* 543–552.

Smith, S. K. (1997a). Women's experiences of victimizing sexualization, Part I: Responses related to abuse and home and family environment. *Issues in Mental Health Nursing, 18,* 395–416.

Smith, S. K. (1997b). Women's experiences of victimizing sexualization, Part II: Community and longer term personal impacts. *Issues in Mental Health Nursing, 18,* 417–432.

Soeken, K. L., McFarlane, J., Parker, B., & Lominack, M. C. (1998). The Abuse Assessment Screen: A clinical instrument to measure frequency, severity, and perpetrator of abuse against women. In J. C. Campbell (Ed.), *Empowering survivors of abuse: Health care for battered women and their children* (pp. 195–203). Thousand Oaks, CA: Sage.

Stevens, P. E., & Richards, D. J. (1998). Narrative case analysis of HIV infection in a battered woman. *Health Care for Women International, 19,* 9–22.

Taggart, L., & Mattson, S. (1996). Delay in prenatal care as a result of battering in pregnancy: Cross-cultural implications. *Health Care for Women International, 17,* 25–34.

Tilden, V. P., Schmidt, T. A., Linardi, B., Chioda, G. T., Garland, M. J., & Loveless, P. A. (1994). Factors that influence clinician's assessment and management of family violence. *American Journal of Public Health, 84,* 628–633.

Torres, S. (1991). A comparison of wife abuse between two cultures: Perceptions, attitudes, nature, and extent. *Issues in Mental Health Nursing, 12,* 113–131.

Torres, S., Campbell, J. C., Ryan, J., King, C., Campbell, D., Stallings, R., & Fuchs, S. (in press). Abuse during pregnancy: An ethnic group comparison. *Violence and Victims.*

Ulrich, Y. (1991). Women's reasons for leaving abusive spouses. *Health Care Women International, 12,* 465–473.

306   WOMEN'S HEALTH AND ILLNESS ISSUES

Varvaro, F. F., & Lasko, D. L. (1993). Physical abuse as cause of injury in women: Information for orthopaedic nurses. *Orthopaedic Nursing, 12*, 37–41.

Walker, L. E. (1979). *The battered woman.* New York: Harper & Row.

Wang, J. F., & McKinney, J. (1997). Battered women's perceptions of loss and health. *Holistic Nursing Practice, 11*, 50–59.

Weingourt, R. (1990). Wife rape in a sample of psychiatric patients. *Image: The Journal of Nursing Scholarship, 22*, 144–147.

Wessel, l., & Campbell, J. C. (1997). Providing sanctuary for battered women: Nicaragua's casas de la mujer. *Issues in Mental Health Nursing, 18*, 455–476.

Wingood, G. M., & DiClemente, R. J. (1997). The effects of an abusive primary partner on the condom use and sexual negotiation practices of African-American women. *American Journal of Public Health, 8*, 1016–1018.

Woodtli, M. A., & Breslin, E. (1996). Violence-related content in the nursing curriculum: a national study. *Journal of Nursing Education, 35*, 367–374.

Wuest, J., & Merritt-Gray, M. (1999). Not going back: Sustaining the separation in the process of leaving abusive relationships. *Violence Against Women, 5,* 110–133.

Yam, M. (1995). Wife abuse: Strategies for a therapeutic response. *Scholarly Inquiry for Nursing Practice, 9,* 147–158.

Chapter 11

Health Decisions and Decision Support for Women

MARILYN L. ROTHERT AND ANNETTE M. O'CONNOR

ABSTRACT

Women are more likely to live longer with chronic illness and have a long-term relationship with their health care provider; this requires a situation in which patients and providers have a role in managing illness. In this chapter, the authors provide a conceptual overview of decision making along with key issues: historical concepts related to patients and providers, consumerism, informed choice/consent, patient rights, shared decision making, patient involvement, as well as an overview of models of patient/provider partnerships. This review builds on the work of O'Connor et al. (1999), which resulted in a Cochrane review of decision aids and focuses the examination of patient decision aids that support women's decisions regarding health treatment or screening. The authors conclude with a look to the future and recommendations for research in the area of shared decision making and health care decision aids.

Key words: clinical decision aids, health care decision making, patient decision support, patient–provider partnership models, shared decision making

Consumers are taking increasing responsibility in managing their health care, requiring them to assume expanded roles in health care decision making. Consumers will continue to play an influential role in the health care industry, and the explosion of information available on the Internet is expected to give them more influence on how care is delivered (Herzlinger, 1999).

307

As information expands, health care, decisions become more complex and difficult. The expansion of treatment and diagnostic options has created more choices. Greater choice has increased the complexity of the decisions and the uncertainty related to outcomes. In many situations, there are no obvious best treatments. Individuals value outcomes differently, and the options available may have both positive and negative outcomes. Further, the studies providing data to support the decision may provide conflicting data adding to the uncertainty.

While availability of information is necessary for optimal decision making, the magnitude and conflicting nature of information can become an additional source of confusion. Historically, there has been a stronger emphasis on the creation and dissemination of knowledge than on strategies to appropriately use knowledge to inform decisions. This is consistent with a national survey on consumers' health care knowledge and satisfaction that reports that patients' satisfaction with their health care depends more on how well informed they are about their diagnosis, treatment, and follow-up than on length of their hospital stay. Patients reporting a good understanding of their diagnosis and follow up treatment gave higher ratings on satisfaction with their care (1999 Survey on Consumer Health Care Knowledge and Satisfaction, 1999).

With recognition of the gap in medical knowledge concerning women's health, major studies are now producing considerable data focused on women's health state, management, and treatment. At the same time, journals, books, internet sites, and lay publications have emerged on women's health. Women are increasingly coming to the health care system with information and expectations of being active consumers in a shared decision making process.

In recent years, various strategies have been identified to support patients and providers with knowledge and skills needed to make the best decisions. This chapter will examine patient decision aids to support women's decisions regarding health treatment or screening. This chapter will build on the work of O'Connor et al. (1999), which resulted in a Cochrane review of decision aids.

SHARED DECISION MAKING

The underlying concepts of shared decision making have been a major focus of concern in the last a decade. Initially, key issues included whether patients could become adequately informed, whether patients wanted to become involved in the decision, and whether providers wanted patients to become more involved in health care decision making (Rothert, 1991). More recently, the rise in consumerism, informed choice, and informed consent have led to changes in the model of provider–patient relationship. The shift from acute care to chronic care with patients in a long-term state of illness has also been a factor. Such patients do not experience sickness on a temporary basis, but illness may become a permanent part of their life leading to a long-term relationship with their provider and fostering a situation where patients and providers have a role in managing the illness (Charles, Gafni, & Whelan, 1997). These factors enhance the concept of patient rights and imply at least a minimum of shared decision making in the form of consent to treatment (Sutherland et al., 1989).

The concept of shared decision making has been used with a variety of meanings in the literature, at times equating sharing information with sharing decisions. Frequently, the concepts of persuasion and shared decision making have been used interchangeably to describe patient involvement. Persuasion includes sharing of information but does not include a range of possible courses of action or outcomes (Rothert, 1991). More recently, three models of provider/patient partnerships have been identified as one way of categorizing varying models. The paternalistic model has been the traditional model of patient acquiescing to professional authority and agreeing to the prescribed treatment. In the informed model, the provider communicates all relevant treatment options, benefits, and risks, providing information adequate for the patient to make an informed decision. In the third model of shared decision making, both provider and patient reveal treatment preferences and agree on the decision to be implemented (Charles, Whelan, & Gafni, 1999).

Characteristics of shared decision-making have been identified as: (1) involving at least two participants— the provider and patient; (2) both parties participating in the process of decision making; (3) information sharing as a prerequisite to shared decision making; and (4) both parties agreeing to the decision (Charles et al., 1997). It is essential that both the consumer and professional share responsibility for health care decisions. While providers have the scientific knowledge, experience, and awareness of the clinical course of a particular health state, patients have the information regarding their response to illness, life experiences, preferences, and values. Thus, both bring essential information necessary to make the best decision for an individual. The sharing of information in the process of making decisions requires sharing the uncertainties about outcomes and exposes the fact that data are often not available or not known. This can be a source of anxiety to the patient and of concern to the provider (Elwyn, Edwards, Gwyn, & Grol, 1999). Understanding the probabilistic nature of data, however, is necessary for the patient to understand that there are no "clear" answers. Moreover, the varying benefit/risk profiles also indicate that values play an important role in identifying the right individual decision.

Many providers are untrained in methods of sharing decision making with patients (Elwyn et al., 1999). The challenge is to create an environment in which the patient feels comfortable to provide candid contributions to the exchange of information and both agree on the decision to implement. In today's health care climate, both time and funding can act as a disincentive for practitioners to explore patients' preferences regarding partnership with clinicians to make the decision (Charles et al., 1999). Carefully constructed interventions can provide patients with information and a way of thinking about treatment decision making to support this process (Charles et al., 1997).

DECISION AIDS

A variety of terms is used to describe products and interventions designed to support patients in making wise health care decisions. Decision support is a broad term used to describe a variety of interventions or strategies to enhance the patient's ability to make wise choices. Decision supports have emerged in a variety of forms and frameworks, many times moving from development to implementation without strong evaluation and research.

The term "Decision Aid" is commonly used to describe materials based on a decision, analytic framework, or decision tree. Structuring a decision tree over time requires identification of the choice over time, identification of the outcomes affected by the choice, identification of the probabilities of outcomes occurring if each decision path is followed, and considering values or utilities for each outcome. For those who use the full decision analytic model, the probability of each outcome is multiplied by the value or utility weight to arrive at the option that maximizes a person's expected value or utility.

Decision aids rarely follow the formal decision, analytic process of combining utilities and probabilities to identify a "correct" path. Instead, they frequently display the elements of the decision and explain the consequences of choosing each option on the outcomes (e.g., mortality and morbidity). In the clinical setting, decision aids are used as a supplement to counseling to assist the patient in treatment decisions. As contrasted with general patient information materials, decision aids are specific to the decision. The elements in decision aids include identification of patient choices, risks and benefits of each option, and identification of values or importance placed on each outcome (O'Connor et al., 1998a). The decision aid is often tailored to an individual's personal risk profile, the information is provided in understandable format, and data are provided in comparable terms. The goal is to assist patients to clarify their values, understand the trade-offs, and hold realistic expectations regarding the likelihood of outcomes. The probabilities used in decision aids are derived from empirical data when available or pooled estimates of outcomes with and without treatment. Personal values for outcomes may be obtained either implicitly or explicitly.

The framework, content, and components of decision aids may vary by the clinical problem, and the explicitness of the framework may vary by study. Examples of common components can be found in two studies of the hormone replacement therapy decision. Rothert et al. (1997) and O'Connor (1998a) developed and evaluated decision aids to assist women to understand the options and outcomes related to the decisions around hormone replacement therapy, to identify personal values, and to incorporate them into the decision. Although the modes differed across the studies, key elements in common included: (a) identification of information consumers want to know; (b) the concept of probability so risks can be understood; (c) population risks and benefits presented in comparable terms so trade-offs between options can be compared; (d) steps for identifying personal risks and benefits; (e) clarifying a woman's personal values related to perceived importance of the risks and benefits; (f) combining risk information and values; (g) identification of preference for participation in decision making; and (h) identification of current health practices in promoting health. The interventions were tested for reading level and content validity.

Evaluation of Decision Aids

Evaluation of decision aids is an important and difficult issue. Frequently the options presented in health care decisions include tradeoffs of positive and negative outcomes. Therefore, there is no "right" or "wrong" decision, and the patient's values become a critical part of the analysis. O'Connor (1995) has defined an effective decision as one that is informed, consistent with personal values, and acted upon. It is important to distinguish between good decisions and good outcomes (O'Connor et al., 1998b). Good decisions can produce both good and bad outcomes due to the probabilistic nature of clinical outcomes. The usefulness of decision aids is to assist the patient to receive clear information on the options and tradeoffs, understand the probabilities, consider personal values, and make a decision designed to give the best chance to achieve the outcome of choice. The process of decision making should be judged separate from the outcome of decisions.

Studies have used a variety of outcome measures in evaluating decision aids. Prominent among outcome measures are knowledge, expectations, decisional conflict, and/or satisfaction with decision. The *knowledge* measures identify the degree to which patients have the essential information with which to make informed decisions. Knowledge measures are usually designed to reflect the content addressed in the specific intervention, including options, risks, and benefits. Expectations elicit a person's perception of the likelihood of outcomes with and without an option. They are usually classified as realistic or unrealistic using the evidence of outcomes associated with a person's clinical risk status. *Decisional conflict* is used as a measure to identify level of uncertainty. A commonly used decisional conflict scale assesses: (1) uncertainty about choosing among alternatives; (2) modifiable factors contributing to uncertainty as being uninformed, unclear about values, and unsupported; and (3) perceived effective decision making (O'Connor, 1995). *Satisfaction* measures are also frequently used. These measures may focus on satisfaction with the decision, satisfaction with the decision making process, and/or satisfaction with the provider (Rothert et al., 1997; Holmes-Rovner et al., 1995).

There are many other measures that have been used to evaluate decision aids, including impact on the patient's decision. This measure may be used when the decision aid is compared to usual care. The impact of the decision aid depends on the situation. As the patient becomes informed, understands the options, and clarifies personal values, the decision may more likely reflect the patient's preferences. For example, rates of use may increase if under-utilization of interventions is due to uninformed practitioners and patients. The impact of the decision aid also depends on the inclination of the patient at baseline. If the patient is undecided, the decision aid will make more impact than if the patient initially has a stated preference (O'Connor et al., 1999).

Literature Search

The search strategy as described in O'Connor (1998a) reviewed electronic databases, personal files, and contents lists of targeted journals between varying periods of 1966 and March/April 1998. Specifically, randomized controlled trials comparing decision aids to controls or alternative interventions were identified from searches of published literature from MEDLINE (1966–April 1998); PsychINFO (1974–March, 1998); CINAHL (1983–February 1998); Aidsline (1980–April 1998); CancerLit (1983–April 1998); and EMBASE (1974–March 1998). The Cochrane Database of Systematic Reviews was also searched as well as contents lists of Health Expectations (1998), Medical Decision Making (January–March 1986—January–March 1998), and Patient Education and Counseling (January 1995–February 1998). Decision aids or decision supports were defined as interventions designed to assist individuals to make choices among screening or treatment options. They included information on the disease or condition, options, and outcomes. Studies of hypothetical choices, decisions regarding lifestyle changes, entry to a clinical trial, general advance directives, educational programs for unspecified decisions, and interventions designed to promote compliance or elicit informed consent were excluded. A systematic process was used to complete the Cochrane review to extract data and analyze the pooled results.

Since the original Cochrane review, screening for studies of the MEDLINE data base has been updated to December 1999 and updates of others are in progress. To date, the search has identified over 10,600 unique citations with 500 focused on patient decision making and 20 meeting the inclusion criteria. Of these 20, 11 studies included women subjects. These studies are the source of data for analysis described in this chapter. *Table 11.1 summarizes the 11 studies that met the criteria and included women participants.* The rigorous literature search and screening process used by O'Connor and colleagues was considered a strong base to examine decision aids for women. Much of the literature related to patient decision support and decision aids lacks scientific design and methodology, presenting descriptive data, opinion, and theoretical constructs. To move the field into a useful tool for evidence based practice, sound data based on randomized trials are essential.

Decision Supports for Women

Among the 11 citations that included women in a clinical trial of decision supports meeting the Cochrane criteria, six involved a treatment decision, four focused on a diagnostic procedure, and one described a preventive strategy. The 11 studies included seven unique decisions, with two studies of menopause and hormone replacement therapy, two studies of ischemic heart disease, two studies of prenatal screening, two studies of breast cancer testing or treatment, and one study each on dentofacial surgery, antithrombotic therapy for atrial fibrillation, and hepatitis vaccine. None of the studies addressed unique needs or characteristics of women decision makers. Among the topics, six of the studies involved totally female populations. Of the five studies with both male and female participants, one had a 2:1 ratio of females to males consistent with the population seeking dentofacial surgery (Phillips, Hill, & Cannac, 1995). Three studies addressed decisions related to heart disease (Morgan, 1997; Bernstein et al., 1998, ManSon-Hing et al., 1999) with only 13%, 21%, and 24% women participants respectively. Demographic data were not provided for one study (Clancy, Cewbul, & Williams, 1998)

Three of the studies focused on women with an average age less than 40 (Michie, Smith, McClennan, & Marteau, 1997; Phillips et al., 1995; Thornton, Hewison, Lilford, & Vail, 1995). Six involved women 40 to 80 (Bernstein et al., 1998; Man-Son-Hing et al., 1999; Morgan, 1997; O'Connor et al., 1998a;

TABLE 11.1   Characteristics of Included Studies

Study	Decision	Comparison intervention #1	Comparison intervention #2	Comparison intervention #3	N	Media
O'Connor '98 Canada	hormone therapy	($n = 84$) options & outcomes-pamphlet			81	Audio-guided workbook
Rothert '97 USA	perimeno-pausal health	($n = 89$) options & outcomes pamphlet	($n = 80$) group lecture/discussion		83	group lecture, hand-outs, personal decision exercise
Morgan '97 Canada	ischemic heart disease	($n = 94$) usual care			86	interactive videodisc + brochure
Bernstein '98 USA	ischemic heart disease	($n = 48$) usual care			61	video
Thornton '95 UK	prenatal screen	($n = 567$) usual care & pamphlet	($N = 563$) class—information + pamphlet		561	individual counseling, pamphlet
Michie '97 UK	prenatal screen	($n = 88$) pamphlet	($N = 93$) pamphlet + decision tree	($N = 76$) pamphlet + video	67	pamphlet, video, decision tree
Street '95 USA	breast cancer surgery	($n = 30$) pamphlet			30	interactive multimedia
Lerman '97 USA	BRCAI gene testing	($n = 164$) waiting list control	($N = 114$) personal education		122	personal education + counseling
Phillips '95 USA	dental surgery	($n = 37$) usual care			37	video imaging facial reconstruction
Clancy '88 USA	Hepatitis B vaccine	($n = 263$) usual care	($n = 264$) mailed handout		753	handout + risks, values, + offer of feedback on personal decision analysis
Man-Son-Hing '99 Canada	Atrial fibrillation	($N = 148$) usual care			139	Audioguided workbook

TABLE 11.1 *(continued)*

			Intensive decision aid intervention			
Options outcomes	Clinical problem	Outcome probability	Others' opinion experiences	Values clarification	Patient role	Guidance coaching
✓	✓	✓ personal	✓	✓	✓	
✓	✓	✓ personal	✓ likely with group discussion	✓	✓	✓
✓	✓	✓ personal	✓			
✓	✓	✓	✓			
✓	✓	✓ age specific				✓
✓	✓	✓		✓		✓
✓	✓	✓	✓		✓	✓
✓	✓	✓ personal		✓		✓
✓	✓					✓
✓	✓	✓ personal		✓		✓
✓	✓	✓	✓	✓	✓	✓

Rothert et al., 1997; Street, Voigt, Geyer, Manning, & Swanson, 1995). One had a broad distribution across the age span of 18 to 75 (Lerman et al., 1997). One study (Clancy et al., 1988) did not provide population demographics.

The studies were all randomized, controlled trials comparing an intensive decision aid intervention with at least one comparison intervention. The unit of randomization varied and included the patient, practitioner, or site. As seen in Table 11.1, the mode of delivery varied across the studies. Comparison of various modes was a common research question with a goal of identifying the most cost effective strategy. The media varied from personal education and counseling to interactive multimedia, audio-guided workbook, group lecture, handouts and exercises, video, and videodisc. Five of the intensive interventions were self-driven strategies with media that could be used independently by patients. This is an important consideration in the current environment of cost containment in health care.

Components of the Decision Aid

All of the intensive decision aid interventions presented information related to the clinical problem and possible outcomes, and all but Phillips et al. (1995) identified the probabilities related to the outcomes. The topic of dental surgery with video imaging of facial reconstruction may account for the absence of outcome probabilities. Of the 10 decision aids with outcome probabilities, six provided women with information based on their personal risk profile and one presented age specific data.

A variety of strategies were used to enable patients to become engaged in the decision, to relate the information to their own situation, and to identify their own preferences and values. One strategy presented personal experiences with various treatment options, giving the women knowledge of the personal experiences of other women in a similar situation as well as the counsel of other providers. The relevance of this strategy may vary by topic. As Table 11.1 identifies, decision aids on menopause, heart disease, and breast cancer surgery included this strategy. The underlying assumption is that women value other women's opinions. Strategies including written mode, group discussion, and media have been used to convey how women with similar conditions have dealt with the situation and the outcomes resulting from their decisions. The use of examples, however, can be argued to bias the decision maker toward one answer rather than remain neutral (O'Connor et al., 1999).

Six of the studies included a values clarification component, giving women exercises and strategies to identify the values or preferences for the options presented. This is a necessary component for the strategies using decision trees.

Women's Participation in Decision Making

Shared decision making requires active participation by the patient. Four of the interventions focused specifically on issues to inform and empower women to participate in decision making and take an active role in communicating with their health care provider. One intervention (Street et al., 1995) was specifically designed to increase women's involvement in choosing treatment for early breast cancer in a comparison study of a brochure and an interactive multimedia program. Findings indicated the method of education did not affect patient involvement. Women younger that 65 years of age who had attended college asked more questions and had more active communication than did less educated or older patients. *In addition to age and education, patient perception of provider facilitation of patient involvement was positively associ ated with patient participation.* In another study comparing decision aids to usual care (Morgan 1997), there was a non-significant trend toward greater active participation in decision making *in the experimental group.*

A study with an intervention to empower and support women to interact positively with their health care provider found that women indicated a positive level of satisfaction with their health care provider postintervention. Health care self-efficacy increased from pre- to postintervention and remained higher than baseline (Rothert et al., 1997). Further, self-efficacy significantly predicted intention to participate in the next health care encounter (Kroll et al., 2000).

Outcome Comparisons

Common measures used to compare interventions are knowledge, expectations, decisional conflict, and satisfaction with the decision, the provider, or the decision making process (Table 11.2). Knowledge was the most common measure found in eight of the 11 studies. Expectations were more realistic in the decision aid groups compared to comparison interventions in two of the studies. In the four studies comparing decision aids to usual care, there was a significant difference in knowledge between the decision aid and comparison intervention. *The other four studies comparing simpler educational strategies to decision aids found significant improvements in knowledge after using either intervention, but no apparent advantage of decision aids over simpler*

TABLE 11.2 Measures Across Studies

Study	Decision	Comparison interventions	Knowledge	Expectations	Decisional conflict	Anxiety	Satisfaction
O'Connor '98 Canada	hormone therapy	less intensive intervention	NS	$p < .001$	$p < .05$		w/hlth care prov. (NS); w/dec (NS)
Rothert '97 USA	perimenopausal health	less intensive intervention	NS		$p < .05$ early NS 6 months later		w/dec mkg process (NS); w/dec (NS); w/Rx (NS)
Morgan '97 Canada	ischemic heart disease	usual care	$p < .005$		$p < .05$ informed subscale only		
Bernstein '98 USA	ischemic heart disease	usual care	$p < .0001$				Satis w/decision (NS) & decision process (NS)
Thornton '95 UK	prenatal screen	usual care				NS	Satisfaction with decision (NS)
Michie '97 UK	prenatal screen	less intensive intervention	NS			NS	w/dec (NS)
Street '95 USA	breast cancer surgery	less intensive intervention	NS				
Lerman '97 USA	BRCAI gene testing	usual care	$p < .001$				
Phillips '95 USA	dental surgery	usual care					
Clancy '88 USA	Hepatitis B vaccine	usual care					
Man-Son-Hing '99 Canada	atrial fibrillation	usual care	$p < .05$	$p < .001$	$p < .05$ informed subscale only		w/decision process (NS)

methods. The decision aids, however, were superior to simpler methods in reducing decisional conflict particularly the "informed" subscale. Post-intervention decisional conflict was significantly better for those exposed to decision aids relative to comparison interventions in four studies, with the most consistent improvement in the "feeling informed" subscale. The one study examining the long-term effects of interventions on decisional conflict found the advantage disappeared at six months. *When decision aids were compared to simpler methods found in usual care, there was no comparative advantage of decision aids in improving satisfaction with the decision, with the decision making process, or with the health care provider.*

OBSERVATIONS AND RECOMMENDATIONS FOR FUTURE RESEARCH

We initially discussed the rising activation of consumers and importance of having more informed participation in the decision making process. This premise underlies the development of decision aids. Given the identified need for well-designed studies of decision supports, this chapter chose to build a review from randomized controlled studies of decision aids selected from an extensive systematic Cochrane review. This is the most rigorous literature available and was chosen without bias for topic or focus.

The studies are consistent in showing that decision aids do a better job than usual care in improving patients' knowledge regarding options and outcomes, however, knowledge gains are comparable when simpler education methods are compared to detailed decision aids, presumably because of the overlap in information. In areas where decision aids do not have overlapping information (e.g., probabilities of outcomes), there is a clear advantage of decision aids in creating realistic (evidence-based) personal expectations. The effect of decision aids on decisional conflict is more apparent in the early, post-intervention phases and in the 'feeling informed' dimensions. Decision aids appear to have no clear advantage over usual care and other interventions in improving satisfaction with decisions or decision making. The few studies examining impact on anxiety show no deleterious effects, *but no extra benefits either.*

It should be noted that of the 20 studies, nine dealt with topics unique to men and one to parents of children. Of the remaining 11 studies involving women, six dealt with women only, one did not describe demographics, one had a 2:1 ratio of women to men, and the other three had only a small proportion of women. Thus, data on differences between men and women on the same measures and within the same study were not available.

Few studies in the literature have examined why and how men and women make treatment decisions. Therefore, data do not exist to identify key characteristics to support women in the decision making process. With the recognition given women's studies, gender variance in treatment response, care seeking behavior, and morbidity and mortality among women, it is of concern that gender differences are not yet a factor in this important research. The one study that acknowledged the preponderance of men as a limitation of the study (Morgan, 1997) indicated that the small number of women was a natural occurrence because women in the target population did not undergo coronary angiography at the same rate as men. Other reasons that studies have not included women at a rate similar to the general population may include: (1) lack of forethought in planning the study to be appropriate and attractive to women and men; (2) lack of interest among women in the participant pool; and (3) recruitment/marketing strategies not appealing to women.

It is not unreasonable to expect gender differences to occur in the decision making process. Gender differences have been documented in utilization of health services (Dempsey, Dracup, & Moser, 1995; Giles, Anda, Casper, Escobedo, & Taylor, 1995; Haas, 1998) and approaches to health care decisions (Dempsey et al., 1995; Young, 1996). In two separate studies, it appears that a shared approach to medical decision making as opposed to a provider-centered approach may be preferred by women who are younger and better educated (Blanchard, Labrecque, Ruckdeschel, & Blancahard, 1988; Degner & Russell, 1988). Although knowledge is the foundation of decision aids, differences in knowledge are not expected to explain gender differences in those using decision aids. No differences were observed in knowledge of those exposed to decision aids in two studies (Engler-Todd, Drake, O'Connor, & Hunter, 1997; Man-Son-Hing et al., 1999). However, Man-Son-Hing did show that being female was an independent predictor of having higher decisional conflict. Moreover, one small study involving 10 men and 10 women with end-stage COPD showed that decisions following a decision aid were significantly different, with all women choosing palliative care and 6 out of 10 men choosing intensive care (Dales et al., 1999).

In spite of the paucity of research, there can be little doubt of the need for gender-related research on health care decision making. In a review of studies exploring lifestyle change in women with coronary heart disease, the lack of data and inconsistent findings were noted in the course, outcomes, and management of CHD among women (Toobert, Strycker, & Glasgow, 1998). An overview of decision making for hysterectomy, oophorectomy, and HRT noted the paucity of data about how women make decisions to seek treatment, who advises women, and the practical aspects of how to deliver information appropriately to assist women in processing the information, weighing benefits and risks, and becoming empowered to interact effectively with the health care systems (Lewis, Groff, Herman, McKeown, & Wilcox, 2000). Gender differences also relate to the providers. In a review of why provider gender matters in shaping the provider-patient relationship, it was noted that different communication patterns exist among providers of different genders. Female providers show greater affinity for collaborative models of patient-provider relationship than their male colleagues, spend more time with the patients, and are more likely to discuss social and psychological issues and deal with emotions (Roter & Hall, 1998). With recognition of the importance of women's values and the interaction between provider and patient in the decision making process, the lack of knowledge regarding the role of gender appears to be significant.

Based on the review of the 11 studies cited, the following areas of future research are suggested:

1. Decision aids should be evaluated in clinical trials with a pool of subjects sufficient for analysis by gender.
2. Studies should focus on contrast with usual care using cost-effective strategies women can use independently, followed by counseling.
3. Key issues in women's health including the leading causes of mortality should be considered for future research with decision aids.
4. Longitudinal studies should assess impact of decision aids on decisions made and long-term adherence behavior.
5. The relation of patient/provider communication, patient participation in the decision making process, and adherence to preferred therapies should be studied.
6. Variables contributing to patient satisfaction with the decision and decisional conflict should be identified across contexts.
7. Decision aids should study the decision making model used by women, including identification of the variables influencing their decision making process.
8. Studies should be done to identify which health care decisions are successfully impacted by decision aids.

In summary, the few studies evaluating decision aids for women show that they improve knowledge, expectations, and some aspects of decisional conflict without increasing anxiety. Simpler methods are just as effective as more complex ones in improving knowledge and satisfaction. Research on women's decision making is understudied, and fruitful areas of inquiry have been identified.

REFERENCES

Bernstein, S. J., Skarupski, K. A., Grayson, C. E., Starling, M. R., Bates, E. R., & Eagle, K. A. (1998). A randomized controlled trial of information-giving to patients referred for coronary angiography: Effects on outcomes of care. *Health Expectations, 1*, 50–61.

Blanchard, C. G., Labrecque, M. S., Ruckdeschel, J. C., & Blanchard, E. B. (1988). Information and decision-making preferences of hospitalized adult cancer patients. *Social Science & Medicine, 27*, 1139–1145.

Charles, C., Gafni, A., & Whelan, T. (1997). Shared decision-making in the medical encounter: What does it mean? (Or it takes at least two to tango). *Social Science & Medicine, 44*, 681–692.

Charles, C., Whelan, T., & Gafini, A. (1999). What do we mean by partnership in making decisions about treatment? *British Medical Journal, 319*, 780–782.

Clancy, C. M., Cewbul, R. D., & Williams, S. V. (1998). Guiding individual decisions: A randomized controlled trial of decision analysis. *American Journal of Medicine, 84*, 283–288.

Dales, R. E., O'Connor, A., Hebert, P., Sullivan, K., McKin, D., & LlewellynThomas, H. (1999). Intubation and mechanical ventilation for COPD: Development of an instrument to elicit patient preferences. *Chest, 116*, 792–800.

Degner, L. F., & Russell, C. (1988). Preferences for treatment control among adults with cancer. *Research in Nursing and Health, 11*, 367–374.

Dempsey, S. J., Dracup, K., & Moser, D. K. (1995). Women's decision to seek care for symptoms of acute myocardial infarction. *Heart & Lung, 24*, 444–456.

Elwyn, G., Edwards, A., Gwyn, R., & Grol, R. (1999). Towards a feasible model for shared decision making: Focus group study with general practice registrars. *British Medical Journal, 319*, 753–756.

Engler-Todd, L., Drake, E., O'Connor, A., & Hunter, A. (in press). Evaluation of a decision aid for prenatal testing for women of advanced maternal age. *Journal of Genetic Counseling*.

Giles, W. H., Anda, R. F., Casper, M. L., Escobedo, L. G., & Taylor, H. A. (1995). Race and sex differences in rates of invasive cardiac procedures in U.S. hospitals: Data from the National Hospital Discharge Survey. *Archives of Internal Medicine, 155*, 318–324.

Haas, J. (1998). The cost of being a woman. *New England Journal of Medicine, 338*, 1694–1695.

Herzlinger, R. A. (1999, September 17). Consumers: Wield more power in health care market. *American Health Line* [On-line serial]. Available: www.national journal.com

Holmes-Rovner, M., Kroll, J., Rothert, M., Schmitt, N., Breer, L., Padonu, G., Talarczyk, G., & Rovner, D. (1995). Patient satisfaction with health care decisions: The satisfaction with decision scale. *Medical Decision Making, 16*(1), 58–64.

Kroll, J., Rothert, M., Davidson, II, W., Schmitt, N., Holmes-Rovner, M., Padonu, G., & Reischl, T. M. (2000). Predictors of participation in health care at menopause. *Health Communication, 12*, 339–360.

Laupacis, A., Hing, M., O'Connor, A., Biggs, J., Hart, R., & the Stroke Prevention in Atrial Fibrillation III (SPAF 3) Investigators. (1998). A randomized trial of an audiobooklet (AB) decision aid in patients with atrial fibrillation (AF). *Proceedings of the 14th Annual Meeting of the International Society for Technology Assessment in Health Care (ISTAHC), Ottawa, Ontario, Canada.* 41.

Lerman, C., Biesecker, B., Benkendorf, J. L., Kerner, J., Gomez-Caminero, A., Hughes, C., & Reed, M. M. (1997). Controlled trial of pretest education approaches to enhance informed decision-making for BRCA1 gene testing. *Journal of the National Cancer Institute, 89,* 148–157.

Lewis, C. E., Groff, J. Y., Herman, C. J., McKeown, R. E., & Wilcox, L.S. (2000). Overview of women's decision making regarding elective hysterectomy, oophorectomy, and hormone replacement therapy. *Journal of Women's Health and Gender-Based Medicine, 9*(Suppl. 2), S5–S13.

Man-Son-Hing, M., Laupacis, A., O'Connor, A., Biggs, J., Drake, E., Yetisir, E., Hart, R., & SPAF# Investigators (1999). A randomized trial of a decision aid for patients with atrial fibrillation. *Journal of the American Medical Association, 282,* 737–743.

Michie, S., Smith, D., McClennan, A., & Marteau, T. M. (1997). Patient decision making: An evaluation of two different methods of presenting information about a screening test. *British Journal of Health Psychology, 2,* 317–326.

Morgan, M. W. (1997). *A randomized trial of the ischemic heart disease shared decision making program: An evaluation of a decision aid.* Unpublished master's thesis, University of Toronto, Toronto, Canada.

The 1999 Survey on Consumer Health Care Knowledge and Satisfaction. (1999). Special supplement: Preparing consumers for the new world of health care. The state of health care in America. *Business & Health,* 4–7.

O'Connor, A. M. (1995). Validation of a decisional conflict scale. *Medical Decision Making, 15,* 25–30.

O'Connor, A. M., Fiset, V., Degrasse, C., Graham, I. D., Evans, W., Stacey, D., & Laupacis, A. (1999). Decision aids for patients considering options affecting cancer outcomes: Evidence of efficacy and policy implications. *Journal of the National Cancer Institute Monograph, 25,* 67–80.

O'Connor, A. M., Rostom, A., Fiset, V., Tetroe, J., Entwistle, V., Llewellyn-Thomas, H., Holmes-Rovner, M., Barry, M., & Jones, J. (1999) Decision aids for patients facing health treatment or screening decisions: Systematic review. *British Medical Journal, 319,* 731.

O'Connor, A. M., Tugwell, P., Wells, G. A., Elmslie, T., Jolly, E., Hollingworth, G., McPherson, R., Bunn, H., Graham, I., & Drake, E. (1998a). A decision aid for women considering hormone therapy after menopause: Decision support framework and evaluation. *Patient Education and Counseling, 33,* 267–279.

O'Connor, A. M., Tugwell, P., Wells, G. A., Ehnslie, T., Jolly, E., Hollingworth, G., McPherson, R., Drake, E., Hopman, W., & Mackenzie, T. (1998b). Randomized trial of a portable, self-administered decision aid for postmenopausal women considering long-term preventive hormone therapy. *Medical Decision Making, 18,* 295–303.

Phillips, C., Hill, B. J., & Cannac, C. (1995). The influence of video imaging on patients' perceptions and expectations. *Angle Orthodontist, 65*, 263–270.

Roter, D. L., & Hall, J. A. (1998). Why physician gender matters in shaping the physician-patient relationship. *Journal of Women's Health, 7*, 1093–1097.

Rothert, M. L. (1991). Perspectives and issues in studying patients' decision making. In M. L. Grady (Ed.), *Primary care research: Theory and methods.* (AHCPR Pub. No. 91-0011). Rockville, MD: Agency for Health Care Policy and Research.

Rothert, M. L., Holmes-Rovner, M., Rovner, D., Kroll, J., Breer, L., Talarczyk, G., Schmitt, N., Padonu, G., & Wills, C. (1997). An educational intervention as decision support for menopausal women. *Research in Nursing & Health, 20*, 377–387.

Street, R. L. J., Voigt, B., Geyer, C. J., Manning, T., & Swanson, G. E. (1995). Increasing patient involvement in choosing treatment for early breast cancer. *Cancer, 76*, 2275–2285.

Sutherland, H. J., Llewellyn-Thomas, H. A., Lockwood, G A., Tritchler, D. L, & Till, J. E. (1989). Cancer patients: Their desire for information and participation in treatment decisions. *Journal of the Royal Society of Medicine, 82*, 260–263.

Thornton, J. G., Hewison, J., Lilford, R. J., & Vail, A. (1995). A randomized trial of three methods of giving information about prenatal testing. *British Medical Journal, 311*, 1127–30.

Toobert, D. J., Strycker, L. A., & Glasgow, R. E. (1998). Lifestyle change in women with coronary heart disease: What do we know. *Journal of Women's Health, 7*, 685–699.

Young, R. (1996). The household context for women's health care decisions: Impacts of U.K. policy changes. *Social Science & Medicine, 42*, 949–963.

Chapter 12

Female Troubles: An Analysis of Menstrual Cycle Research in the NINR Portfolio As a Model for Science Development in Women's Health

NANCY KING REAME

ABSTRACT

The National Institute for Nursing Research (NINR) has been active in developing a research portfolio of investigator-initiated studies in addressing the cause and consequences of menstrual cycle and menopause-related health problems. This chapter provides an overview of the nature and level of research activity funded by NINR since its inception in 1986, major findings generated by the most successful award recipients, the impact on the broader field of women's reproductive health and directions for future research. Presented here is an analysis of research designs and methodologies framed within the context of 4 stages of scientific development in the field: exploratory, descriptive studies in well women; illness as a biobehavioral phenomenon; knowledge generation in understudied populations; and the development and testing of clinical therapeutics for symptom management and health promotion strategies. Nursing science contributions to the NINR portfolio of women's health research has been focused primarily on the definition and management of the symptoms of premenstrual syndrome and menopause. The increasing numbers of intervention studies suggests a coming-of-age in nursing science with respect to the development of evidence-based outcome data for the management of menstrual cycle and menopause-related symptoms. Clearly, the range and diversity of NINR grant-funded activity suggest that menstrual cycle research is a strong area of interest in nursing science.

Key words: menopause, menstrual cycle, menstruation, perimenopause, premenopause, premenstrual syndrome

In response to a number of congressional mandates over the last decade to enhance understanding of women's health and disease, the National Institute of Health (NIH) has been actively supportive of research addressing the cause and consequences of menstrual cycle and menopause-related health problems. Although one of the smallest and newest NIH institutes, the National Institute for Nursing Research (NINR) has been especially active in developing a research portfolio of investigator-initiated studies in this area. This chapter provides an overview of the nature and level of research activity funded by NINR since its inception in 1986, major findings generated by the most successful award recipients, the impact on the broader field of women's reproductive health and directions for future research.

The research programs of selected nurse-scientists are used to demonstrate how the body of knowledge has developed in scope, sophistication and scientific rigor. An analysis of research designs and methodologies is presented within the context of 4 stages of scientific development in the field: exploratory, descriptive studies in well women; illness as a biobehavioral phenomenon; knowledge generation in understudied populations; and the development and testing of clinical therapeutics for symptom management and health promotion strategies. Recommendations address the need for evidence-based outcome research and intervention studies that focus on the special needs of women across the lifespan.

METHODS FOR PORTFOLIO ANALYSIS

This chapter is limited to a review of research studies funded by the National Institute for Nursing Research from its inception in 1986 through 1999. From the beginning, menstrual cycle studies have been prominent in the NINR portfolio, but until now, no systematic analysis has documented the impact of this knowledge on the field of women's health or as the foundation for improved health care. To better characterize this body of work, a year-by year search of the NINR grant archives located on the NIH web site (www.nih.gov/grants.crisp) was conducted. Key search words were limited to the following: "menstrual cycle," "menopause," "perimenopause," "premenopause," "premenstrual syndrome," "PMS," "menstruation." Unless the menstrual cycle was identified as a study variable in the abstract or thesaurus, studies that focused on pregnancy, breast cancer, gender-specific health issues (such as domestic violence), or non-reproductive conditions of women (such as diabetes, HIV) were excluded from the analysis. Both research and career development awards (research training) were included. The portfolio was evaluated for the award types, duration and recipient institutions, the level of sophistication of the research designs (from descriptive, exploratory to controlled intervention protocols), the use of a biobehavioral framework and the incorporation of under-represented minority women as research participants. An analysis of the NINR budget commitment to menstrual cycle research or productivity of the individual awardee could not be performed, as information on award costs and publications was not provided on the web site, and budgetary constraints prohibited efforts by NINR staff to retrieve these data.

NINR AWARD MECHANISMS AND ACTIVITY IN MENSTRUAL CYCLE RESEARCH

A total of 24 extramural, investigator-initiated grants was awarded by the NINR for studies on the menstrual cycle over the 13-year interval of 1987 and 1999 (Table 12.1). Two-thirds of the 24 grant awards were for investigator-initiated RO1 support. Of the 16 RO1 awards, 6 received continued support through competitive renewal applications for durations ranging from 7 to 16 years (one had been funded prior to the inception of the NINR in 1986). Other funding mechanisms included three FIRST awards (R29), one Shannon award (R55), one high-risk award (R15) and two technology transfer or small business

TABLE 12.1 NINR Extramural Grant Awards for Menstrual Cycle Research, 1986–1999

Number of grants	Grant mechanism	Duration of funding (years)
16	RO1 (6 renewals for 7–16 yrs)	102
3	R29-FIRST Award	15
2	R55-Shannon Award	4
1	R15-High Risk, New Investigator	1
2	R41/43-Science Technology Transfer/Small Business Invention Awards	2
Total grants = 24		**Total grant years = 124**

research grants (R41/43). Taken together, these awards totaled 124 grant-years of federal support over the 13-year interval.

In addition to these research projects, five career development awards supporting four predoctoral trainees (F31) and one new investigator (K07) were granted for training in menstrual cycle research. The school of nursing at the University of Washington with 8 of the 24 awards was the most active in procuring research support for studies on the menstrual cycle through a variety of research and training mechanisms, followed by the University of California and the University of Michigan (Table 12.2).

Between 1989 and 1999, the last year for which archive data were available, three special grant mechanisms were used by NINR to support menstrual-cycle-related research. In 1989, a P50 Center grant was awarded to the University of Washington School of Nursing (Nancy Woods, Principal Investigator) to support the Center for Women's Health Research. This funding established six research and training cores with emphasis on minority recruitment and training and launched a series of six biobehavioral studies to develop and test therapeutic strategies for nursing practice to promote women's health across the lifespan. The Center has just completed its 10th year of NIH support with Margaret Heitkemper as Center Director. Funded from 1991–97 by a P30 mechanism, the Center for Symptom Management at UCSF School of Nursing has funded several pilot studies on perimenstrual symptom relationships to women's health and illness (Golding & Taylor; Kennedy & Taylor). At the University of Michigan (UM) School of Public Health, a UO1 mechanism has supported an epidemiologic study of perimenopause, bone and arthritis in African Americans as part of the multi-site NIH SWAN project, the Study of Women Across the Nation. The UO1 mechanism is designed to carry out NIH-initiated research mandates through contractual arrangements with extramural investigators who successfully compete for participation in response to an RFA (research funds announcement). The UM site is the only

TABLE 12.2   Top Three Institutions Receiving NINR Grants for Menstrual Cycle Research

Institution	Awards
University of Washington School of Nursing	4 ROIs, 1 R29, 1 R55, 1KO7, 1P30
University of California, San Francisco	2 ROIs, 2 R29s, 1 R41
University of Michigan Schools of Nursing and Public Health	1 RO1, 1UO1, 2 F31s

one of the seven data collection sites to be sponsored by the NINR and include two nurse-scientists from the School of Nursing as co-investigators (the other sites are funded by the National Institute on Aging).

MENSTRUAL CYCLE EFFECTS ON WOMEN'S HEALTH

The bulk of studies funded by the NINR have used an exploratory, descriptive approach to examine the effect of the menstrual cycle on a variety of physical and psychological phenomena and conditions (Table 12.3). Even the rat model has been used by a KO7-funded investigator to examine estrous cycle effects on muscle physiology (E Bond, PI; University of Washington, 1995–1999). Noteworthy is the fact that many of these projects were undertaken well before the federal government mandates of the early 1990's to include women as research subjects.

MODELS AND METHODS USED IN MENSTRUAL CYCLE AND MENOPAUSE STUDIES

Study Populations

The medicalization of women's menstrual function has predominated in biomedical research, with little attention to the interaction of psychological, sociocultural, lifestyle and health factors. Nursing science has focused on defining these influences on the range and diversity of menstrual cycle experi-

TABLE 12.3   Health Phenomena, Conditions, and Diseases Studied for Menstrual Cycle Effects by NINR-Sponsored Investigator

Sleep architecture, quality, insomnia
Fibromyalgia, fatigue
GI/bowel function, irritable bowel syndrome
Brain function, imaging, neurocognition
Depression, mood states, stress responsivity
LH pulsatility
Circadian rhythms, body temperature, pain, analgesia
Bone density, bone biomarkers, arthritis
Postsurgical metastasis

ences, moving beyond those of gynecologic patient populations to the broader spectrum of community samples. Depending on the study aims, participants of NINR-funded studies have included those responding to media advertisements, random-sampling telephone solicitations, public service announcements or personal contacts through church groups, athletic events, patient advocacy organizations and other community health-based programs.

Menstrual Symptoms and Premenstrual Syndrome

The etiology of premenstrual syndrome (PMS) has been the topic of particularly keen interest among nurse researchers. A number of nurse scientists have helped characterize the biopsychosocial context of menstrual symptoms and its impact on women's lives. Healthy volunteers drawn from community samples as well symptomatic recruits (e.g., women with dysmenorrhea, obesity, or sleep disturbances, elite runners with irregular cycles, oral contraceptive users, women in recovery) have been the focus of nursing research.

For nearly two decades, Nancy Woods, her students, and colleagues have focused on the development of explanatory models that incorporate family, psychosocial, and cultural predictors of perimenstrual symptoms. Using a daily health diary and symptom analysis method that have now been tested by nurse researchers in the US and other countries, their body of work defined three types of symptom patterns in healthy menstruating women: (a) low intensity, acyclic symptoms; (b) a PMS pattern; and (c) high-intensity symptoms that increase in severity during the premenstrual week (premenstrual magnification) (Woods et al., 1982; Mitchell et al., 1991, 1994). These symptom patterns are related to a number of psychosocial correlates, such as psychological stress level, years of education and maternal symptom pattern, as well as age, laboratory-induced arousal, and stress responsivity (Woods et al., 1994, 1998a, 1998b).

Given the diverse features of PMS, it is not surprising that nursing studies have been guided by a variety of theoretical underpinnings, including family systems theory, psychosocial concepts, health promotion paradigms and hypotheses grounded in the psychoneuroendocrinology of stress. In general, these theories have served as the basis for studies that can be grouped into three categories, describing (a) incidence rates, symptom patterns and distinguishing features of women with PMS; (b) biological characteristics such as physiological arousal, sleep quality, and endogenous opioid activity; and (c) the effects of nursing interventions, including self-care strategies, and patient support groups.

In keeping with the challenge of Lentz and Woods (1989) for nursing research to consider the dynamic and multidimensional nature of women's health phenomena, there has been a trend in funded studies to move away from the concept of the menstrual cycle as a static construct, employing single-occasion measures that fail to address it as an interactive process with evolving symptom patterns. A by-product of the analyses of the serial data sets obtained from daily diaries and serial hormone assessments has been the refinement and adaptation of statistical modeling methods for handling the detection of nonrandom rhythms in symptom patterns and hormone secretion (Reame et al., 1992; Shaver & Woods, 1986; Taylor, 1990). Even the case study approach has been used to highlight the important within-subject variability that must be considered when designing treatment protocols and interpreting therapeutic efficacy (Lewis, 1995).

An important improvement in research designs has been the incorporation of biomarkers of ovarian function, such as plasma and salivary measures of sex steroids to confirm ovulatory status and anchor symptom reports to biologically determined phases of the menstrual cycle (Estok et al., 1993; Sveinsdottir & Reame, 1991). Other biomarkers that have been examined as potential PMS mediators include salivary cortisol secretion, LH pulsatility, sleep EEG patterns, and stress responsivity of urinary catecholamines (Woods et al., 1994, 1998a, 1998b).

Menopause Research

Since 1989, Nancy Woods and colleagues Ellen Mitchell and Martha Lentz have conducted longitudinal studies examining the change in menstrual symptoms within the context of aging as well as life transitions, stressors and conflicts in a multiethnic population of middle-aged women (Mitchell et al., 2000; Woods & Mitchell, 1996, 2000). This approach is laudable and one of the first examples in the nursing science community of the kind of long-term team effort required in the creation of a meaningful body of work. This program serves as a model for those investigators undertaking studies that integrate concepts from the social and biological sciences, and require the long-term retention of a highly committed, multiethnic study population for the prospective monitoring of symptoms and hormonal data. Now in its 10th year of data collection, most of the sample are still participating. Findings to date suggest that there are three hormonally defined and symptom-distinct stages within the menopause transition and that factors other than menstrual cycle-related ones affect the mood and perceived stress level of midlife women.

NINR Studies of Women of Color

Only a few NINR-funded programs of research have specifically identified ethnicity as a key study variable or over-sampled women of color in menstrual cycle studies. The P50 Center grant at the University of Washington described above was the first, in 1989, to devote a research aim to the training of minority scientists in menopause research.

In 1994 the NINR in conjunction with the National Institute on Aging, cosponsored a longitudinal observational study of the perimenopause transition in women of diverse ethnic and racial backgrounds at seven sites around the country. Known as the SWAN (Study of Women Across the Nation) study, this investigation is for the first time examining an array of physical, emotional, social and behavioral characteristics of some 3,500 participants' ages 40–55 years on a yearly basis as they proceed through menopause. Funded as a U01 mechanism involving seven sites where populations of African Americans, Hispanic Americans, and Asian Americans were oversampled, the goal is to understand better the disparities and scope of the menopause experience in healthy women, especially as it is influenced by socioeconomic, cultural and ethnic factors. Now in its 10th year, the study has recently demonstrated that although symptom types and severity differ by race/ethnicity, most symptoms were reported most frequently among women who had difficulty paying for basics, who smoked, and who rated themselves less physically active than other women their age. Such data suggest that interventions aimed at modifying lifestyle and socioeconomic conditions may hold promise for improved symptom experiences of midlife women (Gold et al., 2000).

Two investigator-initiated projects have recently focused specifically on midlife women of color as the population of interest. In 1995, a 5-year, RO1 study was launched at UCSF (K. Lee, PI) designed to longitudinally assess the menopause experience using an array of biobehavioral health indicators (e.g., sleep, body temperature, body composition, social support) and outcomes (symptoms) in African, Hispanic, and European American volunteers drawn from church-attendees and relatives of public school children. In 1997, to develop a woman-centered, grounded theory of menopause, investigators at Rutgers University (G. Dickson, PI) were funded by an R15 grant to conduct serial open-ended interviews with 25 African American or Hispanic inner-city apartment residents.

Testing Interventions for Menstrual Cycle and Menopause Symptom Management

Intervention research for the management of menstrual cycle or menopause symptoms is the most recent focus of nursing investigations. The search of the NINR Web site revealed 8 awards for experimental studies testing strategies to reduce symptom distress or metabolic dysfunction related to the menstrual cycle. Beginning in 1991, nursing interventions have included a personalized decision-making aid for women considering hormone replacement therapy (Rothert, RO1), behavioral techniques to reduce symptom severity and stress in PMS patients (Taylor, R29; Taylor, 1996, 1999, 2000), a weight-bearing exercise to decrease lipids in postmenopausal women (Christopherson, F31; Christopherson, 1994), self-management strategy for improved perimenstrual bowel function in patients with irritable bowel syndrome (Heitkemper RO1; Heitkemper et al., 1995, 1996), a walking program in sedentary midlife women (Wilbur RO1; Wilbur et al., 1999), and environmental conditioning for meno-pause-related insomnia (Shaver, RO1; Shaver, 1994; Shaver & Zenk, 2000). Using the rat model, Wendy Blakely at Johns Hopkins University began testing in 1998 the effects of reducing postoperative pain as a way to ameliorate surgery-enhanced cancer metastasis specific to the estrous cycle (F31). Also in that same year, Diana Taylor was awarded a Science Technology & Transfer Grant (R41) to develop and test the efficacy of an acupressure garment (the Relief Brief) for the symptoms of dysmenorrhea. Several of these studies make use of a clinical trial design lasting from one month (or menstrual cycle) to as long as 24 months.

IMPRESSIONS, FUTURE DIRECTIONS, AND RECOMMENDATIONS

The use of NINR Web site information as a means to characterize the body of the work devoted to menstrual cycle studies serves at best as a crude yardstick with which to measure progress and productivity in nursing research. For example, no information about supplemental awards funded by other NIH units (such as the Office for Research on Women's Health) was available, thus potentially underestimating the number of studies focusing on women of color. Productivity of the scientists could only be inferred when a subsequent competing renewal application was specifically identified. A future analysis of the NINR portfolio should include not only the amount of total direct costs, but also a description of the resulting published manuscripts.

Having said that, however, a few important themes emerge that may serve as guideposts for future research agendas. Although White males are no longer the norm when undertaking studies of health and illness, the striking use of White women in nursing studies seems to follow the conventional process of how science in general and health in particular generates new knowledge. Despite these drawbacks, the range and diversity of grant activity suggest that menstrual cycle research is a strong area of interest in nursing science. The NINR should undertake a systematic examination of their portfolio in other areas where there is similar evidence of a critical mass of knowledge generation.

It is also noteworthy that the students of the principal investigators of these grants were frequently the recipients of the training grants and research awards at other institutions as well, suggesting a developing critical mass of investigators seeded throughout the country. Moreover, several investigators followed up an NRSA or first award project with an RO1 or other advanced funding mechanism, pointing to the emergence of sophisticated theoretical models and methods in menstrual cycle research.

Nursing science contributions to the NINR portfolio of women's health research has been focused primarily on the definition and management of the symptoms of premenstrual syndrome and menopause. There is now a body of descriptive nursing studies available on the etiology and characteristics of women with PMS that begs for further scrutiny via the systematic application of meta-analysis. Such analysis could greatly enhance the integration and synthesis of this work into a more meaningful picture of the PMS syndrome and its impact on women's health. At the same time, a small but growing list of nursing intervention studies were identified in the most recent awards from NINR, suggesting a coming-of-age in nursing science with respect to the development of evidence-based outcome data for the management of menstrual cycle and menopause-related symptoms. Given the existing theory-based data that supports the value of social support, self-care measures, peer support groups, and lifestyle modifications for other chronic health problems, the time is ripe for large, multi-site clinical trials of these same nursing strategies for the management of PMS as well as menopause distress.

In its re-assessment of the NIH women's health research agenda in 1999, a prominent new direction for research in the 21st Century for the Office for Research on Women's Health was the emphasis on a better understanding of sex-based differences in biology and their influences on treatment and health outcomes (ORWH, 1999). Clearly, the attention by nurse-scientists to the impact of the menstrual cycle on such difficult-to-treat disorders as depression, irritable bowel syndrome, fibromyalgia, breast cancer, and post-surgical pain can only further this important new priority for NIH-funded research.

In conclusion, a major nursing contribution to the body of NIH-sponsored work on women's health has been the application of biobehavioral research strategies to better contextualize the biology of the menstrual cycle and menopause within a woman's lived experience. The time is right for an NINR-sponsored workshop to bring together the experts in the field to suggest the research gaps and future directions to maximize the productivity from these efforts. At the very least, a compilation of all the products and publications generated could be used to enhance the visibility of the NINR as well as provide further justification for a greater allocation of the NIH budget to the NINR. Future studies of gender-based biology and clinical intervention trials across NIH institutes should capitalize on this rich data source as a starting point for generating hypotheses about underlying mechanisms and treatments for women's health problems and conditions. Finally, nurse-scientists should be encouraged to enter the field, given the availability of experienced mentors, the existing rich data bases at numerous institutions across the country, and the continuing high priority of women's health in the research agenda of the NIH.

ACKNOWLEDGMENT

Supported in part by NIH grants NR07309 and AG15083. The author wishes to thank postdoctoral fellow Jane Lukacs, MSN, PhD for assistance with the MEDLINE search and Diana Taylor and Nancy Woods for their careful reviews, suggestions, and editing of the manuscript. An earlier version of this work was presented at the 25th Annual Meeting of the Society for Menstrual Cycle Research in Tucson, June 11, 1999.

REFERENCES

Christopherson, D. J. (1994). *The effect of a 6 kg weight load on functional capacity, body, composition, and the lipid profile in middle-aged women*. PhD dissertation, the University of Michigan.

Gold, E. B., Sternfeld, B., Kelsey, J. L., Brown, C., Mouton, C., Reame, N., Salamone, L., & Stallato, R. (2000). Relation of demographic and lifestyle factors to symptoms in a multi-racial/ethnic population of women 40–55 years of age. *American Journal of Epidemiology, 152,* 463–473.

Golding, J. M., & Taylor, D. (1996). Sexual assault and premenstrual distress in two general population samples. *Journal of Women's Health, 5,* 143–152.

Golding, J. M., & Taylor, D. (2000). Prevalence of sexual assault in women experiencing severe PMS. *Journal of Psychosomatic Obstetrics & Gynecology, 21,* 69–80.

Heitkemper, M., Jarrett, M., Cain, K., Shaver, J., Bond, E., Woods, N. F., & Walker, E. (1996). Increased Urine Catecholamines and Cortisol in Women With Irritable Bowel Syndrome. *American Journal of Gastroenterology, 91,* 906–913.

Heitkemper, M. M., Jarrett, M., Cain, K. C., Shaver, J., Walker, E., & Lewis, L. (1995). Daily gastrointestinal symptoms in women with and without a diagnosis of Ibs. *Digestive Diseases and Sciences, 40,* 1511–1519.

Lee, K. A., Shaver, J. F., Giblin, E. C., & Woods, N. F. (1990). Sleep patterns related to menstrual cycle phase and premenstrual affective symptoms. *Sleep, 13,* 403–409.

Lentz, M., & Woods, N. F. (1989). Women's health research: implications for design, measurement and analysis. In I. L. Abraham, D. M. Nadzam, & J. J. Fitzpatrick (Eds.), *Statistics and quantitative methods in nursing: Issues and strategies for research and education* (pp. 84–93). Philadelphia: Saunders.

Lewis, L. (1995). One year in the life of a woman with premenstrual syndrome: A case study. *Nursing Research, 44,* 111–116.

Mitchell, E. S., Woods, N. F., & Lentz, M. J. (1991). Recognizing PMS when you see it: Criteria for PMS sample selection. In D. Taylor & N. Woods (Eds.), *Menstruation, health and illness* (pp. 89–102). Washington, DC: Hemisphere.

Mitchell, E. S., Woods, N. F., & Lentz, M. J. (1994). Differentiating women with premenstrual syndrome and premenstrual magnification of symptoms: The development of a predictive model. *Nursing Research, 43,* 25–30.

Mitchell, E. S., Woods, N. F., & Mariella, A. (2000). Three stages of the menopausal transition from the Seattle Midlife Women's Health Study: Toward a more precise definition. *Menopause, 7,* 334–349.

National Institutes of Health. (1999). *Agenda for research on women's health for the 21st century* (NIH Publication No. 99-4385). Bethesda, MD: Author.

Reame, N. E., Marshall, J. C., & Kelch, R. P. (1992). Pulsatile LH secretion in women with premenstrual syndrome (PMS): Evidence for normal neuroregulation of the menstrual cycle. *Psychoneuroendocrinology, 17,* 205–213.

Reame, N. E., Kelch, R. P., Beitins, I. Z., Yu, M. Y., Zawacki, C., & Padmanabhan, V. (1996). Age effects of FSH and pulsatile LH secretion across the menstrual cycle of premenopausal women. *Journal of Clinical Endocrinology & Metabolism, 81,* 1512–1518.

Rothert, M., Holmes, M., Rovner, D., Kroll, J., Breer, L., Talarczyk, G., Schmitt, N., Padonu, G., & Wills, C. (1997). An educational intervention as decision support for menopausal women. *Research in Nursing & Health, 20,* 377–387.

Rothert, M., Padonu, G., Holmesrovner, M., Kroll, J., Talarczyk, G., Rovner, D., Schmitt, N., & Breer, L. (1994). Menopausal women as decision makers in health care. *Experimental Gerontology, 29,* 463–468.

Rothert, M., Rovner, D., Holmes, M., Schmitt, N., Talarczyk, G., Knoll, J., & Gogato, J. (1990). Women's use of information regarding hormone replacement therapy. *Research in Nursing and Health, 13,* 355–366.

Shaver, J. L. F., Giblin, E., Lentz, M., & Lee, K. (1988). Sleep patterns and stability in perimenopausal women. *Sleep, 11,* 556–561.

Shaver, J., & Woods, N. F. (1986). Consistency of perimenstrual symptoms across two cycles. *Research Nursing Health, 8,* 313–319.

Shaver, J. L. F. (1994). Beyond hormonal therapies in menopause. *Experimental Gerontology, 29*(3-4), 469–476.

Shaver, J. L. F., & Zenk, S. N. (2000). Sleep disturbance in menopause. *Journal of Womens Health & Gender-Based Medicine, 9*(2), 109–118.

Sveinsdottir, H., & Reame, N. E. (1991). Symptom patterns in women with premenstrual syndrome complaints: A prospective assessment using a marker for ovulation and screening criteria for adequate ovarian function. *Journal of Advanced Nursing, 16,* 689–700.

Taylor, D. (1990). Time-series analysis: Use of autocorrelation as an analytic strategy for describing symptom pattern and change. *Western Journal of Nursing Research, 12,* 254–261.

Taylor, D. (1994). Evaluating therapeutic change in symptom severity at the level of the individual woman experiencing severe PMS. *Image: Journal of Nursing Scholarship, 26,* 25–33.

Taylor, D. (1996). The perimenstrual symptom management program: Elements of effective treatment. *Capsules & Comments in Perinatal/Women's Health Nursing, 2*(2), 140.

Taylor, D. (1999). Effectiveness of professional-peer group treatment: Symptom management for women with PMS. *Research in Nursing and Health, 22*(6), 496–511.

Taylor, D. (2000). More than personal change: Effective elements of symptom management. *NP Forum, 11*(2), 1–10.

Woods, N. F., Most, A., & Dery, G. K. (1982). Prevalence of perimenstrual symptoms. *American Journal of Public Health, 72,* 1257–1264.

Woods, N., Lentz, M., Mitchell, E., Heitkemper, M., Shaver, J., & Henker, R. (1998a). Perceived stress, physiologic stress arousal, and premenstrual symptoms: Group differences and intra-individual patterns. *Research in Nursing and Health, 21,* 511–523.

Woods, N., Lentz, M., Mitchell, E., Shaver, J., & Heitkemper, M. (1998b). Luteal phase ovarian steroids, stress arousal, premenses perceived stress, and premenstrual symptoms. *Research in Nursing and Health, 21,* 129–142.

Woods, N. F., Lentz, M. J., Mitchell, E. S., & Kogan, H. (1994). Arousal and stress response across the menstrual cycle in women with three perimenstrual symptom patterns. *Research in Nursing Health, 17,* 99–110.

Woods, N. F., & Mitchell, E. S. (1996). Patterns of depressed mood in midlife women: Observations from the Seattle Midlife Women's Health Study. *Research in Nursing and Health, 72,* 1257–1264.

Woods, N., & Mitchell, E. (2000) Anticipating menopause: Observations from the Seattle Midlife Women's Health Study.

Index

risk factors, 277–278, 280
women's responses:
  active resistance, 281–283
  physical, 279–280
  psychological, 280–281
Irritable bowel syndrome (IBS), 13

Job burnout, 95
Job satisfaction, 94, 96, 110
Joint pain, menopause and, 41–42
Journal of Health Care for Women International, 11
Journal of Lesbian Studies, 146
Journal of Obstetrics & Gynecologic and Neonatal Nursing, 11
Journal of Transcultural Nursing, 45

Korean women, menopause experience in, 46–47

Labor and delivery, 256–257, 265
Lead levels, implications of, 204
Leadership, feminist scholarship and, 6–7
Length of stay, 308
Lesbian health:
  access to care, 147–148
  cancer screening, 152–154
  future research directions, 168
  health care interactions:
    disclosure, 149–151
    types of, generally, 148–149
  health care professionals' attitudes, 148
  health care providers:
    interventions with, 151, 168
    preferences for, 151
  health risk/health screening, 152
  information retrieval methods, 146–147
  mental health concerns:
    alcohol use, 162–164
    childhood sexual abuse, 164
    substance use, 162–163
    suicide, 166–167
    therapy, use of, 162
    types of, generally, 161–162
    violence, 164–166

motherhood, 155–156
osteoporosis screening, 154
parenting, 155–156
physical health concerns:
  AIDS, 158–160
  body image, 156–157
  eating disorders, 156–157
  HIV, 158–159
  interventions, generally, 160–161
  pregnancy, 155–156
  sexually transmitted infections (STIs), 157–158
  weight, 156–157
Life history, significance of, 231
Life satisfaction, 91–92
Life span studies, 32–33
Life stress:
  illness and, 230–233
  maternal role and, 69, 74
  menopause and, 40–41, 43
  working women, 89–90
Lifestyle, maternal, 67, 78
Limbic system, 234
Literature review, *see* specific types of studies
  feminist scholarship, 7–10
  maternal role, 64, 78
  menopause, 39–40, 51
Loneliness, 196
Longitudinal studies:
  historical perspective, 11, 13
  pregnancy and postpartum, 100
Low-birthweight infants, 72, 103, 108, 203, 286
Lung cancer, 98, 241–242
Luteal phase, 238–239
Lymphedema, 99

MacPherson, Kathleen, 5, 11, 31–32, 34, 37
Major Mood Disorder, 235–236
Mammograms, 154, 192
Mania, 237
Marriage:
  abuse in, *see* Battered women; Intimate partner violence
  maternal employment and, 108–109
Massachusetts Youth Risk Behavior Survey, 167

Contents of Previous Volumes

ORDER FORM

Save 10% on Volume 20 with this coupon.

____ Check here to order the *Annual Review of Nursing Research*, Volume 20, 2002 at a 10% discount. You will receive an invoice requesting prepayment.

Save 10% on all future volumes with a continuation order.

____ Check here to place your continuation order for the *Annual Review of Nursing Research*. You will receive a prepayment invoice with a 10% discount upon publication of each new volume, beginning with Volume 20, 2002. You may pay for prompt shipment or cancel with no obligation.

Name _____

Institution _____

Address _____

City/State/Zip _____

Examination copies for possible adoption are available to instructors "on approval" only. Write on institutional letterhead, noting course, level, present text, and expected enrollment (include $3.50 for postage and handling). Prices slightly higher overseas. Prices subject to change.

Mail this coupon to:
SPRINGER PUBLISHING COMPANY
536 Broadway
New York, NY 10012